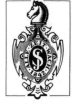

H. Ishikura   K. Kikuchi (Eds.)

Intestinal Anisakiasis in Japan

Infected Fish, Sero-Immunological
Diagnosis, and Prevention

With 109 Figures, 27 in Color

Springer-Verlag
Tokyo Berlin Heidelberg
New York London Paris
Hong Kong Barcelona

HAJIME ISHIKURA
Honorary Member of the Japanese Society of Clinical Surgery
Director, The Ishikura Hospital
Iwanai, 045 Japan

KOKICHI KIKUCHI
President and
Professor, Department of Pathology
Sapporo Medical College
Sapporo, 060 Japan

ISBN-13:978-4-431-68301-8   e-ISBN-13:978-4-431-68299-8
DOI: 10.1007/978-4-431-68299-8

Library of Congress Cataloging-in-Publication Data
Intestinal anisakiasis in Japan : infected fish, sero-immunological diagnosis,
  and prevention / H. Ishikura, K. Kikuchi (eds.). p.   cm. Includes bibliog-
  raphical references. Includes index. ISBN-13:978-4-431-68301-8 :
  DM234.00   (approx.) 1. Anisakiasis. 2. Intestines—
  Infections. I. Ishikura, H. (Hajime), 1914– . II. Kikuchi, Kōkichi.
  [DNLM: 1. Immunologic Tests. 2. Intestinal Diseases, Parasitic—
  diagnosis. 3. Intestinal Diseases, Parasitic—prevention & control—
  Japan. 4. Nematode Infections—diagnosis. 5. Nematode Infections—
  prevention & control—Japan. WC 850 I61]. RC840.A56I58 1990.
  616.9'654—dc20. DNLM/DLC. 90-10120

This work is subject to copyright. All rights are reserved, whether the whole
or part of the material is concerned, specifically the rights of translation,
reprinting, reuse of illustrations, recitation, broadcasting, reproduction on
microfilms or in other ways, and storage in data banks.

© Springer-Verlag Tokyo 1990
Softcover reprint of the hardcover 1st edition 1990

The use of registered names, trademarks, etc. in this publication does not
imply, even in the absence of a specific statement, that such names are ex-
empt from the relevant protective laws and regulations and therefore free for
general use.

Product liability: The publisher can give no guarantee for information about
drug dosage and application thereof contained in this book. In every individual case the respective user must check its accuracy by consulting other
pharmaceutical literature.

Typesetting: Asco Trade Typesetting Ltd., Hong Kong

Preface

This monograph follows the previously published "Gastric Anisakiasis in Japan." As is well-known from experimental examination, the pathogenic species of Anisakidae larvae are *Anisakis simplex, Anisakis physeteris, Pseudoterranova decipiens,* and *Contracaecum osculatum sp.,* but only *Anisakis simplex* larvae get into the human intestinal wall by the consumption of raw paratenic host fish and squid. Normally, this larva is not only paratenic in the tissue of the gastrointestinal tract but may also invade the peritoneal or thoracic cavity, causing extra-gastrointestinal anisakiasis.

The fulminant form of gastric anisakiasis is diagnosed by gastrofiberscopy with larvae easily removed endoscopically. The mild form of gastric anisakiasis which produces a tumor (granuloma) is diagnosed by biopsy using a gastrofiberscope.

However, intestinal anisakiasis is hard to diagnose, and when the fulminant form of intestinal anisakiasis is clinically suspected, roentgenographic, ultrasonographic or seroimmunological examination should be performed.

Intestinal anisakiasis may produce severe symptoms of ileus due to an Arthus-type allergic reaction. However, an emergency laparotomy is not always necessary.

There are rare mild cases in which the tumor is found in the intestinal wall by roentgenography, and is sometimes misdiagnosed as a neoplasm.

The total number of intestinal anisakiasis cases reported in Japan is 567, with most of these of the fulminant form.

This monograph explains intestinal anisakiasis from several viewpoints. Recent morphological findings and advances in larvae identification have helped in warning of new causative species.

We hope to deal with the different kinds of paratenic hosts which are captured in the neighboring waters of Japan.

Histopathological and seroimmunological findings with improved technology have helped to establish the specific monoclonal antibody of *Anisakis simplex* larva as a new method of immune diagnosis.

Studies on eosinophilia and lymphokine are included to further clarify the subject.

Finally, we hope this book will be of help to doctors who are interested in intestinal anisakiasis and Anisakidae itself.

HAJIME ISHIKURA
KOKICHI KIKUCHI

Table of Contents

Introduction
H. ISHIKURA 1

Epidemiological Aspects of Intestinal Anisakiasis and Its
Pathogenesis
H. ISHIKURA 3

Anisakis Larvae in Intermediate and Paratenic Hosts in Japan
K. NAGASAWA... 23

The Life Cycle of *Anisakis simplex:* A Review
K. NAGASAWA... 31

Prevalence of Larval Anisakid Nematodes
in Fresh Fish from Coastal Waters of Hokkaido
K. MIYAMOTO 41

Infection Rate of Anisakinae Larvae in Fish Taken from the
Offing of Ishikawa Prefecture
Y. OIKAWA, T. IKEDA... 45

Anisakinae in Sanin Waters of the Japan Sea
J. MAEJIMA... 49

Anisakinae in the Seto Inland Sea
T. AJI, T. FUKUDA, Y. TONGU 57

Survey of Anisakidae Larvae from Marine Fish Caught in the
Sea Near Kyushu Island, Japan
Y. TAKAO 61

Surface Ultrastructure of Anisakidae Larvae
Y. TONGU, T. FUKUDA, T. AJI 73

Restriction Endonuclease Analysis of *Anisakis* Genome
K. SUGANE... 81

Clinical Features of Intestinal Anisakiasis
H. ISHIKURA 89

Table of Contents

Radiographic Features of Intestinal Anisakiasis
T. Matsui, M. Iida, M. Fujishima, T. Yao 101

Diagnosis of Intestinal Anisakiasis by Ultrasonography
T. Yamamoto, K. Minami 109

Differential Diagnosis of Intestinal Anisakiasis
H. Ishikura 119

Pathology of Intestinal Anisakiasis
Y. Kikuchi, H. Ishikura, K. Kikuchi 129

Clinical Patho-Parasitology of Extra-Gastrointestinal
Anisakiasis
H. Yoshimura 145

Immunodiagnosis for Intestinal Anisakiasis
M. Tsuji 155

Skin (Intradermal) Testing Using Several Kinds of *Anisakis*
Larva Antigens
H. Ishikura, Y. Kikuchi, O. Toyokawa, H. Hayasaka,
K. Kikuchi 159

Passive Hemagglutination Test (Boyden)
K. Asaishi, C. Nishino, H. Hayasaka 167

Immune Adherence (IA), Sarles Phenomenon (SP) and
Diffusion Chamber Method (DC)
H. Ishikura, Y. Kikuchi, O. Toyokawa, H. Hayasaka,
K. Kikuchi 173

Ouchterlony Test and Immunoelectrophoresis
M. Tsuji 183

Immunodiagnosis for Anisakiasis with Detection of IgE
Antibody to Human Anisakiasis by Enzyme-Linked
Immunosorbent Assay
Y. Takemoto, M. Tsuji, Y. Iwanaga 187

Detection of Cellular Immunity by Migration Inhibition Test
on Rabbits and Guinea Pigs Immunized with *Anisakis* Larval
Antigens
Y. Kikuchi, H. Saeki, H. Ishikura 191

Measurement by ELISA of *Anisakis*-Specific Antibodies of
Different Immunoglobulin Classes in Paired Sera of Gastric
Anisakiasis
N. Akao 199

Detection of Anti-*Anisakis* Antibody of IgE Type in Sera of
Patients with Intestinal Anisakiasis
Y. Yamamoto, H. Nakata, Y. Yamamoto 205

Development of Monoclonal Antibodies Reacting with
Anisakis simplex Larvae
S. Takahashi, A. Yagihashi, N. Sato, K. Kikuchi............ 217

Serodiagnosis of Intestinal Anisakiasis Using Micro–ELISA—
Diagnostic Significance of Patients' IgE
S. Takahashi, A. Yagihashi, N. Sato, K. Kikuchi............ 221

Mechanism of Eosinophilia in Parasitic Infection with Special
Emphasis on the Eosinophil Chemotactic Lymphokines
Directed Against Different Maturation Stages of Eosinophils
Y. Nawa, M. Owhashi, H. Maruyama 225

Antigenicity of the Cuticle with Emphasis on the Immuno-
cytochemical Approach
Y. Takahashi, T. Araki 239

Immune Response to *Anisakis* Larvae in Healthy Humans
C. Nishino, K. Asaishi, H. Hayasaka....................... 251

Conclusion
H. Ishikura, K. Kikuchi 257

Subject Index 259

List of Contributors

*AJI, TOSHIKI — Department of Parasitology, Okayama University Medical School, Okayama, 700 Japan

*AKAO, NOBUAKI — Assistant Professor, Department of Parasitology, School of Medicine Kanazawa University, Kanazawa, 920 Japan

ARAKI, TSUNEJI — Professor, Department of Parasitology, Nara Medical University, Kashihara, Nara, 634 Japan

*ASAISHI, KAZUAKI — Assistant Professor, The First Department of Surgery, Sapporo Medical College and Hospital, Sapporo, 060 Japan

FUJISHIMA, MASATOSHI — Professor, The Second Department of Internal Medicine, Faculty of Medicine, Kyushu University, Fukuoka, 812 Japan

FUKUDA, TOMIO — Okayama Fisheries Experimental Station, Okayama, 700 Japan

HAYASAKA, HIROSHI — Honorary Professor, The First Department of Surgery, Sapporo Medical College and Hospital, Sapporo, 060 Japan

IIDA, MITSUO — Lecturer, The Second Department of Internal Medicine, Faculty of Medicine, Kyushu University, Fukuoka, 812 Japan

IKEDA, TERUAKI — Assistant Professor, Department of Medical Zoology, Kanazawa Medical University, Uchinada, Kahoku, Ishikawa, 920–02 Japan

*ISHIKURA, HAJIME — Honorary Member of Japanese Society of Clinical Surgery, Director, The Ishikura Hospital, Iwanai, Hokkaido, 045 Japan

xii   List of Contributors

IWANAGA, YUZURU — Assistant Professor, Department of Parasitology, School of Medicine, Hiroshima University, Hiroshima, 734 Japan

KIKUCHI, KOKICHI — President and Professor, Department of Pathology, Sapporo Medical College, Sapporo, 060 Japan

*KIKUCHI, YUKO — Director, Sapporo City Institute of Public Health, Sapporo, 003 Japan

*MAEJIMA, JOJI — Lecturer, Department of Medical Zoology, Tottori University, School of Medicine, Yonago, 683 Japan

MARUYAMA, HARUHIKO — Department of Parasitology, Miyazaki Medical College, Kiyotake, Miyazaki, 889–16 Japan

*MATSUI, TOSHIYUKI — Assistant Professor, Fukuoka University School of Medicine, Chikushi Hospital, Chikushino, 818 Japan

MINAMI, KOUHEI — Section of Internal Medicine, Niwa Hospital, Odawara, 406 Japan

*MIYAMOTO, KENJI — Assistant Professor, Department of Parasitology, Asahikawa Medical School, Asahikawa, 078 Japan

*NAGASAWA, KAZUYA — Hokkaido Fisheries Experimental Station, Yoichi, Hokkaido, 046 Japan

NAKATA, HIROFUMI — The First Department of Internal Medicine, Kochi Medical School, Nangoku, 781–51 Japan

*NAWA, YUKIFUMI — Professor, Department of Parasitology, Miyazaki Medical College, Kiyotake, Miyazaki, 889–16 Japan

*NISHINO, CHISATO — Assistant Professor, The First Department of Surgery, Sapporo Medical College and Hospital, Sapporo, 060 Japan

*OIKAWA, YOSABURO — Department of Medical Zoology, Kanazawa Medical University, Uchinada, Kahoku, Ishikawa, 920–62 Japan

OWHASHI, MAKOTO — Department of Parasitology, Miyazaki Medical College, Kiyokake, Miyazaki, 889–16 Japan

SAEKI, HISASHI — Director, Saeki Surgical Hospital, Shiroishi-ku, Sapporo, 004 Japan

List of Contributors

SATO, NORIYUKI — Associate Professor, Department of Pathology, Sapporo Medical College, Sapporo, 060 Japan

SUGANE, KAZUO — Professor, Department of Parasitology, Faculty of Medicine, Shinshu University, Asahi 2-1-1, Matsumoto, 390 Japan

*TAKAHASHI, SYUJI — Department of Pathology, Sapporo Medical College, Sapporo, 060 Japan

*TAKAHASHI, YUZO — Assistant Professor, Department of Parasitology, Nara Medical University, Kashihara, Nara, 634 Japan

*TAKAO, YOSHINORI — Department of Parasitology Kurume University, School of Medicine, Kurume, 830 Japan

*TAKEMOTO, YUMI — Department of Parasitology, School of Medicine, Hiroshima University, Hiroshima, 734 Japan

*TONGU, YASUMASA — Professor, School of Health Sciences, Okayama University, Okayama, 634 Japan

TOYOKAWA, OSAMU — Director, Hokkaido Social Work Society, Iwanai Hospital, Iwanai, Hokkaido, 045 Japan

*TSUJI, MORIYASU — Professor, Department of Parasitology, School of Medicine, Hiroshima University, Hiroshima, 734 Japan

YAGIHASHI, ATSUSHI — Department of Pathology, Sapporo Medical College, Sapporo, 060 Japan

YAMAMOTO, TATSURU — Department of Oriental Medicine, Toyama Medical and Pharmaceutical University and Hospital, Sugitani 2630, Toyama, 930–01 Japan

YAMAMOTO, YASUTAKE — Professor, The First Department of Internal Medicine, Kochi Medical School, Nangoku, 781–51 Japan

*YAMAMOTO, YASURO — Assistant Professor, The First Department of Internal Medicine, Kochi Medical School, Nangoku, 781–51 Japan

YAO, TSUNEYOSHI — Professor, School of Medicine, Fukuoka University, Chikushi Hospital, Chikushino, 818 Japan

*Yoshimura, Hiroyuki   Dean of Ishikawa Prefectural School of Nursing, Minami Shinbo-cho Nu-153, Kanazawa, 920–02 Japan

---

* First author

Introduction

H. Ishikura

The correct diagnosis and treatment of gastric anisakiasis have been facilitated by the popularization of gastrofiberscopy and the remarkable progress in medical electronic techniques. However endoscopic research of intestinal anisakiasis has not progressed as rapidly because of technical difficulty. In addition, when resection of affected foci was carried out in intestinal anisakiasis, larvae were not always found as they sometimes pass through the wall, extending into the abdominal cavity. For the above reasons intestinal anisakiasis is found less frequently than the gastric form.

So far, 567 cases of intestinal aniskiasis have been reported in Japan, most of which were misdiagnosed as ileus caused by other diseases. Recently, however, correct diagnosis on first examination has made remarkably rapid progress.

The differential diagnosis of intestinal anisakiasis is now done in Japan using a combination of clinical symptoms, and information from roentogenography, ultrasonography, abdominoscopy and seroimmunological examination.

Progress in diagnostic methodology for this parasitic disease are described in the following chapters, as well as an analysis of the host immune responses based on clinical features and animal experiments.

The grade of immune response differs in several conditions, that is, 1: The foci (organ) where antigen (larva) invade (less in gastric than intestinal anisakiasis), 2: The quantity of antigens (the larger the number of invading larvae, the stronger the immunity), 3: Frequency of infection (the larger the number of infections, the stronger the immunity.)

In Japan, many people eat raw fish and therefore may already be sensitized to *Anisakis* antigens, although appearing to be healthy. Therefore, when they get intestinal anisakiasis, it can be complicated by a more serious ileus reaction. If the patient shows symptoms of an ileus–like disease, doctors must decide on the necessity of surgical treatment rapidly. It is important therefore that clinician's have sufficient knowledge based upon the inflammation mechanism and a definitive method of differential diagnosis.

The belief that resection of localized lesions should always be done may not be the best treatment, though clinicians must form their own internal medical treatment protocols based on current research.

Anisakiasis results solely from the consumption of raw paratenic host fish and squid. Therefore the first step in diagnosis is simply to ask if such food has been eaten.

Immunobiological examination must include specific antigens which are delivered by the monoclonal antibody.

Since animal experiments have shown that *Pseudoterranova dicipiens* larvae invade the intestinal wall (Croll N.A. et al., 1980, in Canada) and *Contracaecum osculatum sp.* larva invade the gastrointestinal tract (Otsuru M. et al., 1969, in Japan), it is possible that these larva could also invade the human body, showing the need for continued research in these areas.

Epidemiological Aspects of Intestinal Anisakiasis and Its Pathogenesis

H. Ishikura

Introduction

Nationwide surveys of anisakiasis in Japan have been compiled are mainly evaluations of cases with eosinophilic granuloma from pathological labaratories at various universities [1,2,6]. Since 1955 Ishikura has kept a record of acute localized enteritis, and in 1965 determined the need for a separate pathological entity for the majority of such cases [10]. They were evaluated as intestinal anisakiasis, and show that this disorder is common in the north, with the chronic granuloma and phlegmonous acute intestinal type especially common, since many of the marine organisms that act as paratenic hosts are caught in large volumes in that area. Diagnosis of the acute form of intestinal anisakiasis has been increasing rapidly, beginning with the use of the endoscope to establish the presence of larvae in cases of peritonitis displaying acute symptoms [11]. With the increasing use of this method in Hokkaido and across the rest of the nation, the incidence of intestinal anisakiasis has changed. There are still problems in separating cases with intestinal anisakiasis; the impossibility of determining larvae in the intestinal cavity when the wall is perforated; the increase in cases recovering without surgery; and the decrease in parasitologically established cases, leaving the ratio of gastric to intestinal cases at less than 1 to 22 (Table 1), where only 567 of 12,586 are cases intestinal anisakiasis.

Intestinal anisakiasis is different from cancer, where a histopathological diagnosis is possible even when the pathogenic agent has not been established. Acute intestinal anisakiasis may be histopathologically determined without a trace of the larvae, making an epidemiological diagnosis difficult to establish. Diagnosis of probable intestinal anisakiasis is based on rapid advances in clinical experience, X-ray, ultrasonography, and immunosero diagnosis. Discussion of the suitability of such a diagnosis is still going on, and if agreement among researchers can be achieved, the number of cases of intestinal anisakiasis will increase dramatically with the ratio of intestinal to gastric anisakiasis consequently changing.

The main problems with epidemiological statistics for anisakiasis relate to the sources of infection. In the last ten years the incidence in Hokkaido and Kyushu has been reversed, with changes in the cycle of parasites in the host marine organisms. These changes have been most remarkable in Alaska pollack, mackerel, and sardines.

Table 1. Occurrence of anisakiasis in Japan 1989a

Interval from the first case	Gastric anisakiasis	Intestinal anisakiasis	Hetero-anisakiasis	Gastric pseudo-terranovasis	Intestinal pseudo-terranovasis	Unknown	Total	Reference
To 1980	1,524	223	7	68	0	1	1,823	1
To 1987 Jun	4,081	375	11	215	0	0	4,682	2
To 1988 Jun	10,863	524	13	282	0	0	11,682	3
To 1988 Aug	10,920	524	13	312	0	8	11,777	4
To 1989 Jun	11,629	567	45	335	0	10	12,586	This report

References; 1) Ishikura H. et al.: Stomach and Intestine 18: 393–397, 1983, 2) Ishikura H. et al.: Hokkaido J Med. Sci. 63: 376–391, 1988.a, 3) Ishikura H.: Gastroenterol. Endosc. 30: 2731–2733, 1988.b, 4) Ishikura H.: J Jpn. Soc. Clin. Surg. 50: 237–247, 1989.

Epidemiological concerns related to the ability of different *Anisakis* larvae affecting primary and secondary infections as well as mass outbreaks of anisakiasis will be described.

Analysis of Changes in the Occurrence of Gastric and Intestinal Anisakiasis in Japan During the Last 10 Years

Endoscopes were first used in the diagnosis and the treatment of acute gastric anisakiasis in 1968, and from the early 1970s the number of cases of gastric anisakiasis grew explosively while the ratio of gastric to intestinal anisakiasis changed (Table 1.)

Nationally 496 cases were reported in 1974 [8], from 1975 to 1980 1327 cases [9], and from 1981 to 1987 2283 cases [12], with the ration between gastric and intestinal anisakiasis changing from 64.0% gastric and 31.4% intestinal in 1966 [2] through 70.5% gastric and 27.7% intestinal in 1969 [6] to 75.6% gastric and 21.6% intestinal and 73.2% gastric and 25.0% intestinal reported in 1974 [16]. This shows that until 1974 the relative incidence of intestinal anisakiasis was in the 31.4%–21.6% range, with an average of about 25%. This changed after 1980 when Ishikura reported 1823 cases, 83.6% gastric and 12.2% intestinal [9], and in the most recent data for 1989 where the proportions of 12,586 cases are 92.40% gastric anisakiasis and 4.50% intestinal anisakiasis, showing a marked decrease in the relative incidence of intestinal anisakiasis.

A comparison between Hokkaido in the north and Kyushu in the south, shows that Hokkaido had 256 cases over a three-year-period with 94.1% gastric and 4.7% intestinal anisakiasis [13], while in 2278 Kyushu cases 98.1% were gastric and 1.4% intestinal [15]. Therefore despite advances in diagnostic methods of intestinal anisakiasis, these are similar results to the 1969 survey by Ishikura [6].

Future of the Infective Larvae in the Body of Dead-end-hosts

Hitchcock's report in 1950 that anisakid larvae were found in 10% of the stools of Alaskan Eskimos was the first report of anisakid larvae in the human body [17]. It was believed that the larvae came from fresh (raw) fish eaten by the Alaskans, and had passed through the digestive tract, with no discussion of the pathogenesis of the larvae. Since the discovery that larvae migrating from a host to a dead-end-host are pathogenic [18], research into the progress of the disease has advanced rapidly. Initially it centered on where the migrating larvae went in the host, and the following discussion will be divided into observations fom animal experiments and in the human body.

The Fate of Orally Infected Larvae (Animal Experiments)

It has been noted that some orally administered larvae are expelled through the anus, verified by Ruitenberg [19], who considered it important that such larvae were dead and digested at evacuation, with no reports of living evacuated larvae. Ruitenberg did extensive experiments with oral infection, and related them to larval penetration of the walls of the abdominal and intestinal cavities, and also noted experiments on histopathological determinations of infecting larvae migrating into the digestive tract wall [20,21]. Myers (1963) reported orally administered larvae in the abdomen [20], small intestine, large intestine, pancreas, and liver, while Young (1969) found coiled larvae that had penetrated into the mesentery [21].

Their experiments employed guinea pigs, cats, dogs, rabbits, and rats. The rate of infection was high with guinea pigs, recovery of larvae was complex, and penetration was made into the thyroid gland and subcutaneous tissue. Usutani (1966) used cats, but the numbers were small and the rate of infection was poor.

Anisakid larvae in the experiments were obtained from different fish and squid species acting as catanic hosts, and various researchers have pointed out that this may be a reason for the different rates of infection obtained with larvae from different marine organisms. Larvae obtained from *Trichiurus lepturus*, *Todarodes pacificus*, and *Trachurs japonicus* were found to be aggressive in infiltrating the host, but comparisons were difficult as freshness and other larval factors must be considered. There is still a need to compare the effect of larvae from Alaska pollack, *Scomber japonicus*, *Torarodes pacificus*, and others on dogs, rabbits, and rats.

Within three days of parasitic *Scomber japonicus* larvae being orally administered to rats 50% were evacuated through the anus, while 68% of *Dentex tumifrous* were evacuated [24]. Ruitenberg's assumption that all larvae evacuated through the anus were dead is mistaken, but the observation that all larvae in the intestinal cavity were dead is an important pathogenetic finding. Dead larvae in the abdomen have been reported to immunize the animals, but because Ruitenberg did not perform such experiments, any relationship between these two findings is difficult to establish [25]. We found both a cutaneous and agglutination reaction after orally administering freeze dried larvae powder to rabbits, and acute infiltrative allergic changes occurred in surrounding tissue after the introduction of live larvae to the gastric and intestinal walls [26,27]. This leads to the conclusion that larvae, alive or dead, immunize by their passage through the digestive tract.

Anisakis larvae which are not evacuated after passing the digestive tract penetrate into the animals, and may be divided into larvae that die and remain in the walls of the digestive tract or larvae that penetrate the walls and enter the abdominal cavity. It has been shown experimentally that the ability of larvae to embed in tissue varies with experimental animal and host organism [28], in rats, larvae are quickly expelled, but of those that remained more entered the gastric than the intestinal wall. A high proportion of larvae obtained from *Trachurus japonicus* took part in perforation, in agreement with Okimura's (1967) experiments [24]. With *Scomber japonicus*, the penetration of the gastric wall starts within two hours, and while a similar number of larvae move from the gut to the small intestine, there is no penetration of the small intestine at this point, all larvae in the small intestine remain in the intestinal cavity. Movement of the larvae that had reached the cavity of the large intestine within 10 days was determined to have started from the abdominal cavity 10 hours after administration. The experiments found several times more larvae penetrating the abdomen than in the small intestine, corroborating the situation in humans, where gastric anisakiasis occurs more than ten times more often than intestinal anisakiasis.

Epidemiological Aspects of Intestinal Anisakiasis and Its Pathogenesis 7

Intraperitoneal infection with *Anisakis* larvae. There is considerable difficulty in comparing experimental results due to the complexity of determining fish species, the freshness of the raw fish, and differences in experimental animals and experimental procedures. However, the number of larvae penetrating the intestinal tract wall and entering the abdonminal cavity is similar to the number that stop in the wall of the intestinal tract and die there. Larvae are found in practically all organ tissue, the caul, mesentery, abdominal wall, liver, pancreas, spleen, uterus, urinary bladder, testicles, ovaries, sperm duct, thyroid gland, muscle, fat, and other tissue [24].

Yoshimura reported on 13 cases from Honshu with what he termed extra-gastro intestinal anisakiasis in which larvae were found in the digestive wall [29], and the author has recognized 45 such cases as well [59]. These larvae had penetrated the gastric and intestinal walls and reached the abdominal cavity. Where the digestive tract wall is perforated, experiments have shown that larvae disappear into the gastric wall within 10 minutes, and from endoscopic examinations perforation has been reported within seconds [30]. Penetration takes place within a very short time with the physical stimulation resulting in subjective symptoms which soon subside and may not be paid attention to explaining the frequently found assymptomatic cases where larvae are identified of autopsy [6].

The invasive course of larvae into the abdominal cavity. Larvae administered orally pass through the wall of the digestive tract and enter the abdominal cavity, where they reach the serous membranes of organs and often produce numerous eosinophilic cell granuloma. Compared with other fish and squid, a large proportion of larvae from the blood of *Trachurus japonicus* penetrate into the abdominal cavity [23,24], while *Scomber japonicus* larvae were found to enter the abdominal cavity after 10 hours, and in order of incidence concentrated in the omentum, mesentary, and various organs. No penetration of the small intestine was found with larvae from *Theragra chalcogramma*, only perforation of the gastric wall; larvae were found in omentum, muscle, and fat tissue. Reports of *Todarodes pacificus* state that the parasitic larvae behave in much the same manner, entering the abdominal cavity via the gastric wall, but rather than concentrating in the omentum and mesentery, many were found in muscle and fat tissue or scattered in the serous membrane of organs. There was no clear indication that the seriousness of the infection in different experimental animals was dependent upon the host species, however, this may be due to differences in the time from infection until examination. The experimental results indicate that the number of larvae penetrating the abdominal cavity are between 1/3 and 1/4 of the total.

Extra-gastrointestinal anisakiasis cases are those where the ailment was diagnosed outside the gastric and intestinal canal, although recently there have been more discoveries of larvae penetrating into the abdominal cavity [29], with larvae being found just after perforation of the small intestine menbrane [34,35], or in the abdominal cavity after penetration of the small intestine [36,48]. Yoshimura et al. reported one case with stomach penetration and eosinophilic cell granuloma in the caul, and another with perforation in the end section of the ileum [29], and there are more reports of such cases. Many physicians have verified the perforation of the mucous membrane from bleeding observed endoscopically while, Mizugaki et al. has shown histological experimental results with

8 H. Ishikura

a strong cell reaction at second infection and perforation outside the stomach and intestine with extensive bleeding and internal bleeding in the mucous membrane [32]. This is considered to be a result of localized reactions to secretion and excrement (ES antigen).

The first infection, re-infection and double infection of larvae. Experimental studies on rabbits have been conducted [37], where they were subjected to a subcutaneous first infection with *Anisakis* larvae, which stayed alive for seven days and caused a foreign body reaction in the tissue. At re-infection dead larvae appeared from the second day, the surrounding edema and flare was clearly histologically acute exudative inflammation with infiltration of immune cell neutrocytes and eosinophilic cells. The exudative inflammation quickly subsided and there was abscess and granuloma formation around the dead larvae. When the re-infection used soluble fraction fluid instead of live larvae, supernatant fluid generally produced an instantaneous allergic reaction, and caused a delayed allergic reaction with sedimented antigen. This brought antigen directly to the stomach and intestinal walls, and even when live larvae were buried there, the stomach reaction was weaker than in the intestine. The proportion of larvae entering the stomach and intestinal walls at the first and later infections were determined in separate experiments, with more larvae found to penetrate the walls of immunized animals. This experiment did not study larvae that had penetrated into the abdominal cavity an aspect which requires further investigation.

In the Netherlands, attention has been drawn to the "double hit" theory, which is that acute exudative inflammation caused by intestinal anisakiasis results from penetration by a single larvae offering immunization for only about 4 months [36]. This local hypersensitivity was quickly questioned by Ruitenberg who considered it to be acute allergic reaction at re-infection [19].

Together with anisakiasis, so-called skip lesions occur in great numbers. To study this phenomena we orally administered larvae to rabbits which then showed abcess and granuloma morbidity (symptoms of the first infection) in their digestive tracts [32]. After 3 weeks *Anisakis* larval antigens were injected in the ear vein of the rabbits, causing acute exudation in the vicinity of the re-infection, showing that the inflammation in the area of the first infection has became infected again. With skip lesions there is a simultaneous elective outbreak of the ailment similar to the localized morbidity, however, when the site of the first infection and the re-infection are different, it is differentiated from a skip lesion. The experiments also showed that tissue morbidity at re-infection was most severe where the greatest penetration had taken place, indicating that the strongest changes occurred in the earliest affected parts. Changes in the vicinity of the remains of intrusions into the abdominal cavity were weak (light bleeding and edema), and although clinical observation of repeated *Anisakis* infections have been reported [39–43], more details will be established when a thorough survey of the abdominal cavity is made at surgery.

Complications with bacillus infection. It is estimated that one-third of the *Anisakis* larvae eaten with marine organisms are evacuated through the anus, one-third die in the walls of the stomach and intestine, and one-third die forming granuloma or after penetrating the abdominal cavity. To enter the abdominal cavity, the wall of the digestive tract must be penetrated, and this is more com-

Epidemiological Aspects of Intestinal Anisakiasis and Its Pathogenesis

mon in the intestinal than the gastric form studies in which laparotomy was performed because of acute stomach ailments report abdominal fluid present in about 70% of cases. In early stages the abdominal fluid is lemon yellow and clear, becoming opaque then yellow and turbid as the illness worsens. This leads experienced physicians to suspect secondary infection, but microscopic observations do not show bacteria in the sediment of the abdominal fluid [44,45].

Ishikura [44] described 2 cases out of 132 subjects with bacteria in the histopathological samples, a further 5 cases with accumulation of neutrocytes or necrotic areas between the mucous and serous membranes which were also considered to show bacterial infection. Agglomeration of bacteria in the tissue of one of 6 cases was reported by Saito [45], though these cases did not show ulcerated necrosis of the mucous membrane and the bacterial infection must have taken place from the intestine via larval perforations. Naka reported on bacterial cultivation revealing mucous in the abdominal fluid and intestinal serous membrane and found 7 cases out of 65 with coli baccillus and staphylococcus, and of 23 cases with fibrous fur 4 had bacteria in the mesentary [46].

We injected 30 *anisakis* larvae into the abdominal cavity of rabbits, and injected antigen into the ear vein three months later [47]. The immunized rabbits had antigen injected in the lymphatic cavity under the serous membrane of the ileum by Fisher's method and simultaneously nonpathogenic coli baccilla were injected at the same site before closing off the abdomen. These rabbits were later subjected to repeated laparotomy and tissue from the intestinal wall was observed under the microscope. The observations were conducted for 40 days and revealed ulceration of the mucous membrane, necrosis, and necrotic abcesses with numerous neutrocytes under the mucous membrane; the appearance of giant cells was accelerated and necrotic perforations were apparent. This coincides with observations of acute anisakiasis in humans, but more comprehensive observations are necessary to determine whether the pathogenic changes appear as Crohn's disease when it becomes chronic.

The immune mechanisms in *Anisakis* larvae infections in humans. Based on immune response experiments with animals, infections of the abdominal cavity were found to create immunity and led to speculation that the immunity created by larvae that had penetrated into the abdominal cavity was stronger than that created by larvae that had entered the digestive tract wall and died there, and that this may be the situation wih human cases of anisakiasis [31]. This hypothesis is supported by the increasing number of laparotomies performed as a result of acute symptoms of the primary infection in which intestinal anisakiasis has been determined. The increase appears to be due to more thorough examinations of the stomach by surgeons performing laparotomies on intestinal anisakiasis cases.

Primary infections of the digestive tract walls are rarely diagnosed since they are often assymptomatic but may be discovered during laparotomies performed for other ailments or at post mortems. Re-infection with anisakiasis larvae cause violent immune reactions leading to acute symptoms (mainly ileus) that result in laparotomy which then leads to the discovery of signs of the primary infection. As described in another section (with the pathology of the mild form of intestinal anisakiasis), this activation of the first infection may mistakenly be interpreted as the appearance of a wave-like phenomenon or a relapse change.

Simultaneous Multiple Infections and Larvae Species Specific Differences in the Place of Infection

As explained under the section on animal experiments and skip lesion symptoms in humans, larvae occasionally cause multiple infections occurring when large numbers of larvae are consumed with the paratenic host, and are always the result of eating fresh (raw) fish. The ability of different species of *anisakis* larvae to perforate is different for larvae from different intermediate paratenic hosts.

Simultaneous Multiple Infections

During the season when intestinal anisakiasis is common in Iwanai, Hokkaido, one specimen of *Theragra cholocogramma* (pallas), the main species caught, contained up to 495 *Anisakis* type 1 larval parasites. In areas where gastric anisakiasis is common, the greatest source of infection is *Scomber japonicus* Houttuyn which has been reported to hold up to 631 *Anisakis* type 1 larva in one specimen. In Takao (in this volume) and in southern areas, *Trachurus japonicus* is common and has been recorded to hold an average of 113.5 parasites per specimen. The larvae from various fish species show differences in the ratio that penetrate into organs in animal experiments: a high proportion of *Trachurus japonicus* parasitic larvae penetrate. As a result, multiple infections of humans even after only one intake of fresh fish are not rare, shown clearly in Table 2, and except for one case by Hayasaka et al. [61] all the 120 cases were of gastric anisakiasis.

All the cases of gastric anisakiasis were observed endoscopically with 0.04% showing multiple infections, the highest number a surprising seven. Such cases are especially common in southern areas such as Kyushu, and in recent years the number of specimens of infecting marine organisms has shown an increase.

The small number of multiple intestinal anisakiasis reported is not due to the rarity of such multiple infections, but rather to the difficulty of substantiating the diagnosis.

A skip lesion–like phenomenon has been occasionally reported together with intestinal anisakiasis, however, no larvae have been discovered in the area of the pathological changes. When histopathological indicators point to anisakiasis there are many more cases where no larvae are found than those where larvae are identified. This is thought to be due to the large number of cases where

Table 2. Simultaneous infection by multiple larvae

Locality	No. of Anisakiasis	No. of Removed Larvae						Authors
		7	6	5	4	3	2	
Kyushu	2,252	1	3	1	10	16	59	Iino H. (1985)
Honshu	269			2	1	5	11	Koyama T. et al. (1982)
							6	Koyama T. et al. (1982)
Hokkaido	495						4	Shibata O. et al. (1984)
							2	Ishibashi S. et al. (1984)
							1	Hayasaka H. et al. (1969)
Total	3,016	1	3	3	11	21	83	4%
				121				

Epidemiological Aspects of Intestinal Anisakiasis and Its Pathogenesis 11

infecting larvae have penetrated the walls entering the abdominal cavity, and recent reports of this corroborates have supported this assumption.

Differences in Place of Penetration for Different Larvae Species

There are reports of *Anisakis simplex* larvae being spat out from the oral cavity before they enter the digestive tract (five cases in Yoshimura 1978 [49]) but among a total of 4682 reported cases they are very rare.

Vomiting or attachment to the throat in human infection by *Terranova dicipiens* larvae (3 cases in Yoshimura 1978 [49]) and one in Ishikura et al. [50]) are more common than for *anisakis* larvae; this is also reported from Hawaii by Desowilz [57]. There is a lack of experimental results but it appears that *Terranova* larvae are weaker than *Anisakis* larvae in infecting and penetrating into humans.

Terranovasis in Japan

The clinical symptoms of *Terranova decipiens* larvae type A infections in humans are weaker than for *Anisakis simplex* type 1, and may even be assymptomatic, with the infection only be discovered when patients are being examined for other ailments [4].

They have been found attached to the oral, pharynx, and digestive mucosa or released in the stomach, and discovered by endoscopy. The infection is milder than with *Anisakis* type 1 and there are no reports of penetration of the digestive tract walls. This type of infection has been reported with 335 cases at present diagnosed in Japan (Table 1) [52,58]. This is about 3.0% of the 11,629 cases of *Anisakis* type 1 reported for the same period, and include one case of gastric anisakiasis in Karasawa where *Anisakis* type 1 and *Terranova* A larvae were determined.

Terranova has not been found in the intestinal tract though there are reports of evacuation through the anus and separated larvae found in the rectum, and may fall outside the scope of this report. However, intestinal anisakiasis occurs in distinct geographical areas, and is related to migratory host organisms caught at distinct times (Table 3). These host organisms are spreading to the southern parts of the Japan Sea, and anisakiasis cases now occur in southern Kyushu. A detailed epidemiological discussion of infections with *Terranova* will not be attempted here.

Why Intestinal Anisakiasis is Diagnosed Less Frequently than Gastric Anisakiasis

According to the animal experiments reported [24,28,53] one-third of the administered *Anisakis* larvae were ejected through the anus and one-third penetrated the intestinal cavity. The remaining one-third perforated the stomach and intestinal walls, and while more perforated the stomach than the intestinal walls there is no proof that the ratio is 1 to 10. At the same time only 0.3% of human

Table 3. Terranovasis in Japan

Locality (District)	No. of cases	No. of anisakiasis caused by *Anisakis* Type I Larvae	Authors
Bihoro	11	25	Doi K. (1973)
Asahikawa	60	127	Karasawa Y. et al. (1984)
Hakodate	9	19	Nagano K. et al. (1975)
Other areas of Hokkaido	59	290	Koyama T. et al. (1982)
(Total No. in Hokkaido)	139	461	Ishikura H. et al. (1987)
Hirosaki	21	Unknown	Tsushima K. et al. (1984)
Goshogawara	31	28	Chiba T. et al. (1986)
Toyama	1	Unknown	Sakaguchi et al. (1978)
Ishikawa	18	103	Koyama T. et al. (1982)
Fukui	1	113	Koyama T. et al. (1982)
Tokyo	2	24	Koyama T. et al. (1982)
(Total No. in Honshu)	74	268 + x	
Fukuoka	1	857	Iino H. (1985)
Ooita	1	533	Takao Y. et al. (1985)
(Total No. In Kyushu)	2	1,490	
Total no. in Japan	215	2,219 + x	

anisakiasis cases are of the intestinal type, the reasons for which are thought to be the following.

1) Larval penetration of the intestinal wall is often assymptomatic in the primary infection, probably because the pain is short and soon disappears, so few cases are brought to the hospital. Even with bacterial infection, the infiltrated parts heal and a diagnosis of intestinal anisakiasis requiring treatment is rare.

2) The diagnosis of gastric anisakiasis has become possible through endoscopic developments which unfortunately are technically more difficult to perform in intestinal anisakiasis. However, clinical aspects of intestinal anisakiasis are also not sufficiently analysed, and there are few X-rays done on patients suspected of having this ailment, with ultrasonic diagnostic techniques also not well developed. Intestinal endoscopy and abdominal perforation though technically complex should be performed in greater numbers, and if done the number of diagnoses would increase substantially, indicating this lag in the use of the gastro endoscope, as being the most serious cause of discrepancies in numbers between gastric and intestinal cases.

3) Anisakiasis is a parasitic ailment and the diagnosis is established by determining the presence of the Anisakidae larvae. The difficulty in discovering larvae in tissue arises from its histopathologically similarity to the *Anisakis*. The author has analysed 122 cases of anisakiasis (Table 4) [54]. In Japan there is a general consensus that even in the absence of parasitic larvae, it is acceptable to diagnose anisakiasis when an ailment is pathologically similar. It is still difficult to accept this as a final diagnosis and the reasons for the absence of larvae must be investigated. To remedy this, we have to continually investigate areas with high exudative eosinophilic cell infilration and many immune cells (high lymph follicle and parts where the mucosal membrane is ejected), to raise the ratio of cases where larvae are found.

With different approaches to the diagnosis, it has been possible to cure the

Epidemiological Aspects of Intestinal Anisakiasis and Its Pathogenesis

Table 4. Diagnostic foundation of intestinal anisakiasis[a]

Method of diagnosis	No. of cases
Anisakis larva type I itself	66
Anisakia like larva	3
Visceral larva migrans	1
Cuticle or charcolyden cristal	8
histopathologic (non-parasite)	44
Total	122

[a] From [54]

majority of fulminant type intestinal anisakiasis with conservative internal treatment and without surgery, as has been reported elsewhere [54,55]. In these cases the diagnosis has been probable intestinal anisakiasis [55]. As confidence in the diagnosis grows, it will become possible to term it simply as intestinal anisakiasis and win approval from professional organizations for this diagnosis, the number of these diagnoses will then increase and approach to the number of gastric anisakiasis cases.

There is further proof that the number of intestinal anisakiasis cases is larger than statistics would lead us to believe.

At hospitals where researchers have shown interest in localized enteritis, and further investigated these, there is a large number of reports of cases of probable intestinal anisakiasis. A survey of seven hospitals with histological tests of 641 cases of localized enteritis, showing that *anisakis* larvae and similar Anisakidae were located in 35 cases and that intestinal anisakiasis was histologically verified in 292 cases (Table 5).

From the above the number of intestinal anisakiasis cases is much larger than appears in Table 1. To improve the internal and clinical diagnosis of probable anisakiasis, immunosero–diagnosis will be necessary. We have produced monoclonal antibodies of *Anisakis simplex* larva and with these measured immunoglobulin in the sera of patients using the ELISA method establishing a very convenient method of diagnosis.

Changes in Infecting Marine Organisms and in the Incidence of Infecting Larvae

In the early days of research on anisakiasis the fulminant type was common in Hokkaido. This northern orientation was strengthened with the endoscopic verification of larvae by Namiki et al. [11], and with the increasing use of endoscopic diagnosis for gastric anisakiasis, a few cases have been diagnosed in Kyushu. These were thought to be due to the improved diagnostic method, but the number of cases has continued to decrease in Hokkaido while here together with the Tohoku area anisakiasis caused by *Pseudoterranova decipiens* larvae (type A) and terranovasis have multiplied rapidly, being different from infections with *Anisakis simplex* larvae (type 1). There is evidence of changes in the infection rates of anisakid larvae of the *Anisakis* family in marine organisms, and changes in catch volumes and areas for the intermediate hosts.

Table 5. Collective outbreak of intestinal anisakiasis

Locality	Name of Hospital	No. of Int. Anisakiasis	By Larva	By Histopathologic	Authors
			Base of Diagnosis		
Iwanai	Ishikura Surg. Clinic	132	22	106	Ishikura H. (1968)
Hirosaki	I. Dep. Int. Med. Hirosaki	64	1	47	Oouchi S. et al. (1971)
Kanazawa	Seiryo Hospital	174	11	17	Naka T. et al. (1970)
Tokyo	Shinohara Hosp.	120	1	Unknown	Furukawa A. et al. (1972)
	I. Dep. Surg. Nippon Uni.	5	0	5	Saito K. et al. (1966)
Tyugoku	Gyohoku Hospital	26	0	Clinical Findings	Hara K. et al. (1955)
Kyushu	Amakusa Cent. Hosp.	120	3	117	
	Total	641	38	292(26)	

Table 6. Survey of Anisakinae in paratenic host fishes and squid caught in the sea near Japan (1987)

Province	Names and infection rate of the paratenic host fishes and squid			
	Anisakis simplex larva		*Pseudoterranova decipiens* larva	
Hokkaido (by Miyamoto K.)	1. *Myoxocephalus polyacanthocephalus*	100	1. *Myoxocephalus polyacanthocephalus*	100
	2. *Atheresthes evermanni*	100	2. *Hexagrammos otakii*	42.9
	3. *Pleurogrammus azonus*	66.7	3. *Osmerus epelanus mordax*	34.6
	4. *Clupea pallasi*	66.3	4. *Paralichthys olivaceus*	33.3
	5. *Hipploglossus stenolepis*	25.0	5. *Gadus macrocephalus*	23.8

▽

Epidemiological Aspects of Intestinal Anisakiasis and Its Pathogenesis

Kanazawa (by Oikawa Y.)

	Anisakis (%)	Pseudoterranova
1. Scomber japonicus	100	
2. Gadus macrocephalus	100	
3. Theragra chalcogramma	90	
4. Cleisthenes pinetorum herzensteini	40	
5. Sardinops melanostictus	28	

Pseudoterranova Larva was not found in this area

Sanin (by Maejima J.)

	Anisakis (%)
1. Trachurus japonicus	10
2. Sardinops melanostictus	4
3. Engraulis japonica	0
Doryteuthis kensaki	0

(Todarodes pacificus: Hysterothylacium sp. 71%)
*Scomber japonicus
*(Bring in from Shizuoka Prefecture 85, and Chiba 91%)

Pseudoterranova Larva was not found in this area

Seto Inland Sea (by Aji T.)

	Anisakis (%)
1. Saridinops melanostictus	0
2. Mugil cephalus	0
3. Scomberomorus niphonius	0
4. Hexagrammos otakii	0

(Engraulis japonica: Thynnascaris 1/41)
*Scomber japonicus 28.89
*Trachrus japonicus 42.85 from the Open Sea

Pseudoterranova Larva was not found in this area

Kyushu (by Takao Y.)

	Anisakis (%)	Pseudoterranova (%)
1. Scomber japonicus (AII 47.5)	100	1. Scomber japonicus 5.1
2. Scomber australasicus (AII 4.9)	97.6	2. Sebastiscus marmoratus 4.3
3. Decapterus muroadsi	73.7	
4. Trachurus japonicus	44.2	
5. Sardinops melanostictus	5.9	
6. Etrumeusteres	1.09	

Survey of Anisakiasis Larvae Hosts and the Catch Areas where Infections Originate

There are detailed reports of marine organisms infected by *Anisakis* larvae from Hokkaido, Kanazawa, Shimane, the Seto Inland Sea, and Kyushu. Table 6 shows the five main infecting agents from these areas. For Hokkaido, the incidence of *Anisakis simplex* larvae type 1 infection is the highest in great scalopin, followed by arrow-toothed halibut, arabesque greeling, herring, and chicken halibut; in Kanazawa it is chul mackerel, codfish, Alaska pollack, plaice, and sardine; in San-In (Shimane) it is horse mackerel, sardine (Japanese pilchard), half-mouthed sardine, squid, and Japanese chub mackerel; in the Seto Inland Sea there are no infected fish species, but parasites are found in the half-mouthed sardine which was introduced from other sea areas; in Kyushu there are parasites in all chub mackerel followed by slim mackerel, brownstriped mackerel, horse mackerel, Japanese pilchard, and big-eye sardine. This is the situation today, but in the 1970s the infection ratio was very high in Alaska pollack, squid, and chub mackerel in Hokkaido. At that time the author found parsites in all Alaska pollack, while today about one-third have no parasites; Ishikura had found a maximum of 495 parasites in a single fish while in 1986 he found an average of 4.7 parasites in 450 fish. In 1987, fewer fish were investigated, but no parasites were found in 30 squid (*Todarodes pacificus*), indicating changes in the kinds of marine organisms infected with *Anisakis* type 1 larvae.

Survey of Infecting Marine Organisms

Marine organisms that patients have listed as sources of anisakiasis infection are shown (Table 7). This has been noted previously, showing the changes in infecting species. The numbers in the table indicate the infecting species which are listed in the order of number of infected cases.

The marine organisms that caused *Anisakis* infection in humans in the 1970s in Hokkaido were chub mackerel, Alaska pollack, arabesque greeling, tunny tuna, and squids, and in Kyushu chub mackerel, Japanese mackerel, and squids; Recently the order in Hokkaido has changed to Pacific halibut, chub mackerel, arabesque greelings, squid, and codfish, and in Kyushu, chub mackerel, sardine, Japanese mackerel, and squid. In the north Alaska pollack has disappeared as an infecting agent and codfish has increased in incidence, while in Kyushu sardines have rapidly become important infecting agents. Due to the different sea conditions it is natural that there are differences in the types of marine organisms, and here chub mackerel, squid, and sardines migrate with warm currents and move around with temperature and sea currents. *Anisakis* larvae become parasites in dolphins and attain the first to third stages in *Euphausia pacifica* and *Euphasia vallentini* infecting 166 species of marine organisms in the third stage. The northern most infect species showing decreases in infection ratios of *Anisakis simplex* larvae (type 1) are Alaska pollack and squids while chub mackerel and sardines show decreases, and the migrations of southern dolphins are probably related to their appearance here. The author has shown that squid development as they travel north through the Japan Sea is retarded, and the numbers of parasites of *Anisakis simplex* larvae have shown dramatic decreases.

Table 7. Survey of the paratenic host fish and squid responsible for anisakiasis (*Anisakis simplex* larva)

○ The Numeral of this table means the occurence-grade of infection to patients of Anisakiasis	Nation-wide (1)[a]	Nation-wide (2)[b]	Iwanai[c]	Bihoro[d]	Asahikawa[e]	Hokkaido[f]	Kizukuri[g]	Odate[h]	Tokyo[i]	Shinshu[j]	Kanazawa[k]	Yamaguchi[l]	Sanin 1[m]	Sanin 2[n]	Kyushu 1[o]	Kyushu 2[p]	Kyushu 3[q]
Scomber japonicus	4[o]		1		2	5			1	1	1	1	1	1	1	1	1
Hippoglossus stenolepis	1	1		1	1												
Trachurus japonicus															2	2	3
Todarodes pacificus	2	2	5	4	4	1	3		2	2	3				3	3	4
Gadus macrochephalus		3		2	5	3	1				2						
Paralichthys olivaceus		5			4												
Thunnus thynnus	3	4	4														
Theragra chalocogramma	5		2			2											
Hexagrammos otakii																	
Saridinops melanostictus		(18)												2			2
Scomberomorus nophonius											4						
Pleurogrammus azonus			3	4	3												
Sebastes schlegeli				2	4						3						
Seriola quinqueradiata							2				4	5	2	2	4		
Sebastes matsubarae																	
Pleuronectidae				4													
Tribolodon sp.				4													
Lamma ditropis								1									
Euthynnus palamis												3	3				
Takifugu rubripes												4					
Shellfish										3							
Salmo sp.											5						
Zeus japonicus														3			

[a] Iwano H. (1974) 138 cases; [b] Ishikura H. (1983) 448 cases; [c] Ishikura H. (1968) 132 cases; [d] Doi K. (1973) 25 cases; [e] Karasawa Y. (1983) 54 cases; [f] Kawauchi H. (1973) 46 cases; [g] Chiba T. (1986) 28 cases; [h] Suzuki T. (1983) 21 cases; [i] Hirata F. (1984) 20 cases; Kato. K. (1987) 71 cases; [j] Omachi K. (1985) 47 cases; [k] Yoshimura H. (1978) 82 cases; [l] Hatano Y. (1985) 29 cases; [m] Fukumoto S. (1984) 222 cases; [n] Ishida A. (1986) 208 cases; [o] Iino H. (1977) 250 cases; [p] Iino H. (1980) 387 cases; [q] Iino H. (1984) 1615 cases.

Monthly Catch and Monthly Case Numbers Coincide

Japan is surrounded by water, and as the Japanese like fresh (raw) seafood. Japan has the most cases of anisakiasis. There are seasonal as well as regional differences in dietary habits. Fresh fish are transported to areas where fish catches are small, ensuring a supply of fresh fish to all areas of the nation. The author has found that the number of patients closely parallels the fishing seasons [40], and this finding has been verified by numerous researchers. Knowledge of the seasons in which particular fish are caught is an indispensable tool in the diagnosis and treatment of anisakiasis.

Summary

The author has made an epidemiological study and analysis of the nationwide occurrence of anisakiasis since 1968, with the 1989 results now included. In 1989 Ishikura counted 12,586 cases; terranovasis totaled 335 cases.

Now, the analysis has given the following results:

1. Parasitologically and histopathologically 567 cases of intestinal anisakiasis have been identified 0.3% of the 11,629 were cases of gastric anisakiasis.

2. Animal experiments corroborate the finding that intestinal cases form less than 0.3/1 of the gastric cases.

3. Animal experiments show that about 1/3 of orally administered larvae die and are evacuated through the anus, and except for the few that are presumed to die in the digestive tract the remaining 2/3 penetrate and remain in the wall of the digestive tract or perforate into the abdominal cavity.

4. Multiple gastric infections are common in human anisakiasis, but in chronic cases multiple granuloma are not observed. It is surmised that larvae penetrate the abdominal cavity in acute cases.

5. Recently, cases of intestinal anisakiasis where perforation by larvae is determined by laparotomy have increased. Cases where bacteria were identified in abdominal fluid have also multiplied due to infections from bacteria after the perforation.

6. Immunity after infection is strong after the primary infection of the abdominal cavity.

7. It is concluded that the slow development of diagnostic techniques for intestinal anisakiasis is the reason for the relatively few cases.

8. Acute abdominal pains in the majority of the 641 cases during mass outbreaks reported from six hospitals were due to larvae moving about in the intestine and abdominal cavity.

9. *Pseudoterranova decipiens* larvae (type A) is less pathogenic than *Anisakis simplex* larva, and has not been identified in the digestive tract wall or anywhere else. Only 333 cases had been reported for the northern part of Japan, but now, however, there are two cases of *Terranova decipiens* larvae in the south, suggesting that it is spreading.

10. The major species acting as hosts in the north and south were surveyed. Identifying the infecting agent in anisakiasis requires knowledge of fishing seasons, areas, dietary habits, and transportation routes.

11. This report showed that Alaska pollack, squid, and chub mackerel are decreasing as sources of infection in the north, while chub mackerel, horse mack-

Epidemiological Aspects of Intestinal Anisakiasis and Its Pathogenesis

erel, and sardines are increasing in Kyushu. With the increasing incidence of human anisakiasis the importance of sardines needs to be stressed.

References

1. Yokogawa M, Yoshimura H (1965) *Anisakis*-like larvae causing eosinophilic granulomata in the stomach of man. Am J Trop Med Hyg 14: 770–773
2. Yoshimura H (1966) Clinicopathological analysis on *Anisakis*-like larva infection in the digestive apparatus of man. Jpn J Parasitol 15: 283–284 (in Japanese)
3. Yoshimura H (1966) Clinic of parasitic gramuloma of human digestive tract and its entity. Stomach Intestine 1: 803–811 (in Japanese)
4. Yoshimura H (1966) A case of acute abdomen due to provable penetration of *Anisakis*-like larva into the intestinal wall. Surgical Treatment 15: 626–630 (in Japanese)
5. Ishikura H, Kikuchi Y, Hayasaka H, Miyagi H, Ueno T (1968) Anisakiasis in Hokkaido. Jpn J Clin Surg Soc 29: 49–60 (in Japanese)
6. Ishikura H (1969) Occurrence of anisakiasis and its presentation Saishin Igaku 24: 357–365 (in Japanese)
7. Iwano H, Ishikura H, Hayasaka H (1974) Statistical analysis of anisakiasis in Japan during the last five years. Geka Shinryo 16: 1336–1342 (in Japanese)
8. Koyama T, Araki J, Machida M, Karasawa Y (1982) Current problems on the anisakiasis. Modern Media 9: 434–443 (in Japanese)
9. Ishikura H, Kikuchi Y, Ishikura H (1983) Enteritis acuta caused by *Anisakis* larvae (Intestinal anisakiasis). Stomach and Intestine 18: 293–297 (in Japanese)
10. Ishikura H (1965) Feature of regional enteritis which frequently occurred at Iwanai district-proposal of the pathological entity. Hokkaido J Surg 10: 29–38 (in Japanese)
11. Namiki M, Morooka T, Kawauchi H, Ueda N, Sekiya C, Nakagawa K, Furuta T, Ooguro T, Kamada H (1970) Diagnosis of acute gastric anisakiasis. Stomach and Intestine 5: 1437–1440 (in Japanese)
12. Ishikura H (1985) Anisakiasis, Review of the literature. (suppl) 6: 1–40. Sapporo, (printed privately, in Japanese)
13. Asaishi K, Nishino C, Totsuka M, Hayasaka H, Suzuki T (1980) Studies on the etiologic mechanism on anisakiasis-2 Epidemiological study of inhabitants and questionaire survey in Japan. Jpn Soc Gastroenterol 15: 128–134
14. Karasawa Y, Kawakami Y, Hirafuku I, Hoshi K, Koyama T (1983) Studies on anisakiasis and terranovasis of the digestive tract. Jpn Med J 3099: 30–34 (in Japanese)
15. Iino H (1985) Occurrence of Anisakiasis in Kyushu (6th examination). Jpn J Gastroenterol Endosc 27: 630 (in Japanese)
16. Totsuka M (1974) II Human anisakiasis 3. Epidemiology: Fishes and *Anisakis* (No. 7 fishes scientific series). The Japanese Society of Scientific Fisheries, Koseisha Koseikaku, Tokyo, pp. 44–57 (in Japanese)
17. Hitchcock DJ (1950) Parasitological study on the Eskimos in the Bethel area of Alaska. J Parasit 36: 23–234
18. van Thiel PH, van Kuipers FC, Roskam RTh (1960) A nematode parasitic to herring causing acute abdominal syndromes in man. Trop Geogr Med 12: 97–115
19. Ruitenberg EJ (1970) Anisakiasis. Pathogenesis, serodiagnosis and prevention; Doctor thesis in Rijks University, Utrecht. (Translation into Japanese by Ooishi K et al.)
20. Myers BJ (1963) The migration of *Anisakis*-type larvae in experimental animals. Canad J Zool 45: 147–148 (1963)
21. Young PC (1969) Larval nemotodes from fish of the subfamily Anisakinae and gastro-intestinal lesions in mammals. J Comp Path 79: 301–313
22. Usutani T (1966) Histological studies on experimental animals administered with *Anisakis*-like larvae from marine fish (Studies on larva migrans, Part 3). Shikoku Acta Med 22: 486–503 (in Japanese)

23. Oyanagi T (1967) Experimental studies on the visceral migrans of gastro-intestinal walls due to *Anisakis* larvae. Jpn J Parasitol 16: 470–493 (in Japanese)
24. Okumura T (1967) Experimental studies on the anisakiasis. J Osaka City Med Center 16: 465–499 (in Japanese)
25. Matsuoka Y (1966) Studies on peripheral blood picture and serum protein in experimental anisakiasis (Studies on larva migrans Part 4). Shikoku Acta Med 22: 12–36 (in Japanese)
26. Ishikura H, Hayasaka H, Miyagi H, Ueno T, Uchiumi A, Saeki H (1968) Studies on anisakiasis (7) Allergic reaction by oral administration of frozen Anisakis *larvae* in rabbits, Jpn J Parasitol 17: 266 (in Japanese)
27. Suzuki T, Shiraki T, Sekino S, Otsuru M, Ishikura H (1970) Studies on the immunological diagnosis of anisakiasis. III Intradermal test with purified antigen. Jpn J Parasitol 19: 1–9 (in Japanese)
28. Inamoto T (1972) Experimental Studies on the Tissue Invasion and Ecdysis of *Anisakis* Larvae. J Osaka City Med Center 21: 243–269 (in Japanese)
29. Yoshimura H, Kondo K, Akao N, Onishi Y, Watanabe K, Shinno T, Akikawa K (1979) Two cases of eosinophlic granulomas formed in the large omentum and mesentery by the penetrated *Anisakis* larva through the gastrointestinal tract. Stomach and Intestine 14: 519–522 (in Japanese)
30. Ishikura H (1981) Anisakiasis, Review of the literature. (suppl) 4: 1–16. Sapporo, (printed privately, in Japanese)
31. Suzuki T, Ishikura H (1974) Pathogenic mechanisms, symptoms and diagrams of anasakiasis. Fishes and Anisakis (No. 7 fishes scientific series). The Japanese Society of Scientific Fisheries, Koseisha Koseikaku, Tokyo, pp. 58–72 (in Japanese)
32. Mizugaki H, Asaishi K, Ishikura H, Hayasaka H (1970) Studies on enteritis regionatis (VI)-Experimental study on skip lesion. Hokkaido J Surg 15: 47–52 (in Japanese)
33. Ishikura H, Mizugaki H, Hayasaka H (1971) Studies on regional enteritis (7)—Experimental studies on enteritis regionalis exsudativa acuta with bacillus infection. Hokkaido J Med Sci 46: 374–381 (in Japanese)
34. Ishikura H, Kikuchi Y, Hayasaka H (1967) Pathological and clinical observation on intestinal anisakiasis. Arch Jpn Chir 36: 663–679 (in Japanese)
35. Fukuda S, Hachisuga K, Yamaguchi A et al. (1984) Three cases of anisakiasis causing acute intestinal obstruction. Clin Surg 39: 707–711 (in Japanese)
36. Sasaki M, Aoki Y, Syoji M, Matsumoto K, Okamoto S, Katsumi M (1979) A case report of perforation of small intestine by penetrated *Anisakis* larva, Jpn J Surg 80: 288 (in Japanese)
37. Kikuchi Y, Ueda T, Yoshiki T, Aizawa M, Ishikura H (1967) Experimental immunopathological studies on intestinal anisakiasis. Igakuno Ayumi 62 (11): 731–736 (in Japanese)
38. Kuipers FC, Kampelmacher EH, Steenbergen F (1963) Onderzoekingen over harinawormziekte dij Konijen. Ned T Geneesk 22: 990–995
39. Ishikura H, Kanemoto T, Goto T, (1960) Acute abdomen caused by ileitis terminalis: A case accompanied skip areas and invaginations ileus. Jpn J Gastroenterol 58: 867 (in Japanese)
40. Ishikura H, Tanaka M, Goto T et al. (1965) Studies on regional enteritis: I. Epidemiology of 87 cases at Iwanai district in Hokkaido. Geka chiryo 13: 144–154 (in Japanese)
41. Ishikura H. Kikuchi K, Tsuji Y (1961) Several clinico-pathological appearances on Crohn's disease. J Clin Digestive Disease 3: 662–675 (in Japanese)
42. Inoue J, Shimizu N, Yoshida K, Fugii S, Adachi H (1974) Clinical studies on 6 cases of intestinal anisakiasis, particularly cases accompanied by skip lesion. Clin Surg 29: 809–814 (in Japanese)
43. Sasaki K, Sasaki T, Nagamine Y (1984) A case report of intestinal anisakiasis with skip lesion and mesenteric granulima formation. J Jpn Soc Clin Surg 45: 1183–1187 (in Japanese)

Epidemiological Aspects of Intestinal Anisakiasis and Its Pathogenesis

44. Ishikura H, Mizugaki H, Asaishi K, Sato K, Hayasaka H (1970) Studies on enteritis regionalis (4)—Histo-pathological studies on regional enteritis acuta in Japan. J Jpn Soc Clin Surg 31: 79–91 (in Japanese)
45. Saito K, Okino M (1966): Enteritis regionalis; Clin & Ex Med 43: 1818–1823 (in Japanese)
46. Naka T, Aikawa K, Shinno T, Kuranishi H (1969) Experiences with acute nonspecific regional enteritis. Clin Surg 24: 129–133 (in Japanese)
47. Ishikura H, Mizugaki H, Hayasaka H (1971) Studies on regional enteritis (7)—Experimental studies on enteritis regionalis exsudative acuta with bacillus infection. Hokkaido J Med Sci 46: 374–381 (in Japanese)
48. Furukawa A (1974) Anisakiasis—Its history and a case of acute ileitis, attributable to a living larva of *Anisakis* in a peritoneal cavity. J Jpn Soc Clin Surg 35: 63–69 (in Japanese)
49. Yoshimura H, Kondo K, Oonishi Y, Akao N, Tsubota N (1978) Statistical observation on Anisakiasis of our department during the last 3 years, especially on its clinico-pathology and immunodiagnostics. Jpn Med J 2837: 29–32 (in Japanese)
50. Ishikura H, Kobayashi Y, Yagi K, Fujita O, Nakajima O, Miyamoto K (1987) Current topics of terranovasis in Japan Proceedings of the 34th North Japan regional meeting 39pp. in Sapporo City, Hokkaido, Sept 11 (in Japanese)
51. Karasawa Y, Takahara K, Hirafuku I, Hoshi K (1984) Experience of anisakiasis and terranovasis of digestive tracts. Gastroenterol Endosc 26: 2134–2135 (in Japanese)
52. Suzuki H, Oonuma H, Karasawa Y (1972) *Terranova* larva infection in human stomach wall. Saishin Igaku 29: 521–526 (in Japanese)
53. Nishimura T (1969) Ecological appearance on *Anisakis* larvae. Sai-shin Igaku 24: 405–412 (in Japanese)
54. Ishikura H, Hayasaka H (1974) Current problems on anisakiasis in Japan. Surg 36: 887–892 (in Japanese)
55. Ishikura H (1969) Anisakiasis, especially treatment of intestinal anisakiasis. Jpn Med J 2375: 133 (in Japanese)
56. Hara K, Yokoyama T (1985) A clinical study on possible anisakiasis intestinalis causing acute intestinal obstruction. J Jpn Soc Clin Surg 46: 416–421 (in Japanese)
57. Desowitz RS: Human and experimental anisakiasis in the United States (1986) Hokkaido J Med Sci 61: 358–371
58. Kagei N, Yanagawa I, Nagano K, Oishi K (1972) A larva of *Terranova sp.* causing acute abdominal syndrome in woman. Jpn J Parasitol 21: 262–265
59. Ishikura H (1989) New findings concerning Anisakis larva and anisakiasis. Jpn Soc Clin Surg 50: 237–247 (in Japanese with English abstract)
60. Ishikura H. Namiki M (Eds) (1989) Gastric anisakiasis in Japan-Epidemiology, Diagnosis, Treatment. Springer-Verlag Tokyo 140pp.
61. Hayasaka H, Takagi R, Iwano H, Asaishi K, Ishikura H, Mizugaki H (1969) A case of anisakiasis caused by two *Anisakis* larvae penetration. Hokkaido J Med Sci 14: 141–146 (in Japanese with English abstract)

Anisakis Larvae in Intermediate and Paratenic Hosts in Japan

K. Nagasawa

Introduction

In 1972, Oshima [1] published an excellent and comprehensive review, "*Anisakis* and anisakiasis in Japan and adjacent area", based on widely scattered information in numerous Japanese publications. This is still one of the most important and useful reviews of the general biology of *Anisakis* and human anisakiasis in the world. In recent years, however, our knowledge on the life cycle and host relationships of *Anisakis* has increased considerably in Japan and it is now worthwhile to assemble new information. This paper introduces current knowledge on the occurrence of larval *Anisakis* in intermediate and paratenic hosts in Japan. As reviewed by Nagasawa [2], marine invertebrates (especially euphausiids) are the intermediate hosts of *A. simplex* and a wide variety of fish and squid serve as its paratenic hosts.

Anisakis Larvae in Intermediate Hosts

There are three records of natural infection of euphausiids with *Anisakis* larvae in the waters around Japan. Shimazu and Oshima [3] found a larva from *Euphausia pacifica* collected in the western North Pacific off Onagawa, Miyagi Prefecture. Kagei [4] recovered two larvae in *E. pacifica* from the East China Sea and recently Shimazu [5] found a larva in *E. nana* from the same area. In all cases, one larva was found in each infected euphausiid. The site of infection was the cephalothoracic hemocoel of the hosts. Prevalences of these infections were extremely low, ranging from 0.002% (= 1/54,000) [3] to 0.007% (= 2/28,219) [4]. Additionally, Shimazu [6] examined over 35,000 specimens of *E. similis* collected in Sagami and Suruga Bays in central Honshu, but failed to find any larval *Anisakis* in them. Kagei [4] also examined about 220 specimens of *E. similis* from the same waters with negative results.

The larvae reported from Japanese euphausiids were all morphologically identical with *Anisakis* sp. larvae type I of Berland [7], which is a larval form of *A. simplex*. According to Kagei [4] and Shimazu [6], the larvae ranged in body length from 2.70 to 17.70 mm. The boring tooth was present at the anterior extremity of the body, and the oesophagus consisted of the anterior muscular portion (preventriculus) and the posterior glandular portion (ventriculus). The ventriculus was long (0.15–0.67 mm) and connected obliquely with the intestine, with the excretory pore located between the subventral lips on the head. The

24 K. Nagasawa

rounded tail was 0.05–0.08 mm long and had a mucron at the posterior end. Genital organs were not observed.

Euphausia pacifica is principally a cold-water species, being widely distributed in the northern North Pacific region including the southern Bering Sea, the southern Sea of Okhotsk, and the Sea of Japan [8]. This euphauiid often forms dense shoals and surface swarms in the waters off Sanriku and Joban districts in northeastern Honshu, where a commercial fishery to exploit its patches or swarms exists [9,10]. *Euphausia pacifica* is one of the major food items of the most frequent teleosts of *Anisakis* larvae, such as chub mackerel (*Scomber japonicus*) [11,12] and walleye pollock (*Theragra chalcogramma*) [13,14], and it seems to play an important role in the transmission of *Anisakis*. On the other hand, *E. nana* is the most dominant species of euphausiid occurring in the East China Sea, especially within the shallow continental shelf [15]. Since fish from this sea have high prevalences of infection with larval *Anisakis* [16], *E. nana* may serve as an important intermediate host there.

Despite the intensive field surveys, only three euphausiid species belonging to the genus *Euphausia* (*E. pacifica*, *E. nana*, and *E. similis*) have been examined for larval *Anisakis* in Japan. However, there are a number of euphausiid species in this country. For example, 9 genera and 39 species have been recorded from Sagami Bay [17] and 8 genera and 35 species from the East China Sea and its adjacent waters [15]. Thus, it is necessary to examine as many species as possible to assess their role as intermediate hosts in the life cycle of *Anisakis*.

Shiraki et al. [18] examined two species of caridean prawns, *Pandalus borealis* and *P. kessleri*, from the Sea of Japan and the Sea of Okhotsk, respectively, and found larval *Anisakis* in them. Prevalences were 0.01% (= 5/5,046) in *P. borealis* and 0.3% (= 2/724) in *P. kessleri*. The larvae closely resembled *Anisakis* sp. larvae type I of Berland [7]. They had three pseudolabia on the head and a rounded tail with a mucron and a conical boring tooth was present at the anterior tip of the body. The junction between the ventriculus and intestine was oblique. Nagasawa [2] stated that benthic inveterbrates may be of little importance in the transmission of *A. simplex*.

Anisakis Larvae in Paratenic Hosts

Larval types of *anisakis*. Four larval types of *Anisakis* have been recorded from fish and squid in Japanese waters. Of these, type I and type II larvae were described in detail by Koyama et al. [19] and Shiraki [20], and the surface ultrastructure of these larvae observed by Fukuda et al. [21]. Morphological features of both types were also summarized by Koyama [22]. Furthermore, Aihara [23] made detailed morphological and morphometric observations on type I larvae and Weerasooriya et al. [24] and Ishii et al. [25] have recently reported the external morphology of this type based on a scanning electron microscope study. Type I larva has a relatively long ventriculus with an oblique ventriculus-intestinal junction and a short rounded tail with a mucron, whereas type II larva possesses a short ventriculus with a horizontal ventriculus-intestinal junction and a long, conical, tapering tail without a mucron. According to Shiraki [20], the average sizes of type I and type II larvae from fish in the northern coastal waters of Japan are 28.4 × 0.49 mm and 25.7 × 0.61 mm, respectively. However, there is a marked difference in size between geographical locations: type I larvae from

Anisakis Larvae in Intermediate and Paratenic Hosts in Japan

fish in the East and South China Seas are apparently smaller than those of Shiraki [20], measuring 17.0×0.41 mm on average [16].

Koyama et al. [19] and Shiraki [20] stated that *Anisakis* type I and type II larvae of Japan are identical with *Anisakis* larvae type I and II of Berland [7] respectively from Norwegian fish. In Japanese waters, type I larva is one of the most common parasites of marine fish, occurring in 164 fish species and one squid species [26], and type II larva has been recorded from 26 fish species (excluding coelacanth) and two squid species [26]. Based on hemoglobin analyses of larvae and adults of *Anisakis*, Suzuki and Ishida [27] suggested that type I larvae from walleye pollock and type II larvae from skipjack tuna (*Katsuwonus pelamis*) are *A. simplex* and *A. physeteris* respectively. Agatsuma [28] also stated that both larval types are distinguished from each other by enzyme electrophoresis. Recently, Oshima et al. [29] reared type I larvae from chub mackerel and walleye pollock to adult worms *in vitro*, which were identified as *A. simplex*. They also tried to rear type II larvae but failed to get adults.

Type III and type IV larvae were described by Shiraki [20]. The former type is characterized by a stout body (28.9×0.84 mm on average), a short ventriculus, and a short rounded tail lacking a mucron, and has been recorded from walleye pollock, Pacific cod (*Gadus macrocephalus*), and longfin cutthroat eel (*Synaphobranchus affinis*). Type IV larvae are relatively small (20.1×0.54 mm on average) and possess a short ventriculus and a short, conical, pointed tail without a mucron. This type has been found only in walleye pollock. No *in vitro* cultivation of these larval types has been made and the relationships between the types and adults are unknown.

Paratenic hosts as important sources of human anisakiasis

Chub mackerel (*Scomber japonicus*). There is increasing evidence that chub mackerel are the most important source of human anisakiasis in Japan with a report from Fukuoka Prefecture that most cases (85.2%) of acute gastric anisakiasis found were caused by eating raw or lightly cooked chub mackerel [30]. Kanemitsu et al. [31] detected the first case of this disease in Okinawa, the southernmost prefecture of Japan, and stated that the causative fish was chub mackerel caught in Kyushu waters. Hatano et al. [32] and Omachi et al. [33] also emphasized that raw or vinegared chub mackerel was important as a source of *Anisakis* infections of man in Yamaguchi and Nagano Prefectures, respectively. According to unpublished data of Iino, 1,370 of 1,625 cases (84.8%) of human anisakiasis found in Kyushu during 1980–1984 were attributed to chub mackerel.

There are many published reports of the occurrence of *Anisakis* larvae in Japanese chub mackerel, from which two types (I and II) have been recorded (for references prior to 1970, see Oshima [1]). Most investigations demonstrated high prevalences of infection with type I larvae and a rare occurrence of type II larvae. In Sagami Bay, for example, type I larvae occurred in 43.9% (mean intensity: 3.88) of chub mackerel examined, while type II larvae were found in only 6.3% (1.36) [34]. *Anisakis* larvae are commonly found encapsulated or free among the mesenteries and in the body cavity, viscera and musculature, although type II larvae have never been reported from the musculature. Yamada [35] stated that over 70% of type I larvae found in chub mackerel were located in the body cavity.

The level of infection with *Anisakis* larvae is closely associated with the size (age) of chub mackerel with prevalence and mean intensity of infection steadily rising with increasing host length [34,35].

Regarding seasonal changes in the occurrence of larval *Anisakis*, Kosugi [34] found that type I larvae were most abundant during April and May in chub mackerel from Sagami Bay. Since this fish spends summer and autumn in southeast Hokkaido waters and returns to Sagami Bay in spring for spawning, he suggested that chub mackerel became infected mainly in the Hokkaido waters.

Horse mackerel (*Trachurus japonicus*). Although less important than chub mackerel, horse mackerel is also regarded as an important source of human anisakiasis in Japan, especially in Kyushu. Fujino et al. [30] found that seven of 155 cases (4.5%) of this disease in Fukuoka Prefecture were due to horse mackerel. Iino (unpublished) also mentioned that horse mackerel was responsible for 86 of 1,615 cases (5.3%) of anisakiasis in Kyushu during 1980–1984.

Only type I larvae have been recorded from Japanese horse mackerel. Oshima [1] summarized information prior to 1970 concerning the occurrence of this type in horse mackerel and suggested that infection with *Anisakis* takes place chiefly in the East China Sea. Hirayama [36] compared prevalences of type I larvae in horse mackerel from various localities of Japan and found that the fish from Nagasaki Prefecture, near the East China Sea, were most frequently infected. Larval *Anisakis* are found in the viscera or body cavity but not in the musculature, and Kosugi [34] reported that 72.0% of the larvae found in horse mackerel were located in the mesenteries and 15.0% on the pyloric caeca.

There is a positive relationship between the occurrence of *Anisakis* larvae and the host length, with prevalence increasing with an increase in host size reaching a peak (37.5%) at 33–40 cm in body length [34]. In cases of heavy infections, two horse mackerel of 33–35 cm long harbored as many as 164 and 167 larvae each [35].

Japanese flying squid (*Todarodes pacificus*). This squid is responsible for many cases of human anisakiasis in Japan. Omachi et al. [33] reported that Japanese flying squid followed chub mackerel as the most frequent sources of the disease in Nagano Prefecture. Ishikura et al. [37] also found that, at Iwanai on the west coast of Hokkaido, *Anisakis* infections of man were frequently detected in summer and autumn, which are the main fishing seasons for Japanese flying squid there. Additionally, Fujino et al. [30] detected two cases of anisakiasis due to unidentified squid, which were possibly Japanese flying squid.

Type I and type II larvae have been found in Japanese flying squid, the former type more common than the latter [20,34]. The larvae of both types are found in the viscera and under the inner surface membrane of the mantle [34], although Hirayama [36] found the larvae in the musculature of the mantle as well. Within the viscera, the larvae are mostly located on the wall of the stomach [34].

Oshima [1] discussed seasonal occurrence of type I larvae in Japanese flying squid in relation to its migration and suggested that *Anisakis* larvae are acquired mainly in Hokkaido waters during August and October.

Sardine (*Sardinops melanosticus*). This fish has become important as a recent source of human anisakiasis in Japan with two of 155 cases (1.3%) of gastric

Anisakis Larvae in Intermediate and Paratenic Hosts in Japan

anisakiasis in Fukuoka Prefecture reportedly due to sardine [30]. Iino (unpublished) also found that 95 of 1,615 cases (5.9%) in Kyushu were attributed to this fish.

Since the early 1970s, the population of sardine has increased dramatically around Japan with recent annual catches exceeding three million tons, thus, the increase in human cases of anisakiasis due to sardine is in accordance with such a dramatic increase in the catch of the fish. However, little information is available on the occurrence of larval *Anisakis* in Japanese sardine, from which type I larvae have been recorded. Saito and Ishioka [38] conducted a parasitological survey of marine fish caught in the Sea of Japan off Shimane Prefecture and found heavy infections of *Anisakis* in sardine (prevalence: 40.3%, mean intensity: 52.5). Most worms were located on the pyloric caeca and in the body cavity whereas a small numbers of larvae occurred in the musculature.

Walleye Pollock (*Theragra chalcogramma*). According to Ishikura et al. [37], the highest case number of human anisakiasis at Iwanai, Hokkaido, occurs in the winter season (November to March), when walleye pollock is the most abundantly caught fish there.

Although three larval types (I, III and IV) have been recorded from walleye pollock, type I larvae are the most commonly found. Shiraki [20] reported that type I larvae occurred in 94.7–100% of walleye pollock from the northern waters of Japan while type III larvae were found in 1.3–2.4% of them. He also stated that nine worms of type IV larvae were collected together with several thousands of type I larvae and 16 worms of type III larvae from a large quantity of viscera (about 100 kg) of walleye pollock caught near Otaru, Hokkaido.

Sasaki [39] and Suzuki and Oishi [40] reported that the larvae were mostly found on the liver and to a lesser extent on the pyloric caeca. However, Shiraki [20] stated that muscular infections were found in over 10% of the walleye pollock.

References

1. Oshima T (1972) *Anisakis* and anisakiasis in Japan and adjacent area. In: Morishita K, Komiya Y, Matsubayashi H, (eds) Progress of medical parasitology in Japan, Vol. 4. Meguro Parasitological Museum, Tokyo, pp 301–393
2. Nagasawa K (1990) The life cycle of *Anisakis simplex*: a review. Ishikura H, Kikuchi K (eds) Intestinal anisakiasis in Japan. Springer-Verlag, Tokyo, pp 31–40
3. Shimazu T, Oshima T (1972) Some larval nematodes from euphausiid crustaceans. In: Takenouti Y et al. (eds) Biological oceanography of the northern North Pacific Ocean dedicated to Shigeru Motoda. Idemitsu Shoten, Tokyo, pp 403–409
4. Kagei N (1974) Studies on anisakid Nematoda (Anisakidae) (IV). Survey of *Anisakis* larvae in the marine Crustacea. Bull Inst Publ Health 23: 65–71 (in Japanese with English summary)
5. Shimazu T (1982) Some helminth parasites of marine planktonic invertebrates. J Nagano-ken Junior Coll 37: 11–29
6. Shimazu T (1974) I. Larvae of Anisakinae. 2. Ecology. Jpn Soc Sci Fish (ed) Fish and *Anisakis*, Fish Sci Ser 7. Koseisha Koseikaku, Tokyo, pp 23–43 (in Japanese)
7. Berland B (1961) Nematodes from some Norwegian marine fishes. Sarsia 2: 1–50
8. Mauchline J, Fisher LR (1969) The biology of euphausiids. Adv Mar Biol 7: 1–454
9. Komaki Y (1967) On the surface swarming of euphausiid crustaceans. Pac Sci 21: 433–438

10. Odate K (1979) A euphausiid Crustacea exploited along the Sanriku and Joban Coast. Bull Tohoku Reg Fish Res Lab 40: 15–25 (in Japanese with English summary)
11. Nishimura S (1959) Foods and feeding habits of the Pacific mackerel in the coastal waters of Niigata Prefecture, Japan Sea, in 1958. Ann Rep Jap Sea Reg Fish Res Lab 5: 77–87 (in Japanese with English summary)
12. Sato Y, Iizuka K, Kotaki K (1968) Some biological aspects of mackerel, *Pneumatophorus japonicus* (Houttuyn), in the northeastern sea of Japan. Bull Tohoku Reg Res Fish Lab 28: 1–50 (in Japanese with English summary)
13. Iizuka A, Kurohagi T, Ikuta K, Imai S (1954) Composition of the food of Alaska pollack (*Theragra chalcogramma*) in Hokkaido with special reference to its local differences. Bull Hokkaido Reg Fish Res Lab 11: 7–20 (in Japanese with English summary)
14. Maeda T, Takahashi T, Ueno M (1983) Behavior in each life period of adult Alaska pollack in the adjacent waters of Funka Bay, Hokkaido. Bull Jpn Soc Sci Fish 49: 577–585 (in Japanese with English summary)
15. Nemoto T, Hara K, Kamada K (1970) Euphausiids in the East China Sea and its adjacent waters. The Kuroshio II, Proc 2nd CSK Symposium. Sakon Publ Co Ltd, Tokyo, pp 273–283
16. Sakaguchi Y, Katamine D (1971) Survey of anisakid larvae in marine fishes caught from the East China Sea and the South China Sea. Trop Med 13: 159–169 (in Japanese with English summary)
17. Hirota Y, Nemoto T, Marumo R (1982) Seasonal variation and horizontal distribution of euphausiids in Sagami Bay, Central Japan. Bull Plankton Soc Japan 29: 37–47 (in Japanese with English summary)
18. Shiraki T, Hasegawa H, Kenmotsu M (1976) Larval anisakid nematodes from the prawns, *Pandalus* spp. Jpn J Parasitol 25: 148–152
19. Koyama T, Kobayashi A, Kumada M, Komiya Y, Oshima T, Kagei N, Ishii T, Machida M (1969) Morphological and taxonomical studies on Anisakidae larvae found in marine fishes and squids. Jpn J Parasitol 18: 466–487 (in Japanese with English summary)
20. Shiraki T (1974) Larval nematodes of family Anisakidae (Nematoda) in the northern sea of Japan—as a causative agent of eosinophilic phlegmone or granuloma in the human gastro-intestinal tract. Act Med Biol 22: 57–98
21. Fukuda T, Aji T, Tongu Y (1988) Surface ultrastructure of larval Anisakidae (Nematoda: Ascaridoidea) and its identification by mensuration. Acta Med Okayama 42: 105–116
22. Koyama T (1974) I. Larvae of Anisakinae. 1. Morphology and taxonomy. Jpn Soc Sci Fish (ed), Fish and *Anisakis*, Fish Sci Ser 7. Koseisha Koseikaku, Tokyo, pp 9–19 (in Japanese)
23. Aihara Y (1973) Morphological studies on *Anisakis* larvae Type I. J Osaka City Med Cent 22: 197–235 Pls 1–5 (in Japanese with English summary)
24. Weerasooriya MV, Fujino T, Ishii Y, Kagei N (1986) The value of external morphology of larval anisakid nematodes: a scanning electron microscope study. Z Parasitenkd 72: 765–778
25. Ishii Y, Fujino T, Weerasooriya MV (1989) Morphology of anisakine larvae. In: Ishikura H, Namiki M (eds), Gastric anisakiasis in Japan: epidemiology, diagnosis, treatment. Springer-Verlag, Tokyo, pp 19–29
26. Kagei N (1974) A list of fish infected with larval nematodes of the subfamily Anisakinae. Jpn Soc Sci Fish (ed), Fish and *Anisakis*, Fish Sci Ser 7. Koseisha Koseikaku, Tokyo, pp 98–107 (in Japanese)
27. Suzuki T, Ishida K (1979) *Anisakis simplex* and *Anisakis physeteris*: physicochemical properties of larval and adult hemoglobins. Exp Parasitol 48: 225–234
28. Agatsuma T (1981) Electrophoretic studies on glucosephosphate isomerase and phosphoglucomutase in two types of *Anisakis* larvae. Int J Parasitol 12: 35–39
29. Oshima T, Oya S, Wakai R (1962) In vitro cultivation of *Anisakis* Type I and Type II

Anisakis Larvae in Intermediate and Paratenic Hosts in Japan 29

larvae collected from fishes caught in Japanese coastal waters and their identification. Jpn J Parasitol 31: 131–134

30. Fujino T, Ooiwa T, Ishii Y (1984) Clinical, epidemiological and morphological studies on 150 cases of acute gastric anisakiasis in Fukuoka Prefecture. Jpn J Parasitol 33: 73–92 (in Japanese with English summary)
31. Kanemitsu K, Takara M, Torigoe Y, Satoh Y (1984) A case of anisakiasis in Okinawa. Saishin Igaku 39: 138–141 (in Japanese)
32. Hatano Y, Uchida Y, Hirota K, Ezaki T, Harada H, Kawahara K, Okazaki Y, Takemoto T, Fujii Y (1985) Clinical and endoscopic features in gastric anisakiasis. Gasteroenterol Endosc 27: 2306–2313 (in Japanese with English summary)
33. Omachi K, Omachi T, Maruyama Y (1985) Anisakiasis of gasterointestinal tract in Nagano Prefecture. Shinshu Med J 33: 42–56 (in Japanese with English summary)
34. Kosugi K (1972) Seasonal fluctuation of the infestation with the larvae of *Anisakis* and of related species of nematodes in fishes from Sagami Bay. Yokohama Med J 23: 285–316 (in Japanese with English summary)
35. Yamada G (1971) Studies on the prevention of *Anisakis* larva infection. J Osaka City Med Cent 20: 131–159 Pls 1–2 (in Japanese with English summary)
36. Hirayama T (1974) Prevalence of infection with larval *Anisakis* in horse mackerel and Japanese flying squid at the Tokyo Central Market. In: Jpn Soc Sci Fish (ed), Fish and *Anisakis*, Fish Sci Ser 7. Koseisha Koseikaku, Tokyo, pp 91–97 (in Japanese)
37. Ishikura H, Hayasaka J, Kikuchi Y (1967) Acute regional ileitis at Iwanai in Hokkaido—with special reference to intestinal anisakiasis. Sapporo Med J 32: 183–196
38. Saito K, Ishioka 2 (1970) Survey of *Anisakis* larvae in marine fish in Shimane Prefecture. J Shimane Med Assoc 4: 547–551 (in Japanese)
39. Sasaki M (1973) Survey of parasites of walleye pollock *Theragra chalcogramma*. J Hokkaido Fish Exp St (Hokusuishi Geppo) 30: 14–34 (in Japanese)
40. Suzuki M, Oishi K (1974) III. Infections of fish. 9. Parasites of walleye pollock, *Theragra chalcogramma*. Jpn Soc Sci Fish (ed), Fish and *Anisakis*, Fish Sci Ser 7. Koseisha Koseikaku, Tokyo, pp 113–125 (in Japanese)

The Life Cycle of *Anisakis simplex*: A Review

K. NAGASAWA

Introduction

Anisakis simplex (Rudolphi, 1809, det. Krabbe, 1878) in its larval stage is a common nematode parasite of marine fish, with the adult parasite widely distributed in marine mammals, particularly in colder temperate and polar waters [1]. This parasite causes eosinophilic granuloma in the alimentary tract of man when raw or inadequately cooked fish with live larvae are ingested [2,3]. To determine its medical significance with regard to human infection, called "anisakiasis" or "anisakiosis", various aspects of the parasite have been studied to date. This review focuses on the life cycle of *A. simplex* (Fig. 1), based on information from surveys which were conducted mainly in the North Pacific Ocean and North Sea.

The recent recovery of two sibling species within *A. simplex* in European waters [4–7] has complicated the identification of the parasite. In this review, however, *A. simplex* is treated as a single species because further information is not available on the taxonomy and identification of the *A. simplex* complex from other areas including the North and South Pacific Oceans. In addition, the formerly described *Anisakis* type I larvae [8–10] are regarded as *A. simplex* larvae on the basis of morphological [11] and *in vitro* cultivation studies [12–17].

Eggs and Hatched Larvae

The eggs of *A. simplex* are passed with the faeces of marine mammalian final hosts and embryonate in the sea. Banning [12] and Grabda [14] succeeded in obtaining egg-laying adults of *A. simplex* during their *in vitro* culture studies and according to Banning [12], the eggs have transparent and smooth shells, are round to oval and measure 40×50 μm on average. It takes the larvae 4–8 days at 13–18°C and 20–27 days at 5–7°C to emerge from the eggs after embryonic development in sea water.

The first moult takes place within the eggs and hatched free-living larvae, ensheathed in the cast cuticle of the moult, are in the second stage [2,18,19]. The average length of the hatched *A. simplex* is 355 μm with the sheath and 230 μm without it [12]. The larvae bear a boring tooth at the anterior extremity and show a nerve ring. They are very active in sea water and can survive for 3–4 weeks at 13–18°C and 6–7 weeks at 5–7°C [12]. A hatched second-stage larva of *A. simplex* (or *A. typica*) is finely illustrated by Shimazu [18].

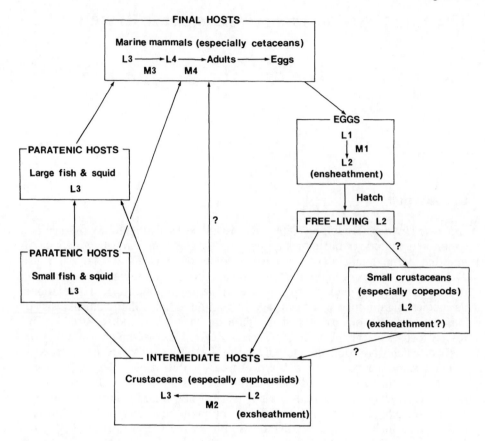

Fig. 1. Life cycle of *Anisakis simplex*. L1: first-stage larva, L2: second-stage larva, L3: third-stage larva, L4: fourth-stage larva, M1: first moult, M2: second moult, M3: third moult, M4: fourth moult

Intermediate Hosts

Uspenskaya [20] was the first scientist to discover *Anisakis* larvae in marine crustaceans. She found larval *Anisakis* in the amphipod *Caprella septentrionalis*, the decapod *Hyas araneus* and the euphausiid *Thysanoessa raschii* in the Barents Sea. Also in European waters, Smith [21] reported *Anisakis* sp. larvae in three euphausiid species (*T. inermis, T. longicaudata,* and *Meganyctiphanes norvegica*) from the northern North Sea and North-East Atlantic. Subsequently, Smith [22,23] identified both these and newly collected larvae from two more euphausiid species (*Nyctiphanes couchi* and *T. raschii*) in the same region as *A. simplex*. Sluiters [24] also obtained an *Anisakis* larva which was emerging from *T. raschii* in the stomach of a North Sea herring (*Clupea harengus*).

Japanese parasitologists have conducted intensive field surveys to find the intermediate hosts of *A. simplex* and have contributed greatly to the understanding of the importance of euphausiids in its life cycle. Oshima et al. [25] and Shimazu and Oshima [26] went as far as the northern North Pacific and Bering Sea to

The Life Cycle of *Anisakis simplex*: A Review

collect euphausiids which were suspected to be the most probable intermediate hosts. Kagei [27] examined over 67,000 marine invertebrates belonging to Crustacea (Calanoida, Euphausiacea, Decapoda), Coelenterata (Scyphozoa) and Chaetognatha (Sagittoidea) collected from various localities in the North Pacific, East China Sea, Sea of Okhotsk, Bering Sea, and Antarctic Ocean. Later, Kagei [28] reported the results of an examination of over 170,000 euphausiids from several oceans in the northern and southern hemispheres. Shimazu [29] also examined large samples of marine planktonic invertebrates representing Chaetognatha (Sagittoidea) and Crustacea (Euphausiacea, Decapoda) taken from Japanese waters, and the East and South China Seas. These authors all succeeded in finding larval *Anisakis* in their euphausiid samples, such as in *T. raschii*, *T. longiceps* [25,26], *Euphausia pacifica* [26,27], *E. vallentini* [28], and *E. nana* [29]. Furthermore, Shiraki et al. [30] examined two species of caridean prawns (*Pandalus borealis* and *P. kessleri*) from the Seas of Japan and Okhotsk and recovered *Anisakis* larvae from both species. The larvae which these Japanese workers found in the euphausiids and prawns were all identified as *A. simplex*. In addition, Hurst [31] has recently found *A. simplex* larvae in the euphausiid *Nyctiphanes australis* from the coastal waters of New Zealand.

Experimental infections of euphausiids with the second-stage larvae of *A. simplex* were carried out by Japanese parasitologists. According to Oshima [2,32], *E. similis* and *E. pacifica* became infected when these were exposed to numerous hatched ensheathed larvae, and some of the larvae exsheathed within 8 days after exposure. Moreover, Smith [23] has recently suggested that the second-stage larvae of *A. simplex* may be transferred to euphausiids or other crustaceans by copepods or other small crustaceans.

As shown by these field and experimental studies, euphausiids definitely appear to play an important role as the intermediate hosts of *A. simplex* [2,18,23]. Euphausiids become infected by feeding on hatched second-stage larvae; such larvae shed their sheath and migrate to the hemocoel, where they moult and develop to the third stage. The larvae are not encapsulated and lie free in the hemocoel [22,25].

Euphausiids are one of the major sources of food for the most frequently *Anisakis*-infected teleosts, such as herring (*Clupea harengus*) in the North Sea [24] and jack mackerels (*Trachurus novaezelandiae* and *T. declivis*) in New Zealand waters [31]. Thus, despite the fact that the prevalence of euphausiid with *A. simplex* larvae is usually quite low [19,33], third-stage larvae are easily acquired by such teleosts in prey-predator relationships. On the other hand, the importance of benthic invertebrates (e.g., decapods and amphipods) as intermediate hosts of *A. simplex* still remains obscure. However, their role appears to be smaller, at least in offshore waters, than that of euphausiids since the most frequent fish hosts of the parasite feed mainly on planktonic animals.

A special comment is necessary on the larval stage and moulting of *A. simplex* in euphausiids. Some Japanese workers (e.g., Oshima et al. [25]; Oshima [32]; Kagei [34]) first considered that euphausiid-infecting larvae are in the second stage. Kagei [34] also indicated that the moult from the second to the third stage occurs in fish, and but not in euphausiids. However, Oshima [2] suggested that the second-stage larvae of *A. simplex* moult to the third stage in euphausiids before they develop to a body size of 6 mm. Shimazu [18] made a similar suggestion that *Anisakis* larvae of roughly 5 mm undergo a moult to grow to the third

34 K. Nagasawa

stage in euphausiids. Recently, based on detailed observations on *A. simplex* larvae from euphausiids in the North-East Atlantic and northern North Sea, Smith [23] has strongly suggested that the moult from the second to the third stage takes place in euphausiids when the larvae are about 4–6 mm long. If these suggestions are correct, small larvae less than 4–6 mm in length could be in the second stage and those larger could be in the third stage. Smith [23] actually identified small larvae, 4.2–5.9 mm long, from euphausiids as the second-stage larvae of *A. simplex*. While Shimazu [29] did not comment on the stage of an *A. simplex* larva, 2.7 mm long, from the euphausiid *E. nana*, it should be regarded as a second-stage larva.

Paratenic Hosts

As pointed out by Smith and Wooten [19], there was confusion in the literature concerning the life cycle of *Anisakis*, particularly the role played by various hosts. For example, Kagei [34] earlier believed that euphausiids and a wide variety of fish and squid serve as the first and second intermediate hosts respectively. However, Shimazu [18] discussed the life cycle of *Anisakis* and the role of various hosts in detail and concluded that euphausiids serve as intermediate hosts but that fish and squid act as paratenic hosts. Kagei [27] also emphasized the importance of fish and squid in this role. Furthermore, Smith and Wooten [19] stated that fish and squid must regarded as "paratenic" hosts if a moult takes place in crustaceans, which can then be regarded as the only obligatory "intermediate" hosts. Smith [23] has recently reviewed the life history and ecology of *A. simplex* and discussed the status of teleosts and squid as hosts of its third-stage larvae.

Anisakis simplex larvae have been recorded from numerous species of marine fish. For example, Oshima [2] and Kagei [35,36] listed 123–164 fish species (mostly teleosts) as hosts of this parasite in Japanese and adjacent waters. Many studies have been made on various aspects of *A. simplex* in commercially important teleosts in different regions: Atlantic herring (*Clupea harengus*) in European and Canadian waters [37–46]; Pacific herring (*C. harengus pallasi*) in the eastern North Pacific [47,48]; Atlantic salmon (*Salmo salar*) in the North Atlantic [42,44,49–52]; chum salmon (*Oncorhynchus keta*) and sockeye salmon (*O. nerka*) in the North Pacific [53–56]; gadoids including cod (*Gadus morhua*), whiting (*Merlangius merlangus*) and haddock (*Melanogrammus aeglefinus*) in the North Atlantic [57–60]; walleye pollock (*Theragra chalcogramma*) in Canadian and Asian Pacific waters [61–63]; and hake (*Merluccius gayi*) in Chilean waters [64,65]. In Japan, Oshima [2] and Nagasawa [33] summarized the occurrence of *A. simplex* larvae in some teleosts, such as chub mackerel (*Scomber japonicus*), horse mackerel (*Trachurus japonicus*) and walleye pollock, which are important sources of human anisakiasis in this country.

Squid are also important paratenic hosts of *A. simplex*, with Japanese flying squid (*Todarodes pacificus*) frequently infected with this parasite [2]. According to Kagei [34], *A. simplex* larvae are most abundant in this squid during the autumn and winter, which is closely associated with the host's northward migration along the coast of Japan. Kosugi [66] also reported the seasonal occurrence of the parasite in Japanese flying squid from Sagami Bay, central Japan.

The Life Cycle of *Anisakis simplex*: A Review   35

In European waters, *A. simplex* larvae have been found in four squid species (*Loligo forbesi, Allotheuthis media, Todarodes saggittatus* and *Todaropsis eblane*) from around Scotland and the northern North Sea [67].

Fish and squid become infected with *A. simplex* by feeding on intermediate hosts (mainly euphausiids) harboring its third-stage larvae. The larvae undergo no moult in these paratenic hosts [18,23]. If small-sized fish or squid are preyed on by large-sized fish or squid, the larvae are capable of re-establishing in the latter hosts without a moult. Such a transfer of larval *Anisakis* from fish to fish was experimentally verified by Smith [68].

The larvae are usually found encapsulated in the viscera and flesh of fish. Smith [69] discussed the difference in the site of *A. simplex* infection between euphausiid-feeding fish (herring, mackerel, blue whiting, walleye pollock) and piscivorous fish (whiting, cod). In the former fish, the larvae are mostly found in the body cavity, while in the latter they occur mainly in the flesh.

Final Hosts

Marine mammals serve as the final hosts for *A. simplex*. Twenty-six cetacean and 12 pinniped species have been recorded to be infected with the parasite in different oceans and seas of the world [70]. Although it is difficult to evaluate the relative importance of these animals as final hosts, pinnipeds may be of less importance than cetaceans. Young [57] stated that seals are not significant hosts of *A. simplex* in British waters, where adult parasites are absent from harbor seals (*Phoca vitulina*) and a few adults occur in grey seals (*Halichoerus grypus*). Smith and Wooten [19] made a similar suggestion. Machida [71,72] also found none or only a few adult *A. simplex* in northern fur seals (*Callorhinus ursinus*) from the North Pacific, Sea of Okhotsk and Bering Sea. On the other hand, cetaceans are considered to be more important final hosts [57], but they are by no means always infected with *A. simplex*. According to Kagei and Kureha [73], entire stomach samples of three whale species (sei whales *Balaenoptera borealis*, fin whales *B. physalus* and pigmy blue whales *B. musculus brevicauda*) from the Antarctic Ocean were completely free from *Anisakis* adults. This is definitely related to the fact that the euphausiid *Euphausia superba*, the major food of these whales in that region, is not infected with larval *Anisakis* [74].

Furthermore, there are considerable differences in prevalence and intensity of *A. simplex* among cetaceans in certain regions. Kagei et al. [75] reported that striped dolphins (*Stenella coeruloalba*) were most frequently infected with *A. simplex* among marine mammals including seven cetacean and one pinniped species mainly from Japanese waters, but this may be influenced by the sampling location, season, and age and size of the hosts. Young [57] also examined the occurrence of *A. simplex* in five cetacean species from British waters.

There are also some records of *A. simplex* from sea birds [19]. However, due to the lack of data, it is impossible to determine the role of such hosts in the life cycle of *A. simplex*. Smith [23] stated that sea birds may be regarded as "accidental" hosts.

Marine mammalian final hosts acquire *A. simplex* by preying on fish and squid harboring third-stage larvae. The main site of infection is the stomach, where the third and fourth moults take place and the parasites develop from the third stage

36 K. Nagasawa

through the fourth stage to sexually mature adults. Because third-stage larvae are infective to final hosts, marine mammals could acquire direct infection by feeding on parasitized crustacean intermediate hosts. Smith [23] suggested such a possibility concerning the infection of blue whales (*B. musculus*) with the parasite.

Summary

The life cycle of *A. simplex* is reviewed based on information from surveys mainly in the North Pacific Ocean and North Sea.

The eggs of *A. simplex* are shed with the faeces of marine mammalian final hosts (mainly cetaceans) and embryonate in the sea. The first moult takes place within the eggs and the embryos develop to second-stage larvae. They hatch or emerge from the eggs, still ensheathed in the cast cuticle of the first moult, and are then free in the sea. The larvae exsheath on being ingested by crustaceans (especially euphausiids) and migrate to the hemocoel, where the second moult occurs and development proceeds to the third stage. They are not encapsulated and lie free in the hemocoel. Copepods or small crustaceans may transfer the second-stage larvae to euphausiids or other crustaceans. Fish (especially teleosts) and squid become infected when they feed on crustaceans harboring the third-stage larvae. If small-sized fish or squid are preyed on by larger fish or squid, the larvae are capable of re-establishing in the latter host without a moult. Marine mammals become infected by feeding on fish and squid parasitized by third-stage larvae, with the third and fouth moults occurring in the stomach of marine mammals, where the larvae grow from the third through the fourth stage to sexually mature adults. As the third-stage larvae are infective to final hosts, marine mammals could acquire direct infections by eating crustaceans harboring such larvae.

References

1. Davey JT (1971) A revision of the genus *Anisakis* Dujardin, 1845 (Nematoda: Ascaridata). J Helminthol 45: 51–72
2. Oshima T (1972) *Anisakis* and anisakiasis in Japan and adjacent area. In: Morishita K, Komiya Y, Matsubayashi H (eds) Progress of medical parasitology in Japan, Vol 4. Meguro Parasitological Museum, Tokyo, pp 301–393
3. Ishikura H and Namiki M (eds) (1989) Gastric anisakiasis in Japan: epidemiology, diagnosis, treatment. Springer-Verlag, Tokyo, 1–144
4. Nascetti G, Paggi L, Orecchia P, Mattiucci S, Bullini L (1981) Divergenza genetica in popolazioni del genere *Anisakis* del Mediterraneo. Parassitologia 23: 208–210
5. Nascetti G, Paggi L, Orecchia P, Mattiucci S, Bullini L (1983) Two sibling species within *Anisakis simplex* (Ascaridida: Anisakidae). Parassitologia 25: 306–307
6. Nascetti G, Paggi L, Orecchia P, Smith JW, Mattiucci S, Bullini L (1986) Electrophoretic studies on the *Anisakis simplex* complex (Ascaridida: Anisakidae) from the Mediterranean and North-East Atlantic. Int J Parasitol 16: 633–640
7. Orecchia P, Paggi L, Mattiucci S, Smith JW, Nascetti G, Bullini L (1986) Electrophoretic identification of larvae and adults of *Anisakis* (Ascaridida: Anisakidae). J Helminthol 60: 331–339

The Life Cycle of *Anisakis simplex*: A Review

8. Berland B (1961) Nematodes from some Norwegian marine fishes. Sarsia 2: 1–50
9. Koyama T, Kobayashi A, Kumada M, Komiya Y, Oshima T, Kagei N, Ishii T, Machida M (1969) Morphological and taxonomical studies on Anisakidae larvae found in marine fishes and squids. Jpn J Parasitol 18: 466–487 (in Japanese with English summary)
10. Shiraki T (1974) Larval nematodes of family Anisakidae (Nematoda) in the northern sea of Japan—as a causative agent of eosinophlic phlegmone or granuloma in the human gastro-intestinal tract. Acta Med Biol 22: 57–98
11. Beverley-Burton M, Nyman OL, Pippy JHC (1977) The morphology, and some observations on the population genetics of *Anisakis simplex* larvae (Nematoda: Ascaridata) from fishes of the North Atlantic. J Fish Res Board Can 34: 105–112
12. Banning P Van (1971) Some notes on a successful rearing of the herring-worm *Anisakis marina* L. (Nematoda: Heterocheilidae). J Cons Int Explor Mer 34: 84–88
13. Pippy JHC, Banning P van (1975) Identification of *Anisakis* larvae (I) as *Anisakis simplex* (Rudolphi, 1809, det. Krabbe 1878) (Nematoda: Ascaridata) J Fish Res Board Can 32: 29–32
14. Grabda J (1976) Studies on the life cycle and morphogenesis of *Anisakis simplex* (Rudolphi, 1809) (Nematoda: Anisakidae) cultured in vitro. Acta Ichthyol Piscat 6: 119–141
15. Carvajal J, Barros C, Santander G, Alcalde C (1981) In vitro culture of larval anisakid parasites of the Chilean hake *Merluccius gayi*. J Parasitol 67: 958–959
16. Oshima T, Oya S, Wakai R (1982) In vitro cultivation of *Anisakis* Type I and Type II larvae collected from fishes caught in Japanese coastal waters and their identification. Jpn J Parasitol 31: 131–134
17. Hurst RJ (1984) Identification and description of larval *Anisakis simplex* and *Pseudoterranova decipiens* (Anisakidae: Nematoda) from New Zealand waters. New Zeal J Mar Freshw Res 18: 177–186
18. Shimazu T (1974) I. Larvae of Anisakinae. 2. Ecology. Jpn Soc Sci Fish (ed) Fish and *Anisakis*, Fish Sci Ser 7. Koseisha Koseikaku, Tokyo, pp 23–43 (in Japanese)
19. Smith JW, Wooten R (1978) *Anisakis* and anisakiasis. Lumsden WHR, Muller R, Baker JR (eds) Advances in parasitology, Vol 16. Academic Press, London, pp 93–163
20. Uspenskaya AV (1963) Parasite fauna of benthic crustaceans from the Barents Sea. Izdatel'stvo Akademiya Nauk SSSR, Moscow and Leningrad, 127 pp (in Russian)
21. Smith JW (1971) *Thysanoessa inermis* and *T. longicaudata* (Euphausiidae) as first intermediate hosts of *Anisakis* sp. (Nematoda: Ascaridata) in the northern North Sea, to the north of Scotland and at Faroe. Nature 234: 478
22. Smith JW (1983) Larval *Anisakis simplex* (Rudolphi, 1809, det. Krabbe, 1878) and larval *Hysterothylacium* sp. (Nematoda: Ascaridoidea) in euphausiids (Crustacea: Malacostraca) in the North-East Atlantic and northern North Sea. J Helminthol 57: 167–177
23. Smith JW (1983) *Anisakis simplex* (Rudolphi, 1809, det. Krabbe, 1878) (Nematoda: Ascaridoidea): morphology and morphometry of larvae from euphausiids and fish, and a review of the life-history and ecology. J Helminthol 57: 205–224
24. Sluiters JF (1974) *Anisakis* sp. larvae in the stomachs of herring (*Clupea harengus* L.). Z Parasitenk 44: 279–288
25. Oshima T, Shimazu T, Koyama H, Akahane H (1969) On the larvae of the genus *Anisakis* (Nematoda: Anisakidae) from the euphausiids. Jpn J Parasitol 18: 241–248 (in Japanese with English summary)
26. Shimazu T, Oshima T (1972) Some larval nematodes from euphausiid crustaceans. In: Takenouti Y et al. (eds) Biological oceanography of the northern North Pacific Ocean dedicated to Shigeru Motoda, Idemitsu Shoten, Tokyo, pp 403–409
27. Kagei N (1974) Studies on anisakid Nematoda (Anisakidae) (IV). Survey of *Anisakis* larvae in the marine Crustacea. Bull Inst Publ Health 23: 65–71 (in Japanese with English summary)

38 K. Nagasawa

28. Kagei N (1979) Euphausiids and their parasites (I). Geiken Tsushin (328): 53–62 (in Japanese)
29. Shimazu T (1982) Some helminth parasites of marine planktonic invertebrates. J Nagano-ken Junior Coll 37: 11–29
30. Shiraki T, Hasegawa H, Kenmotsu M, Otsuru M (1976) Larval anisakid nematodes from prawns, *Pandalus* spp. Jpn J Parasitol 25: 148–152
31. Hurst RJ (1984) Marine invertebrate hosts of New Zealand Anisakidae (Nematoda). New Zeal J Mar Freshw Res 18: 187–196
32. Oshima T (1969) A study on the first intermediate hosts of *Anisakis*. Saishin Igaku 24: 401–404 (in Japanese)
33. Nagasawa K (1990) *Anisakis* larvae in intermediate and paratenic hosts in Japan. Ishikura H, Kikuchi K (eds) Intestinal anisakiasis in Japan. Springer-Verlag, Tokyo, pp. 23–29
34. Kagei N (1969) Life history of nematodes of the genus *Anisakis*. Saishin Igaku 24: 389–400 (in Japanese)
35. Kagei N (1970) List of the larvae of *Anisakis* spp. recorded from marine fishes and squids caught off the Japan and its adjacent islands. Bull Inst Publ Health 19: 76–85
36. Kagei N (1974) A list of fish infected with larval nematodes of the subfamily Anisakinae. Jpn Soc Sci Fish (ed) Fish and *Anisakis*, Fish Sci Ser 7. Koseisha Koseikaku, Tokyo, pp. 98–107 (in Japanese)
37. Khalil LF (1969) Larval nematodes in the herring (*Clupea harengus*) from British coastal waters and adjacent territories. J Mar Biol Assoc U K 49: 641–659
38. Davey JT (1972) The incidence of *Anisakis* sp. larvae (Nematoda: Ascaridata) in the commercially exploited stocks of herring (*Clupea harengus* L., 1758) (Pisces: Clupeidae) in British and adjacent waters. J Fish Biol 4: 535–554
39. Grabda J (1974) The dynamics of the nematode larvae, *Anisakis simplex* (Rud.) invasion in the south-western Baltic herring (*Clupea harengus* L.) Acta Ichthyol Piscat 4: 3–21
40. Smith JW, Wootten R (1975) Experimental studies on the migration of *Anisakis* sp. larvae (Nematoda: Ascaridida) into the flesh of herring, *Clupea harengus* L. Int J Parasitol 5: 133–136
41. Banning P van, Becker HB (1978) Long-term survey data (1965–1972) on the occurrence of *Anisakis* larvae (Nematoda: Ascaridida) in herring, *Clupea harengus* L., from the North Sea. J Fish Biol 12: 25–33
42. Beverley-Burton M, Pippy JHC (1977) Morphometric variations among larval *Anisakis simplex* (Nematoda: Ascaridoidea) from fishes of the North Atlantic and their use as biological indicators of host stocks. Env Biol Fish 2: 309–314
43. Grabda J (1983) Studies on viability and infectivity of *Anisakis simplex* stage III larvae in fresh salted and spiced Baltic herring. Acta Ichthyol Piscat 8: 117–129
44. Threlfall W (1982) In vitro culture of *Anisakis* spp. larvae from fish and squid in Newfoundland. Proc Helminthol Soc Wash 49: 65–70
45. McGladdery SE, Burt MDB (1985) Potential of parasites for use as biological indicators of migration, feeding, and spawning behaviour of northwestern Atlantic herring (*Clupea harengus*). Can J Fish Aquat Sci 42: 1957–1968
46. McGladdery SE (1986) *Anisakis simplex* (Nematoda: Anisakidae) infection of the musculature and body cavity of Atlantic herring (*Clupea harengus harengus*). Can J Fish Aquat Sci 43: 1312–1317
47. Bishop YMM, Margolis L (1955) A statistical examination of *Anisakis* larvae (Nematoda) in herring (*Clupea pallasi*) of the British Columbia coast. J Fish Res Board Can 12: 571–592
48. Hauck AK (1977) Occurrence and survival of the larval nematode *Anisakis* sp. in the flesh of fresh, frozen, brined, and smoked Pacific herring, *Clupea harengus pallasi*. J Parasitol 63: 515–519
49. Nyman OL, Pippy JHC (1972) Differences in Atlantic salmon, *Salmo salar*, from North America and Europe. J Fish Res Board Can 29: 179–185

The Life Cycle of *Anisakis simplex*: A Review 39

50. Beverley-Burton M, Pippy JHC (1978) Distribution, prevalence and mean numbers of larval *Anisakis simplex* (Nematoda: Ascaridoidea) in Atlantic salmon, *Salmo salar* L. and their use as biological indicators of host stocks. Env Biol Fish 3: 211–222

51. Beverley-Burton M (1978) Population genetics of *Anisakis simplex* (Nematoda: Ascaridoidea) in Atlantic salmon (*Salmo salar*) and their use as biological indicators of host stocks. Env Biol Fish 3: 369–377

52. Pippy JHC (1980) The value of parasites as biological tags in Atlantic salmon at West Greenland. Rapp P-v Reun Cons Int Explor Mer 176: 76–81

53. Stern JA, Chakravarti D, Uzmann JR, Hesselholt MN (1958) Rapid counting of Nematoda in salmon by peptic digestion. US Fish Wildlife Service, Spec Sci Rep-Fisheries No 255. 5 pp

54. Novotny AJ, Uzmann JR (1960) A statistical analysis of the distribution of a larval nematode (*Anisakis* sp.) in the musculature of chum salmon (*Oncorhynchus keta* Walbaum). Exp Parasitol 10: 215–262

55. Urawa S (1986) The parasites of salmonid fishes-II. The biology of anisakid nematodes and the prevention of their human infections. Fish and Eggs (156): 52–70 (in Japanese with English summary)

56. Deardorff TL, Throm R (1988) Commercial blast-freezing of third-stage *Anisakis simplex* larvae encapsulated in salmon and rockfish. J Parasitol 74: 600–603

57. Young PC (1972) The relationship between the presence of larval anisakine nematodes in cod and marine mammals in British home waters. J Appl Ecol 9: 459–485

58. Wootten R, Waddell IF (1977) Studies on the biology of larval nematodes from the musculature of cod whiting in Scottish waters. J Conc Int Explor Mer 37: 266–273

59. Wootten R (1978) The occurrence of larval anisakid nematodes in small gadoids from Scottish waters. J Mar Biol Assoc U K 58: 347–356

60. Hauksson E (1984) Prevalence and abundance of larvae of *Phocanema decipiens* (Krabbe) and *Anisakis* sp. (Nematoda, Ascaridata) in cod (*Gadus morhua* L.) from Icelandic waters. Hafrannsoknir 30: 5–26 (in Icelandic with English summary)

61. Arthur JR, Margolis L, Whitaker DJ, McDonald TE (1982) A quantitative study of economically important parasites of walleye pollock (*Theragra chalcogramma*) from British Columbian waters and effects of postmortem handling on their abundance in the musculature. Can J Fish Aquat Sci 39: 710–726

62. Sasaki, M (1973) Survey of parasites of the Alaska pollock, *Theragra chalcogramma*. J Hokkaido Fish Exp St (Hokusuishi Geppo) 30: 14–39 (in Japanese)

63. Suzuki M, Oishi K (1974) III. Infection of fish. 9. Parasites of walleye pollock *Theragra chalcogramma*. Jpn Soc Sci Fish (ed) Fish and *Anisakis*, Fish Sci Ser 7. Koseisha Koseikaku, Tokyo, pp 113–125 (in Japanese)

64. Carvajal J, Cattan PE, Castillo C, Schatte P (1979) Larval anisakids and other helminths in the hake, *Merluccius gayi* (Guichenot) from Chile. J Fish Biol 15: 671–677

65. Cattan PE, Carvajal J (1984) A study of the migration of larval *Anisakis simplex* (Nematoda: Ascaridida) in the Chilean hake, *Merluccius gayi* (Guichenot). J Fish Biol 24: 649–654

66. Kosugi K (1972) Seasonal fluctuation of the infestation with the larvae of *Anisakis* and of related species of nematodes in the fishes from Sagami Bay. Yokohama Med J 23: 285–316 (in Japanese with English summary)

67. Smith JW (1984) Larval ascaridoid nematodes in myopsid and oegopsid cephalopods from around Scotland and in the northern North Sea. J Mar Biol Assoc U K 64: 563–572

68. Smith JW (1974) Experimental transfer of *Anisakis* sp. larvae (Nematoda: Ascaridida) from one fish host to another. J Helminthol 48: 229–234

69. Smith JW (1984) The abundance of *Anisakis simplex* L3 in the body-cavity and flesh of marine teleosts. Int J Parasitol 14: 491–495

70. Dailey MD, Brownell RL, Jr (1972) A checklist of marine mammal parasites. In: Ridgway SH (ed) Mammals of the sea. Biology and medicine. Charles C Thomas, Springfield, Illinois, USA, pp 528–589

71. Machida M (1969) Parasitic nematodes in the stomach of northern fur seals caught in the western Pacific, off the coast of northern Japan. Jpn J Parasitol 18: 575–579 (in Japanese with English summary)
72. Machida M (1971) Survey on gastric nematodes of the northern fur seal on breeding islands. Jpn J Parasitol 20: 371–378 (in Japanese with English summary)
73. Kagei N, Kureha K (1970) Studies on anisakid Nematoda (Anisakinae) (I). Survey of *Anisakis* sp. in marine mammals collected in the Antarctic Ocean. Bull Inst Public Health 19: 193–196 (in Japanese with English summary)
74. Kagei N, Asano K, Kihata M (1978) On the examination against the parasites of Antarctic krill, *Euphausia superba*. Sci Rep Whales Res Inst 30: 311–313.
75. Kagei N, Oshima T, Kobayashi A, Kumada M, Koyama T Komiya Y, Takemura A (1967) Survey of *Anisakis* spp. (Anisakinae, Nematoda) in marine mammals on the coast of Japan. Jpn J Parasitol 16: 427–435 (in Japanese with English summary)

Prevalence of Larval Anisakid Nematodes in Fresh Fish from Coastal Waters of Hokkaido

K. MIYAMOTO

Abstract

Five hundred and forty eight fish consisting of 19 species were purchased from the Kyokuichi (commercial marine fishery) in Asahikawa city, Hokkaido. They were dissected and examined for anisakid larvae in the body muscle and in the viscera.

Five hundred and thirty one anisakid larvae were detected in 109 individuals taken from sixteen species; however, in 3 species no larvae were recovered. The worms were identified as larvae of *Anisakis simplex, Pseudoterranova decipiens* and *Contracaecum osculatum*. The former two species of larvae were found in both muscle and viscera of the fish, but the remainder were recovered only in the viscera.

The majority of larvae were found in the viscera, however, 26 larvae of *A. simplex* and 186 larvae of *P. decipiens* were detected in the muscle of twelve species of fish.

The average number of larvae in the muscle was calculated as 0.05 of *A. simplex* and 0.34 of *P. decipiens*.

In this study, it is suggested that the following seven species of fish are an important source of human anisakiasis: *Gadus macrocephalus, Pleurogrammus azonus, Hexagrammos otakii, Hippoglossus stenolepis, Atheresthes evermanni, Paralichthys olivaceus* and *Sebastes taczanowskii*.

Introduction

Hokkaido was considered to be the endemic area of human anisakiasis in Japan, because it was rich fresh marine products. However, only 489 cases from Hokkaido, compared to 2236 cases of anisakiasis from Kyushu came reported at the 27th meeting of the Japanese Society of Digestive-tract Endoscopy in 1984.

According to Dr. Yazaki (personal communication, 3rd Dept. Internal Medicine, Asahikawa Medical College), the incidence of human anisakiasis in Hokkaido has recently begun to decrease.

In order to investigate this, an up-to-date survey of the source of anisakiasis in Hokkaido was carried out at Asahikawa between February and July, 1987.

42 K. Miyamoto

Two species of larvae, *Anisakis simplex* and *Pseudoterranova decipiens*, were detected in fish muscle, but the infestation rate shown in this study tends to be lower than that reported in previous papers.

Materials and Method

Samples for Examination

A total of five hundred and forty eight fish comprising nineteen species from Hokkaido were purchased at Asahikawa marine fishery. The fish which were examined were chilled but not frozen, and were identified by Drs K. Nagasawa and S. Urawa.

Examination Methood

After the individual fish were measured and weighed, they were eviscerated, then the body muscle and viscera of each fish examined separately. The muscle was sliced in small flesh fillets for examination, each fillet put between glass plates and pressed, and then observed under a dissecting microscope and/or by candling. Larval anisakid nematodes were collected, washed in a saline solution and fixed in 10% formalin solution at 60 C.

The fixed larval specimen was identified by morphological features, especially by the characteristics of their digestive tract.

Results

Larval anisakid nematodes were detected in 109 (19.9%) of the fish examined, consisting of sixteen species (Table 1). The worms were identified as larvae of *Anisakis simplex*, *Pseudoterranova decipiens* and *Contracaecum osculatum*.

Out of 109 fish infested, 80 fish consisting of 14 species were infested with *A. simplex*, 43 fish of 9 species were infested with *P. decipiens* and 3 fish of 2 species were infested with *C. osculatum*.

The infestation rate of the following species; *My. polyacanthocephalus*, *Se. iracundus*, *Pl. azonus*, *Cl. pallasi*, *He. otakii* and *At. evermanni*, was shown to be over 50%.

No larvae were found in 3 species of *Pl. stellatus*, *Li. herzensteini* and *Se. trivittatus*.

A total numer of 531 larvae collected consisted of 264 of *A. simplex* (238 in viscera and 186 in muscle), 198 of *P. decipiens* (12 in viscera and 186 in muscle) and 69 of *C. osculatum* (in viscera of *My. polyacanthocephalus* and *Hi. stenolepis*).

Discussion

In this study, 531 larval anisakid nematods were detected in 109 out of 548 fresh market fish from Hokkaido. The infestation rate of the fish examined was calculated as 19.9% and the mean larval burden as 0.97. These fish harboured three

Table 1. Prevalence of anisakid larvae in the marine fish of Hokkaido, 1987

Host	Locality of host collect	No. fish examine	Weight (Mean, gr.)	No. fish infest	Parasitic larva of									
					A. simplex				P. decipiens				C. osculatum	
					in viscera		in muscle		in viscera		in muscle		in viscera	
					No. fish	No. worm	No. fish	No. worm	No. fish	No. worm	No. fish	No. worm	No. fish	No. worm
Okhotsk sea														
Myoxocephalus polyacanthocephalus	Nemuro	2	4,850	2	2	71	1	3	2	11	2	130	2	68
Atheresthes evermanni	Rausu	4	3,025	4	4	16	1	1	0		0		0	
Hexagrammos otakii	Nemuro	14	570	8	0		2	2	0		6	9	0	
Osmerus mordax dentex	Monbetsu	52	89	22	8	9	1	2	1	1	18	29	0	
Lipidopsetta mochigarei	Nemuro	13	600	2	0		1	1	0		1	1	0	
Sardinops melanosticus	Monbetsu	52	104	2	2	3	0		0		0		0	
Liopsetta obscura	Monbetsu	21	226	1	0		0		0		1	1	0	
Hypomesus pretiosus japonicus	Hiroo	111	63	1	0		1	1	0		0		0	
Liopsetta obscura	Nemuro	80	80	0	0		0		0		0		0	
Platichthys stellatus	Shari	32	264	0	0		0		0		0		0	
subtotal		381		42	16	99	7	10	3	12	28	170	2	68
Pacific ocean														
Sebastes iracundus	Erimo	1	4,500	1	1	31	0		0		0		0	
Pleurogrammus azonus	Kushiro	45	388	32	29	64	5	7	0		8	9	0	
Gadus macrocephalus	Kushiro	21	550	8	0		3	4	0		5	5	0	
Hippoglossus stenolepis	Kushiro	12	488	4	0		3	4	0		1	1	1	1
Sebastes steindachneri	Hakodate	5	682	1	1	1	0		0		0		0	
Sebastes taczanowskii	Hakodate	13	278	1	0		1	1	0		0		0	
subtotal		97		47	31	96	12	16	0		14	15	1	1
Japan sea														
Clupea pallasi	Wakkanai	30	136	19	19	43	0		0		0		0	
Paralichths olivaceus	Tomamae	3	603	1	0		0		0		1	1	0	
Limanda herzensteini	Rumoi	32	153	0	0		0		0		0		0	
Sebastes trivittatus	Wakkanai	5	956	0	0		0		0		0		0	
subtotal		70		20	19	43	0		0		3	12	0	
Grandtotal		548		109 (19.9%)	66	239	19	26	3	12	43	186	3	69

A Oncorhynchus nerka from Canada was infested with two living A. simplex larvae. No larva was found in 30 specimens of Todarodes pacificus (Surumeika squid) from Hakodate.

44   K. Miyamoto

species of larvae, *Anisakis simplex*, *Pseudoterranova decipiens* and *Contracaecum osculatum*. The former two species of larvae were recovered from the viscera and body muscle, but the remainder were found only in the viscera of two species of fish.

Both *A. simplex* and *P. decipiens* larvae are better known as pathogens of human anisakiasis, and were predominant, accounting for 87.0% of larvae harvested in this study.

Since 1979, 18 cases of anisakiasis have been recorded in Asahikawa, and were classified as 7 cases of *A. simplex*, 8 cases of *P. decipiens* and 3 cases undertermined due to broken larvae (unpublished date). The results of this study correlated with the 18 cases of anisakiasis.

According to Saito et al. (1970), *Anisakis* type I (= *A. simplex*) larvae were found in 8 out of 9 species of fish and squid in Hokkaido, while *Terranova* (= *P. decipiens*) larvae were detected only in *Theragra chalcogramma*, and 6 out of 9 species of fish and squid were infested with *Contracaecum* larvae. However, in this study no larvae were found in 30 squid (*Todarodes pacificus*) collected from Hokkaido. Shiraki (1974) reported that *A. simplex* larvae were recovered from all 15 species fish examined, *P. decipiens* from 8 species and *C. osculatum* from 5 species of fish in Hokkaido.

This survey shows a low infestation rate of fish compared with Saito et al. and Shiraki, with no reason for this discrepancy.

Up to the present *A. simplex* and *P. decipiens* larvae have been recovered from 12 species of fish muscle, 7 of the species (*Ga. macrocephalus*, *Pl. azonus*, *He. otakii*, *Hi. stenolepis*, *At. evermanni*, *Pa. olivaceus* and *Se. taczanowskii*) play an important role as a source of human anisakiasis in Hokkaido and are normally consumed as raw fish fillets in the home.

It was interesting to note that one *Oncorhynchus nerka* which was imported from Canada, was infested with two living *A. simplex* larvae in the muscle. Many *On. nerka* have been imported and consumed in Japan. Thus it appears that the source of anisakiasis is related not only to local fish products but also fish imported from foreign countries.

Although the worm infestation rate per single fish is low in this study, the possibility that Japanese people may become infested with anisakid larvae is high, because the Japanese are large consumers of raw fish in home cooking. However, according to Oshima (1987) commercial sushi shops, in which raw fish fillets are prepared by a sushi expert, were evaluated to be safe. The author would like to draw this fact to the attention of consumers who use raw fish in home cooking.

References

1. Saito T, Kitamura H, Tanakawa Y (1970) Frequency of *Anisakis* larvae in marine fish and cuttlefish captured in the area of Hokkaido. Report of the Hokkaido Institute of Public Health 20: 115–122 (in Japanese with English summary)
2. Shiraki T (1974) Larval nematodes of family anisakidae (Nematoda) in the northern sea of Japan as a causative agent of eosinophilic phlegmone or granuloma in the human gastro-intestinal tract. Acta Medica et Biologica 22: 57–98
3. Oshima T (1987) Anisakiasis- Is the Sushi Bar Guilty? Parasitology Today 3: 44–48

Infection Rate of Anisakinae Larvae in Fish Taken from the Offing of Ishikawa Prefecture

Y. OIKAWA and T. IKEDA

The infection rates of Anisakinae larvae were examined in five types of marine fish and two kinds of cuttlefish taken from the offing of Ishikawa Prefecture, during the period of February to April, 1987. The species were walleye pollacks *Theragra chalcogramma* (30 fish), Pacific cod *Gadus macrocephalus* (5), mackerel *Scomber japonicus* (20), plaice *Hippoglossoides dubius* (10), sardines *Sardinops malanosticta* (106), squid *Doryteuthis bleekeri* (15) and sagittated calamary *Todarodes pacificus* (40). Fish were autopsied and Anisakinae larvae were collected from the peritoneal cavity. The infection rate (%) and the number of larvae per larvae-positive fish (larvae/positive fish and larvae/kg of body weight) were calculated. The muscles of the abdomen were digested and the number of larvae in 100g of muscles (larvae/100g muscles) was also calculated. Cuttlefish were autopsied and the muscles were held up to the light after skinning for investigation of parasitized sites. Collected larvae were fixed with hot-70% ethanol, vitrified by glycerin and identified. The result are shown in Tables 1–3.

Infection rates of Anisakinae larvae from the peritoneal cavity of walleye pollacks, Pacific cod and mackerel were high (90–100%), but the rates were low in plaice and sardines (40% and 2.8%). Anisakinae larvae were not observed in the peritoneal cavities of cuttlefish. The number of larvae in the peritoneal cavity per positive fish was 4.8–8.2 in walleye pollocks, Pacific cod and mackerel, and 1.0–1.8 in plaice and sardines. The number of larvae per kg of body weight was high in mackerel (15.1) and sardines (8.8), but low (4.4–5.8) in walleye pollocks, Pacific cod and plaice.

Larvae in abdominal muscles were observed only in Pacific cod (0.8/100g of muscles) and mackerel (1.2/100g of muscles). In sagittated calamary larvae of *Contracaeum* sp. were observed in the muscles, and the infection rate and number of these larvae per positive cuttlefish were 37.5% and 2.2, respectively.

Anisakinae larvae gathered from five kinds of fish had a boring tooth and a mucron but lacked a ventricular appendix or an intestinal caecum. The ratio of body length (B) to the ventriculus length (V), and B to the tail length (T) were 17.8–34.5 (B/V) and 158–429 (B/T) respectively. From these observations the larvae were identified as *Anisakis simplex* larvae. The mean body length of larvae gathered from the peritoneal cavities of walleye pollocks and Pacific cod was 25.6mm and 26.3mm respectively, with the length slightly shorter in larvae from other fish (19.3–21.5mm). The size of larvae in the muscles of Pacific cod and mackerel were larger than when found in the peritoneal cavities of these fish.

Table 1. Infection rates and other indexes of Anisakinae larvae in fish and cuttlefish taken from the offing of Ishikawa Prefecture

Host	Sample		Infection rate (%)	No. of larvae			
	No.	Weight(kg)		Total	Positive fish	kg of body weight	100g of muscles
Walleye pollack	30	20	90	129	4.8	5.8	0
Pacific cod	5	8	100	41	8.2	5.1	0.8
Mackerel	20	8	100	121	6.1	15.1	1.2
Plaice	10	4	40	7	1.8	4.4	0
Sardine	106	12	2.8	3	1.0	8.8	0
Squid	15	3	0	0	0	0	ND
Sagittated calamary	40	9	37.5[a]	33[a]	2.2[a]	11.2[a]	ND

[a] *Contracaecum* sp.

Y. Oikawa and T. Ikeda

Infection Rate of Anisakinae Larvae in Fish

Table 2. Dimensions and indexes of larvae gathered from fish

Host	No. of exam.	Infection site[a]	Body length mm(B)	Ventriculus length mm(V)	Tail length mm(T)	B/V	B/T
Walleye pollack	59	p.c.	25.6 15–31	1.12 0.58–1.42	0.09 0.07–0.13	23.3 17.8–29.4	279 167–429
Pacific cod	17	p.c.	26.3 19–31	1.06 0.68–1.32	0.09 0.07–0.11	25.3 19.8–27.9	294 238–338
	5	m.	28.8 27–31	1.23 1.13–1.29	0.09 0.08–0.10	23.5 22.5–24.6	330 300–363
Mackerel	11	p.c.	21.5 15–30	0.84 0.55–1.42	0.08 0.07–0.11	26.8 20.5–34.5	256 188–375
	10	m.	26.4 19–30	1.12 0.63–1.34	0.08 0.07–0.10	24.3 19.8–30.2	322 271–357
Plaice	7	p.c.	21.0 19–26	0.84 0.66–1.26	0.10 0.09–0.12	26.0 19.4–31.8	204 158–244
Sardine	3	p.c.	19.3 18–20	0.68 0.61–0.76	0.07 0.05–0.08	28.7 26.3–30.3	299 250–360

[a] Infection site, peritoneal cavity (p.c.) and muscle (m.)

Table 3. Dimensions and indexes of larvae from sagittated calamary (Fujita O. 1987)

Sample No.	17[a]	3[b]
Length (mm)	27.41 22.58–31.61	28.50 24.50–32.8
Width(mm)	0.40 0.31–0.47	0.43 0.34–0.48
Ventriculus(mm)	0.31 0.22–0.40	0.32 0.28–0.38
Ventricular appendix(mm)	18.56 13.21–20.94	23.31 20.13–27.86
Intestinal caecum(mm)	1.59 1.04–2.30	1.85 1.56–2.08
v.a/i.c	12.05 9.99–13.89	12.57 11.43–13.39
Tail(mm)	0.19 0.10–0.26	0.18 0.12–0.23

[a] Sample was collected on 24 March 1987
[b] Sample was collected on 23 April 1987

48 Y. Oikawa and T. Ikeda

Larvae of *Contracaecum* sp. gathered from the muscles of sagittated calamaries had a ventricular appendix (v.a), an intestinal caecum (i.c) and a small mucron, but lacked a boring tooth, with the ratio of length of v.a to i.c of 9.9–13.8 (v.a/i.c). These larvae were identified as *Contracaecum* type A larvae reported by Kikuchi S. et al. (1970) (Fujita O., personal letter, 1987).

The larvae of Anisakinae in the muscles of fish are especially important as a cause of anisakiasis. In this study, *Anisakis simplex* larvae were observed in the muscles of Pacific cod and mackerel. There is a custom of eating raw cod as a dish called "Kobumaki" or "Kotsuke" in Ishikawa Prefecture. The meat of raw cod is rolled up with seaweed as "Kobumaki" and is covered with cod eggs as "Kotsuke". It is necessary to examine the pathogenecity of the larvae in these foods. Mackerel is eaten as "Shimesaba" cooked with vinegar and salt, so it is possible that the larvae survive in the muscles of mackerel. Fujino T. et al. (1984) [1] reported that most of the patients with anisakiasis found in Fukuoka Prefecture had eaten mackerel before the onset of their illness. Many larvae were found in 100g of muscles of those mackerel already heavily burdened with larvae in the peritoneal cavity [2]. Mackerel may be the most important fish to be examined in this report, while the pathogenecity of *Contracaecum* sp. larvae in the muscles of sagittated calamary has not been confirmed [3]. Other fish which had no larvae in the muscles may become a cause of anisakiasis when their internal organs or muscles contaminated by larvae from the peritoneal cavity are eaten.

References

1. Fujino T, Ooiwa T, Ishii Y (1984) Clinical, epidemiological and morphological studies on 150 cases of acute gastric anisakiasis in Fukuoka Prefecture. Jpn J Parasitol 33: 73–92 (in Japanese)
2. Oikawa Y, Tani S (1984) Parasitic state of *Anisakis* larvae in mackerel at the market of Kanazawa City. J Kanazawa Med Univ 9: 244–249 (in Japanese)
3. Koyama T (1981) 1. Morphology and classification. In Fishes and *Anisakis*, ed. by Japanese Society of Scientific Fisheries, Koseisha–koseikaku, Tokyo pp 9–19 (in Japanese)

Anisakinae in Sanin Waters of the Japan Sea

J. MAEJIMA

Two hundred and twenty two cases of stomach anisakiasis in the Sanin District were reported by Fukumoto in 1984 [3] at the 27th Meeting of the Japanese Society of Gastroenterological Endoscopy. The Sanin District is one of the most important foci for anisakiasis in Japan, though the incidence can not be clearly determined. Recently the use of endoscopy by medical pracitioners for the diagnosis and treatment of stomach anisakiasis has spread widely in the Sanin District. A total of 49 cases of stomach anisakiasis were reported between 1982 and April 1987 as sample data from a hospital clinic of internal medicine in Yonago City by Shabana and Miura in 1987 [18]. This figure is equal to the total number of cases of stomach anisakiasis which occured in Nagano Prefecture prior to 1984.

A few species of fish and squid which are commonly eaten raw or undercooked by people of the Sanin District, were examined for Anisakinae larvae (Table 1). These fish and squid were bought at a commercial fish market in Yonago City between March 2 to April 28 in 1987. Most of them were caught in coastal waters off the Sanin District, but 33 common mackerel, *Pneumatophorus japonicus japonicus* (Houttuyn) were sent from Shizuoka Prefecture, 46 common mackerel were from Chiba Prefecture, and 25 sardine, *Sardinops meranosticta* (Temminck and Schlegel) were from Fukuoka Prefecture.

Three types of Anisakinae larvae were collected from 50 common mackerel (79 examined), 4 horse mackerel, *Trachurus japonicus* (Temminck and Schlegel) (40 examined), 2 sardine, *S. meranosticta* (50 examined) and 25 squid, *Todarodes pacificus* (Steenstrup) (35 examined). The results were negative for sardine, *Engraulis japonica* (houttuyn) (284 examined) and squid, *Doryteuthis kensaki* (Wakiya and Ishikawa) (30 examined). *Anisakis* type I larvae were found in the muscles of common mackerel and sardine, *S. meranosticta*, and from the viscera of common and horse mackerel.

The incidence of *Anisakis* type I larvae in common mackerel was often high, more than 80% in several area [8,10,17]. A high rate of 20 to 40% of type I larvae were observed in the musculature of common mackerel by several investigators (Oshima, 1972) [15]. The larvae found in the viscera and muscles had a seventy-thirty ratio (Nishimura, 1969) [16]. *Anisakis* type I larvae were found in the muscles of 14 (42%) of common mackerel sent from Shizuoka Prefecture. A high rate was found in the muscles of 36 (78%) and the viscera 42 (91%) of common mackerel B sent from Chiba Prefecture (Table 2). The intensity of type I larval infection in common mackerel, weighing 450–650 g, were 1 to 38 per fish

Table 1. Incidence of Anisakinae larvae in fishes and squids bought in the commercial market at Yonago City

Species name	Location	Data	Body length (cm)	No. examined	No. of infected fishes		No. of collected larvae		Species of larvae
					muscle	viscera	muscle	viscera	
P. japonicus japonicus (common mackerel)	Shizuoka Pr.	3. 2	33–35	33	14(42%)	28(85%)	36	224	*Anisakis* type I
	Chiba Pr.	4.21	30–36	46	36(78%)	42(91%)	179	374	*Anisakis* type I
			(450–650g)		0	3(6%)	0	5	*Anisakis* type II
T. japonicus (horse mackereal)	Shimonoseki City	3. 9	17–18	40	0	4(10%)	—	7	*Anisakis* type I
S. meranosticta (sardine)	Sakaiminato City	4. 3	17–23	25	2(4%)	0	2	—	*Anisakis* type I
	Kyushu Dist.	4. 3	15–18	25	0	0	—	—	
E. japonica (sardine)	Sakaiminato City	4. 7	10–12	60	0	0	—	—	
		4.28	13–14	110	0	0	—	—	
	Matsue City	4.10	10–14	114	0	0	—	—	
T. pacificus (squid)	Yonago City	3. 6		35	25(71%)	0	62	—	*Hysterothylacium* sp.
D. kensaki (squid)	Sanin District	3. 6		30	0	0	—	—	

Anisakinae in Sanin Waters of the Japan Sea

Table 2. The intensity of *Anisakis* type I larvae in common mackerel caught in the coastal waters off Shizuoka Prefecture(A) and Chiba Prefecture(B)

			Habitats of larvae		
				Viscera and muscle	
		Viscera	Viscera	muscle	
No. of infected	A	14(42%)	14(42%)		28(85%)
fish	B	8(17%)	34(74%)		42(91%)
	total	22(22%)	48(61%)		70(87%)
No. of collected	A	1–15(6.9)	1–33(9.1)	1–7 (2.6)	1–
larvae per fish	B	3–15(6.6)	1–21(9.7)	1–15(5.4)	38(11.7)
(average)					2–
					36(15.1)
No. of collected	A	97	128(78%)	36(22%)	260
larvae	B	57	317(64%)	179a(36%)	553
	total	153	445	215	813

aincluding 15 dead *Anisakis* type I larvae, and excluding 23 degenerating nematodes unidentified

(average A, 11.7; B, 15.1), and 11 to 100% (average A, 22%; B, 36%) of the larvae were found in the musculature of fish (Fig. 1). More than 93 (Nishimura, 1969) [16], to 95% (Asami and Tomita, 1967 [1]; Okumura, 1967 [13]) of the larvae were found in the anteroventral musculature. Approximately one half of 36 larvae collected from the musculature of common mackerel A were found in the middle part of the ventral musculature, near the posterior end of the abdominal cavity (Fig. 2A). Most of the larvae in the musculature of fresh common mackerel B were removed from ventral muscles around the abdominal cavity, however more than 20% of the larvae were found in muscles considerably further from the abdominal cavity (Fig. 2B). Degenerating larvae of *Anisakis* type I were frequently found in the muscles of two or three-year-old common mackerel B, 16 (44%). These larvae, surrounded by granulation with black pigments (Fig. 2) fell into two groups, i.e. the degenerating unidentifiable 23 nematodes and the dead or hardly movable *Anisakis* type I larvae. Larvae surrounded by granulation without any pigments and those collected from viscera were shown to have active movement. About 53% [7], 87% [3] and 63% [18] of anisakiasis patients endoscopically treated had eaten dishes containing raw common mackerel before the onset of their illness. This seems to provide evidence that the common mackerel is the most important source of anisakiasis in the Sanin District. The incidence of *Anisakis* type I larvae in common mackerel caught in coastal waters off Sanin District was 67.7% in June and 7.3% in August, and 12.9% of the larvae was found in the muscles [4]. However, common mackerel migrating in the Sanin waters of the Japan Sea in early Spring can not be the object of fishing because of their small size and lack of commercial value.

Anisakis type I larvae in sardines were removed only from viscera of fish such as Japanese anchovies (*E. japonica*), Japanese sardines (*S. meranosticta*) and

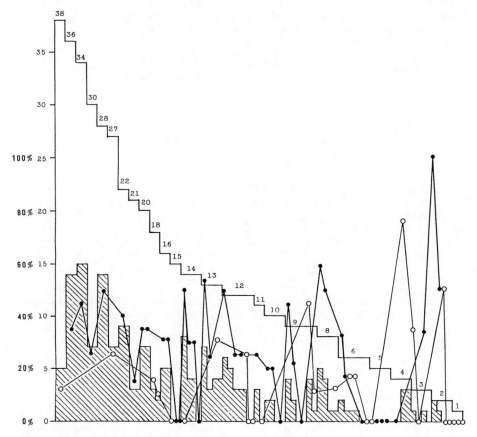

Fig. 1. The number of type I larvae found in the viscera (□), and muscle (▨); and the rate of type I larvae infection in muscle of fish caught in the coastal waters off Shizuoka Prefecture (○) and Chiba Prefecture (●)

round herrings (*Etrumeus microps* Temminck and Schlegel) caught along the coast of Japan [4,5,11,20,21,22,7]. According to Suehiro in 1968 [19], sardines feed on zooplanktons in the young stage, while they live on phytoplanktons after maturity. The infection with *Anisakis* larvae may occur in their young stages. *Anisakis* type I larvae were found for the first time in muscles of Japanese sardines. Two larvae of *Anisakis* type I, about 3cm in length, were buried wholly in the musclature of two out of 25 sardines (4%) examined, caught in the coastal waters off Tottori Prefecture (Fig. 2C). Next to common mackerel, sardines are the most important source of anisakiasis at present in the Sanin District [3,7], as well as in the Kyushu District [12,20]. A catch of fish landed on Sakaiminato port of Tottori Prefecture in 1986 included 472,241 tons of Japanese sardines, 8,170 tons of Japanese anchovies and 8,046 tons of round herrings. These sardines were caught in the coastal waters off the Japan Sea. People in the Sanin District are very fond of small raw Japanese anchovies, prepared in fillets by removal of the spine and head by two fingers without any instrument. The anchovy can be served as sashimi directly. Thus sardines may be

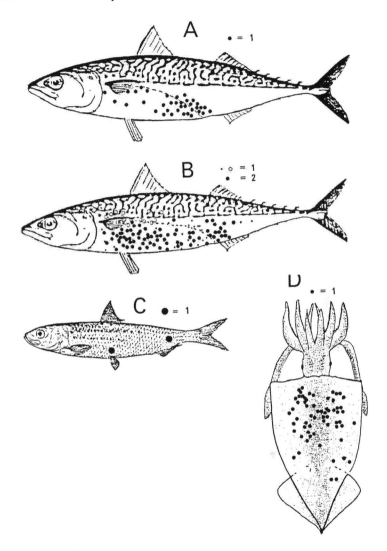

Fig. 2. Distributions of *Anisakis* type I larvae in muscle of common mackerel caught in coastal waters off Shizuoka Prefecture (**A**), Chiba Prefecture (**B**), sardines *S. meranosticta* (**C**) and *Hysterothylacium* sp. larvae of squids *T. pacificus* (**D**)

another cause of human anisakiasis, even though type I larvae are found only in their viscera.

A small number of *Anisakis* type II lavae were found only in the viscera of 3 horse mackerel (Table 1). Another type of larval nematode belonging to *Hysterothylacium-Contracaecum* type B [14] or *Cantracaecum* type A [9] were found in the musculature of squids, *T. pacificus*. Ninety per cent of the larvae were distributed in the anterior half of the musculature of the mantle (Fig. 2D). They are usually parasitic in marine, estuarine and fresh water fish, and no case of human infection has been known, Deardorff and Overstreet [2].

54   J. Maejima

In previous surveys on marine fish and squid caught off the Sanin District, *Anisakis* type I larvae were found in the following: common and horse mackerel, Japanese anchovies, surumeika squid (*T. pacificus*) and dorado (*Coryphaena hippurus* Linnaeus); and not found in the following: round herring, halfbeak (*Hemiramphus sajori* Temminck and Schlegel), young bass (*Lateolabrax japonicus* Cuvier), barracoota (*Sphyraena schlegeli* Steindachner), young yellow-tail (*Seriola quinqueradiata* Temminck and Schlegel), young tunny (*Thunnus thynnus orientalis* Temminck and Schlegel), calamary squid (*Dorytenthis bleekeri* keferstein), sillago (*Sillago japonica* Temminck and Schlegel), saury (*Cololabis saira* Brevoort), sea bream (*Branchiostegus japonicus japonicus* Houttuyn), red sea bream (*Chrysophrys major* Temminck and Schlegel), globefish (*Fugu pardalis* Temminck and Schlegel), bonito (*Katsuworm pelamis* Linnaeus) and flying fish (*Prognichthys agoo* Temminck and Schlegel) [4],[17]. Other important sources of infection with *Anisakis* larvae known in the Sanin District are as follows: horse mackerel, squid, yellow-tail and flounder (*Paralichths olivaceus* Temminck and Schlegel) [6],[13].

References

1. Asami K, Tomita T (1967) Pathogenesis of anisakiasis. Research reports funded by the Japanese Ministry of Education 321 (in Japanese)
2. Deardorff TL, Overstreet RM (1980) Review of *Hysterothylacium* and *Iheringascaris* (both previously *Thynnascaris*) (Nematoda: *Anisakidea*) from the northern gulf of Mexico. Proc Biol Soc Wash 93: 1035–1079
3. Fukumoto S (1984) Parasite and endoscope. Gastroenterological Endoscopy 26(11): 2134 (in Japanese)
4. Hara I (1969) Larval *Anisakis* found in marine fishes collected in coastal waters off Sanin District. Japanese J Med Tech 18: 825–827 (in Japanese)
5. Honda T, Tsubouchi H, Nojiri H (1967) Survey on *Anisakidae* larvae from marine fishes collected in Nagoya City. Reports of Institute of Hygeine, Nagoya City, 14: 79–81 (in Japanese)
6. Ishida A (1976) Acute stomach anisakiasis. Shimane Igaku 5: 649–656 (in Japanese)
7. Ishida S, Higashi T, Ikegami M, Yashiro S, Suwa H, Ikeda Y (1969) Survey on *Anisakidae* larvae from marine fishes. Nihon Juishikai Zasshi 22(8): 371–372 (in Japanese)
8. Kato T, Uminuma M, Ito K, Miura K (1968) On *Anisakinae* from the marine fishes at the Tokyo Central Fish Market. Shokuhin Eisei Kenkyu 18: 31–41 (in Japanese)
9. Kikuchi S, Kosugi K, Hirabayashi H, Hayashi S (1970) Morphological observation of six species of *Contracaecum* larvae found in marine fishes. Yokohama Igaku 21: 421–427 (in Japanese)
10. Kobayashi A, Koyama T, Kumada M, Komiya Y, Oshima T, Ishii T, Machida M (1966) A survey of marine fishes and squids for the presence of *Anisakinae* larvae. Jpn J Parasitol 15: 348–349 (in Japanese)
11. Kuwabata H, Takakuwa M, Shioda T, Atsumi M, Shimakawa T, Kobayashi K (1968) Investigations for the presence of *Anisakis* larvae at Mie Prefecture. Shokuhin Eisei Kenkyu 18: 863–868 (in Japanese)
12. Matsushita H, Sakaguti K, Arima T, Kamikozuru K, Hanamure B, Shibue T, Yamashita Y, Hashimoto S (1984) Investigations for anisakiasis in Kagoshima Prefecture. Gastroenterological Endoscopy 26: 2136 (in Japanese)
13. Okumura T (1967) Experimental studies on anisakiasis. Osaka Shiritsudaigaku Igakuzassi 16: 465–497 (in Japanese)

14. Otsuru M, Shiraki T, Kenmotsu M (1969) On the morphological classification and experimental infection of *Anisakinae* larvae found in marine fishes around the northern sea of Japan. Jpn J Parasitol 18(4): 417–418 (in Japanese)
15. Oshima T (1972) *Anisakis* and anisakiasis in Japan and adjacent area. In: Morishita K, Komiya Y, Matsubashi H (eds), progress of medical Parasitology in Japan. Meguro Parasitol Museum IV: 301–393
16. Nishimura T (1969) The ecology of *Anisakis* larvae. Saishin Igaku 24: 405–412 (in Japanese)
17. Saito K, Ishioka S (1970) A survey on *Anisakidae* larvae from marine fishes in Shimane Prefecture. Shimane Igaku 4: 547–555 (in Japanese)
18. Shabana N, Miura K (1987) Endoscopic figures on stomach anisakiasis. Excerpt of 47th meeting of Chugoku-Shikoku District of Japanese Society of Digestive Tract Endoscopy: 20
19. Suehiro Y (1968) A handbook of Fisheries. Toyo Shinpo Co., Tokyo (in Japanese)
20. Takao Y (1987) Survey on *Anisakidae* larvae from marine fishes (Sardine) caught in the sea near Kyusyu island. Jpn J Parasitol 36(suppl): 81 (in Japanese)
21. Yamaguti S (1935) Studies on the Helminth Fauna of Japan Part 9. Nematodes of Fishes 1. Jap J Zool 6: 337–386
22. Yamaguchi T (1966) The infection and prevention of anisakiasis. Jpn J Parasitol 15: 285–286 (in Japanese)

Anisakinae in the Seto Inland Sea

T. Aji, F. Fukuda, and Y. Tongu

Anisakiasis has been reported from fish cultured in the seto Inland Sea by Aji et al. [1]. However, the infection route in man involves many complicated factors such as parasitic rates and geographical distribution of Anisakinae larvae, the edible portion of the fish and parasitic site of larvae, and the habit of eating raw fish or others [2,3]. To help in the prevention of anisakiasis, we examined the parasitic rate for the 3rd stage of Anisakinae larvae in fish caught in the Seto Inland Sea.

Materials and Methods

Natural infection of Anisakinae larvae was examined in a variety of marine fish caught in the areas near Ushimado, Okayama Prefecture, of the Seto Inland Sea. The examinations were done with fish (20 species, 195 specimens) collected directly by a net or a fishery ship. Twenty specimens of mackerel *Scomber japonicus*, jack mackerel *Trachurus japonicus* caught in the open sea near the South China Sea were examined and compared. Parasitic rates of Anisakinae larvae from the visceral organs in the abdominal cavity were examined. The visceral organs were removed from the fish after the body length and weight were measured, and put into 0.85% physiological saline solution, then on a thin plate for fragmentation. In some specimens, the visceral organs were obtained from a fish market in Ushimado, so the body length and weight measurement could not be performed. Anisakinae larvae were picked up from the fragmented visceral organs and identified under a microscope according to the methods described in the reports of Koyama in 1974 [4], and Koyama et al. in 1969 [5].

Results

Table 1 shows the parasitic rates of Anisakinae larvae in the different fish. *Anisakis simplex* larva was not detected in either the large (mean body length 264 mm) or small (167 mm) mackerel caught in the Seto Inland Sea, whereas 43 larvae from mackerel and 3 larvae from jack mackerel caught in the open sea were detected. In all of the other species of fish taken from the Seto Inland Sea, *Anisakis simplex* larva could not be detected in the visceral organs of the abdo-

58 T. Aji et al.

Table 1. Anisakinae and *Raphydascaris* larvae from various fish caught in the Seto Inland Sea and the open sea

Sea	Host	Nos. Ex- amined	Body Length Average (mm)	Anis akis I	Thynn- ascaris A B C	Contra- caccum B	Terra- nova A	Raphid- ascaris	Total
	Scomber japonicus	29	167[a]	0	0 0 0	0	0	0	0
		9	264[b]	0	1 1 0	0	1	0	3
	Trachurus japonicus	9	248	0	2 5 0	0	0	2	9
	Total	47		0	3 6 0	0	1	2	12
The Seto Inland Sea	*Nibea albiflora*	3	455	0	1 0 0	0	0	0	1
	Engraulis japonica	42	—	0	0 0 1	0	0	0	1
	Takifugu rubripes	3	136	0	0 0 0	25	0	0	25
	Scomberomorus niphonicus	8	700	0	0 0 0	0	0	0	0
	Sardinops melanosticta	40	192	0	0 0 0	0	0	0	0
	Hexagrammos otakii	4	249	0	0 0 0	0	0	0	0
	Pleuronichtys cornutus	2	211	0	0 0 0	0	0	0	0
	Limanda yokohamae	2	186	0	0 0 0	0	0	0	0
	Astruconger myriaster	2	—	0	0 0 0	0	0	0	0
	Takifugu niphobles	1	117	0	0 0 0	0	0	0	0
	Rudarius ercodes	1	47	0	0 0 0	0	0	0	0
	Argyrosomus argentatus	1	—	0	0 0 0	0	0	0	0
	Areliscus joyneri	1	—	0	0 0 0	0	0	0	0
	Areliscus trigtammus	2	395	0	0 0 0	0	0	0	0
	Mugil cephalus	15	—	0	0 0 0	0	0	0	0
	Lateolabrax japonicus	1	250	0	0 0 0	0	0	0	0
	Platycephalous indicus	1	290	0	0 0 0	0	0	0	0
	Mylio macrocephalus	19	299	0	0 0 0	0	0	0	0
	Total	195		0	4 6 1	25	1	2	39
The open sea	*Scomber japonicus*	13	375	43	0 0 0	0	0	1	44
	Trachurus japonicus	7	—	3	1 0 0	0	0	6	10
	Total	20		46	1 0 0	0	0	7	54

[a] Large-sized, [b] Small-sized

minal cavity. *Anisakis* type II was not recognized in any of the fish from either sea. Infection rates of *Thynnascaris* type A, B and C in mackerel and jack mackerel from the Seto Inland Sea were higher than those of the same species from the open sea. One larva each of type A and type B was detected in large-size mackerel, and two and five larvae each of type A and B were detected in jack mackerel from the Seto Inland Sea. However, in the case of the fish caught in the open sea, only one larva of *Thynnascaris* type A was detected in jack mackerel. In the other fish of the Seto Inland Sea, one larva of type A from a croaker *Nibea albiflora* and one larva of type C from an anchovy *Engraulis japonica* were detected. *Contracaecum* was not detected in mackerel and jack mackerel caught in either of the seas. Twenty five larvae of type C were detected in only one species of fish in the Seto Inland Sea, that is, the globe fish *Takifugu rubripes*. Type A larva of *Terranova* was detected in large-size mackerel from the Seto Inland Sea, but not in the other species. In fish that were caught in the open sea, *Terranova* was not detected at all. In addition to Anisakinae larvae, *Raphidascaris* was highly parasitic in jack mackerel caught in both seas.

Discussion

We examined the parasitic rates of Anisakinae larvae in the fish caught in the Seto Inland Sea. The examination was limited to the visceral organs in the abdominal cavity, and was not performed on the muscles. However, it is known that the parasitic rate is higher in the abdominal cavity than in muscles. Nishimura et al. in 1967 [6] reported that the parasitic rate of the *Anisakis*-type worm was 29% in the abdominal cavity alone, 67% in both sites and 3% in the muscle only. Briefly, the positive rate for the abdominal cavity was summed up to be 96%. These results suggest that almost all the positive fish were covered by our method. However, this can not be applied to the genus *Terranova* because the parasitic rate in the muscles was higher than that in the abdominal cavity [7].

Anisakinae larvae were found in various species of mackerel, jack mackerel, croaker, anchovy and globe fish in the Seto Inland Sea. Mackerel and jack mackerel which migrate to a broad area of the open sea during their lifetime, come to the Seto Inland Sea after feeding on *Euphausiacea* or *Thysanoessa* in the open sea. However, these fish were not infected with the genus *Anisakis*. The migration area of mackerel and jack mackerel caught in the Seto Inland Sea seem to be areas other than the South China Sea, because the same species of fish caught in the South China Sea showed high parasitic rates for the genus *Anisakis*. The presence of Anisakinae larvae in non-migratory fish might be due to a secondary infection caused by an interspecific food chain link among the various fish. Takita [8] reported that a croaker has the habit of eating a variety of fish, becoming secondarily infected with Anisakinae larvae after feeding on infected anchovy, immature mackerel or jack mackerel. Globe fish tend to migrate to the open sea and may be infected secondarily by eating anchovy or *Sardinops melanosticta* [9].

In the survey of parasitic rates of Anisakinae larvae in the Seto Inland Sea, Hatada [10] examined fish in the areas near Kobe and Akashi of Hyogo prefecture situated at the other end of the Seto Inland Sea. Mackerel *Pneumatophorus* japonicus japonicus (= *Scomber japonicus*), jack mackerel *T. japonicus*, flathead *Platycephalus indicus*, small yellowtail *Seriola quinqueradiata* and squid of cephapods *Todarodes pacificus* caught in the Japn Sea were examined. All the fish except the small yellowtail and squid were infected with *Anisakis* spp. larvae. However, in 18 species of fish caught in the Seto Inland Sea, *Anisakis* spp. larvae were detected only in mackerel. These results are similar to our survey in the area near Ushimado in the central part of Seto Inland Sea coast. Jack mackerel, anchovy, flathead, *Pleuronichtys cornutus*, *Scomberomorus niphonicus* and *Mugil cephalus* were common species in the survey by Hatada [10] and in the present survey. These fish were not infected with any Anisakinae larvae. Besides these fish, *Anisakis* spp. larvae could not be detected in 21 specimens of cultured small yellowtail. However, a case of intestinal anisakiasis caused by eating small yellowtail sashimi cultured from a fixed net in the Seto Inland Sea has been reported [1]. We considered that the cultured small yellowtail was infected secondarily with *Anisakis simplex* larvae after being fed on fish which were caught in an open sea area near Hokkaido, Tohoku or San-in.

It is confirmed that some species caught in the central part of the Seto Inland Sea were infected with Anisakinae larva. However, it is considered that anisakiasis could not be caused by eating raw non-migratory fish caught in the Seto Inland Sea except for the cultured small yellowtail.

References

1. Aji T, et al. (1982) An intestinal anisakiasis with an ileus. Okayama igakkai Zasshi 94: 775–782 (in Japanese)
2. Fukuda T, Tongu Y, Aji T, Lai J, Ho L, Shimono K, Inatomi S (1982) *Anisakidea* larvae from some fishes in the Seto Inland Sea. Jpn J. Parasitol 31: 171–176 (in Japanese)
3. Smith JW, Wootten R (1978) *Anisakis* and anisakiasis. Advances in Parasitol, Lumusden WHR, (ed) Academic Press, New York, vol.16, pp 93–163.
4. Koyama T (1974) Anisakinae larvae in Fishes and *Anisakis*. Vol. 7, Japanese Society of Scientific Fisheries Koseisha-Koseikaku, Tokyo (in Japanese)
5. Koyama T et al. (1969) Morphological and taxonomical studies on Anisakidae larvae found in marine fishes and squids. Jpn J Parasitol 18: 467–487 (in Japanese)
6. Nishimura T, Okumura T, Abe K, Morishita Y (1967) Studies on *Anisakis*-type worm (8); On the infection mode and distribution of *Anisakis* larvae isolated from various marine fishes. Jpn J Parasitol 16 (suppl): 287 (in Japanese).
7. Ohishi K (1973) Hokke and *Terranova*. Shokuhin-Kogyo 16: 75–84 (in Japanese)
8. Takita T (1974) Studies on early life history of croaker in Ariake Bay. Report of Faculty of Fisheries, Nagasaki University 38: 1–55 (in Japanese)
9. Matsubara K, Ochiai A (1973) Gyoruigaku, Suisangakuzenshu 19, Koseisha-Koseikaku, Tokyo (in Japanese)
10. Hatada T (1970) A survey on *Anisakidae* larvae found in fishes and cephalopods caught in the Seto Inland Sea and the Japan Sea. Report of Public Health Institute of Hyogo Prefecture No.5: 34–43 (in Japanese)

Survey of Anisakidae Larvae from Marine Fish Caught in the Sea Near Kyushu Island, Japan

Y. TAKAO

Introduction

A survey of Anisakidae larvae taken from sardines was reported by Yamaguti S in 1935 [1], Yamaguchi and Kobayashi et al. in 1966 [2,3], Honda et al. in 1967 [4], Katoh et al. and Kuwabara et al. in 1968 [5,6], Ishida et al., Hara and Kagei in 1969 [7,8,9] and Sakaguchi, Katamine in 1971 [10]. In these reports, the authors documented that *Anisakis* type-I larvae (hereafter abbreviated as type A-I) which are the most frequent in man were detected. However, other documents have shown no detection at all. As acute gastric anisakiasis caused by type A-I following ingestion of raw sardines has increased in northern Saga Prefecture and eastern Ooita Prefecture since 1985, a survey was made on Anisakidae larvae from sardines caught in the sea near Kyushu island in the spring and autumn of 1986. This paper presents a report, together with a survey of Anisakidae larvae from *Scomber japonicus* Houttuyn (hereafter abbreviated as *Scomber j.*) and other fish from 1976 to 1986.

Method of Survey (Materials and Methods)

Survey on Sardines (Catchment areas are shown in Fig. 1)

Sardines caught in the following sea areas were packed in icy brine or fresh sea water and delivered directly to the author's laboratory within 12 hours: catchment area—1: Bungo Channel [period—April 27–28 and Nov. 1 in 1986. Kind of paratenic host fishes: *Sardinops melanostictus* (Temminck et Schlegel)].—2: Iki Channel [May 17, 1986, *Sardinops melanostictus* (hereafter abbreviated as *Sardinops m.*), Nov. 21, 1986, *Sardinops m.* and *Etrumeus teres* (DeKay) (hereafter abbreviated as *Etrumeus t.*)]—3: Tsushima Strait [May 31, 1986, *Sardinops m.*].

The length and weight of the sardines were measured individually. The heads were then cut off, intestinal organs removed and the fillets were stored in a refrigerator. The internal organs were individually immersed in tap water in laboratory dishes at room temperature. After examining for the presence of parasites in the digestive tract wall and abdominal cavity, even after renewing the water several times at regular intervals, the number of parasites examined

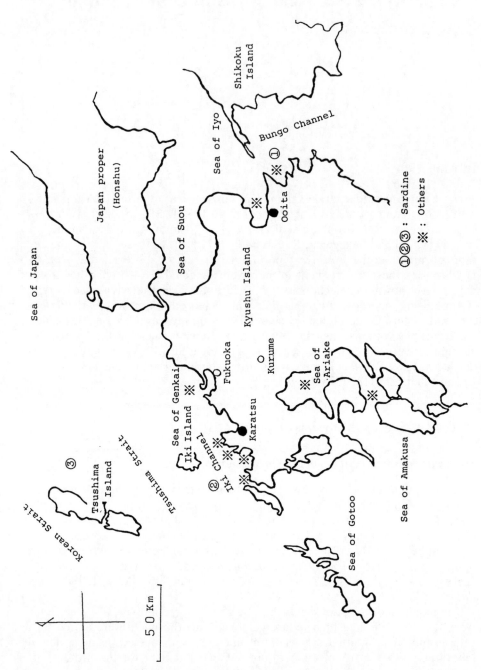

Fig. 1. Map showing the location

Survey of Anisakidae Larvae from Marine Fish

and recorded. Examination of the fillets was carried out in two ways, one with the fillets loosened by tap water and the other in artificial gastric juice.

Survey on *Scomber japonicus* and Other Fishes (catchment area = Fig. 1, Mark*)

Fish were caught by both the author and others in Bungo Channel, Beppu Bay, the coast along Karatsu and Yobuko, on the coast of Hirado, in the Ariake Sea between Amakusa and the peninsula of Shimabara. Only the internal organs of the fish were surveyed. Some fish such as *Decapterus macrosoma* Bleeker (hereafter abbreviated as *Decapterus m.*) were available in the market, and only the internal organs were examined.

Identification of the Parasite

Nematode larvae were collected, classified, examined as to their number and fixed in 10% hot formalin. They were later cleared with lactophenol, and after the body length was recorded with a universal projector, each section was measured with a biological microscope. Sections and measurement values as well as the index were taken according to the method of Koyama et al. [11]. The excretory system was observed according to Hartwich's [12] classification system.

Results of Survey

Survey on Nematode Larvae from Sardines

The number of fish caught in 1: the Bungo Channel, 2: the Iki Channel and 3: the Tsushima Strait are shown in Table 1. A total of 163 type A-I and some Nematode larvae of *Raphidascaris* sp. (hereafter abbreviated as *Raph.* genus) and *Thynnascaris* sp. (hereafter abbreviated as *Thyn.* genus) were detected in the internal organs of 1,429 fishes. No Nematode larvae were detected in the bodies of 92 fillets, and no type A-I were detected in the internal organs of these fish.

All type A-I were found in the abdominal cavity, predominantly in the pyloric appendage, next in the gastric serosa and then in the mesenterium adipose tissue. Among these, small bodied larvae were found free–living on the mesenterium, but not in the peritoneum.

Parasitism of type A-I, differentiated by sea areas is shown in Table 1. The maximum parasitic rate was found in fish from the Tsushima Strait, following by the Iki Channel and then those caught in the Bungo Channel.

The total number of type A-I caught in the Tsushima Strait and Iki Channel was 1,232, with 59 parasitic hostfish identified. The number of type A-I per fish was 1-13 as shown in Table 2. Of these, the number of cases of 1 per fish was the highest at 26 (44.1%) and the number of less than 4 per fish was 53 which is about 90%.

The parasitic rate profile of type A-I in 734 fish caught in the 3 sea areas was as follows: The larger the body length, the higher the parasitic rate (as shown

Table 1. Incidence of type A-I in sardines caught in the sea near Kyushu Island, Japan

Sea area	Season	Fish species	No. of exam.	No. of positive (%)	Total no. of A-I	Mean no.of A-I/1 fish	Mean no.of A-I/fishs 1Kg	Muscles exam.
1. Bungo Chanel	Spring (4/27–28)	S.m.	121	?	12	0.099	0.984	?
	Autumn (11/1)	S.m.	76	0	0	0	0	?
2. Iki Channel	Spring (5/17)	S.m	84	4 (4.76)	10	0.119	1.385	0/10
	Autumn (11/21)	S.m.	693	3 (0.43)	3	0.004	0.197	?
	Autumn (11/21)	E.t.	237	3 (1.27)	3	0.013	0.571	?
3. Tsushima Strait	Spring (5/31)	S.m.	218	49 (22.48)	135	0.619	6.760	0/82
Total			1,429		163	0.114	2.443	0/92

Fish species: S.m.: *Sardinops malanostictus*, E.t.: *Etrumeus teres*, ?: Unexamined.

Survey of Anisakidae Larvae from Marine Fish

Table 2. Parasitizing number of type A-I per fish

Sea area	Season	Fish spec.	No. of exam.	No. of posit.	Number of type A-I 1, 2, 3, 4, 5, 6, 7, · 12, 13,	Total	Mean No. A-I/1 fish
Iki Channel	Spring	S.m.	84	4	1. 1. 1. 1.	10	2.5
Iki Channel	Autumu	S.m.	693	3	3.	3	1.0
Iki Channel	Autumu	E.t.	237	3	3.	3	1.0
Tsushima Strait	Spring	S.m.	218	49	19. 11. 6. 7. 2. 1* 1* . 1* 1*	135	2.76
Total			1,232	59	26. 12. 7. 8. 2. 1. 1. 1. 1.	151	2.56

* 6 larvae : Body length 215mm, Body weight 106g, Female.
* 7 larvae : Body length 225mm, Body weight 126g, Male.
*12 larvae : Body length 215mm, Body weight 120g, Female.
*13 larvae : Body length 206mm, Body weight 124g, Male.

S.m.: = Sardinops malanostictus, E.t.: = Etrumeus teres

Table 3. Parasitizing rate of type A-I by the size of fish

Fishes Body length(mm)	1. Bungo Channel		2. Iki Channel		3. Tsushima Strait		Total	
	No. of exam.	No. of posit. (%)	No. of exam.	No. of posit. (%)	No. of exam.	No. of posit. (%)	No. of exam.	No. of posit. (%)
221–235	0	0	1	1 (100.0)	1	1 (100.0)	2	2 (100.0)
211–220	0	0	1	1 (100.0)	22	9 (40.9)	23	10 (43.5)
201–210	6	0(0)	7	2 (28.6)	52	16 (30.8)	65	18 (27.7)
191–200	18	0(0)	21	0(0)	70	19 (27.1)	109	19 (17.4)
181–190	40	0(0)	25	0(0)	60	4 (6.7)	125	4 (3.2)
171–180	9	0(0)	15	0(0)	12	0(0)	36	0(0)
151–170	3	0(0)	13	0(0)	1	0(0)	17	0(0)
131–150	0	0	61	3 (4.9)	0	0	61	3 (4.9)
121–130	0	0	122	3 (2.6)	0	0	122	3 (2.5)
111–120	0	0	133	0(0)	0	0	133	0(0)
101–110	0	0	41	0(0)	0	0	41	0(0)
Total	76	0(0)	440	10 (2.3)	218	49 (22.5)	734	59 (8.0)

Table 4. The same trend was also observed in the parasitizing number of type A-I

Fish length (mm)	No. of exam.	No. of posit. (%)	Number of type A-I										Total	Infection rate
			1,	2,	3,	4,	5,	6,	7,·	12,	13,		
221–235	2	2 (100.0)			1.		1.					11.	5.50
211–220	23	10 (43.5)	2.		2.	4.		1.		1.		42.	4.20
201–210	65	18 (27.7)	7.	5.	2.	1.	2.				1.	50.	2.78
191–200	109	19 (17.4)	9.	6.	2.	2.						35.	1.84
181–190	125	4 (3.2)	2.	1.	1.							7.	1.75
171–180	36	0 (0)										0	
151–170	17	0 (0)										0	
131–150	61	3 (4.9)	3.									3.	1.0
121–130	122	3 (2.6)	3.									3.	1.0
111–120	133	0 (0)										0	
101–110	41	0 (0)										0	
Total	734	59 (8.0)	26.	12.	7.	8.	2.	1.	1. ·	1.	1.	151.	2.56

Table 5. Dimension and indices of type A-I found in sardines

	1. Bungo Channel	2. Iki Channel	3. Tsushima Strait	Average
No. of Exam.	12	15	60	87
Body length	23.21 (16.40–29.00)	17.72 (13.85–21.25)	17.52 (12.50–20.80)	18.34
Body width	0.49 (0.338–0.626)	0.38 (0.282–0.507)	0.35 (0.211–0.422)	0.37
Oesophagus	2.93 (2.084–3.760)	2.30 (1.817–2.570)	2.36 (1.675–2.822)	2.43
O.muscular	1.89 (1.450–2.380)	1.64 (1.310–1.838)	1.66 (1.196–1.935)	1.69
O.glandular	1.03 (0.634–1.436)	0.65 (0.507–0.746)	0.71 (0.479–0.887)	0.74
Tail	0.10 (0.080–0.129)	0.10 (0.090–0.118)	0.08 (0.070–0.104)	0.09
A	47.15	47.19	50.84	49.52
B	7.93	7.72	7.41	7.55
C	12.25	10.78	10.58	10.87
D	22.48	27.16	24.72	24.66
E	239.77	176.49	210.83	208.40

Legend for all tables: A = Body length / Body width, B = Body length / Oesophagus, C = Body length / O. muscular, D = Body length / O. glandular, E = Body length / Tail. (Measurements in mm)

in Table 3.) With the number of infected larvae having the same tendency (Table 4.).

Of the 163 detected parasitic type A-I the body size of 87 were measured, with results similar to Table 5. In terms of sea areas, type A-I in the Bungo Channel were about 5mm larger in average body length than those of other areas, and those in the Tsushima Strait were the shortest. The length of 52 type A-I detected in *Scomber j.* caught in the open sea of Genkai in June 1986 was compared with these figures. The results and those reported by Koyama et al. [11] and by Sakaguchi et al. [10] are shown in Table 6. The average parasitic rate of type A-I from sardines was not significantly different from those of *Scomber j.*, but the type A-I from *Scomber j.* was a little greater in length in the present

Table 6. Comparison of measurements in type A-I

Fish spec.	Koyama et al. (1969)		Sakaguti et al. (1971)	Present author (1986)	
	Theragra c. and other	*Scomber j.*	*Saurida w.* and other	Sardines	*Scomber j.*
No. of Exam.	139	27	151	87	52
Body length	28.4	26.3	17.0	18.34	20.95
Body width	0.45	0.43	0.41	0.37	0.38
Oesophagus	3.34	3.10	2.28	2.43	2.59
O.muscular	2.22	2.03	1.53	1.69	1.84
O.glandular	1.12	1.07	0.75	0.74	0.76
Tail	0.12	0.12	0.10	0.09	0.10
A	63.21	62.43	41.80	49.52	54.69
B	8.50	8.49	7.50	7.55	8.08
C	12.84	13.07	11.10	10.87	11.41
D	25.51	24.97	22.60	24.66	27.62
E	250.03	229.02	165.10	208.40	219.37

68 Y. Takao

survey. The values of those from sardines were similar to those of *Saurida wanieso* Shindo et Yamada, *Upeneus bensasi* (Temminck et Schlegel) [10] and were smaller than *Theragra chalcogramma* (Pallas) by about 10mm in body length. [11] There was about 5mm difference between those from *Scomber j.* reported by Koyama et al. [11] and those *Scomber j.* in the present survey.

Table 7 compares number of type A-I to body length between 286 bodies (those not damaged in the period from 1977 to 1986) from humans in Ooita, Fukuoka, Saga and part of Nagasaki prefecture, with 87 of those from sardines and 52 from *Scomber j.* in the present survey. Approximately 70% of the length of larvae from humans ranges from 17.55 to 27.5 mm and about 90% of those from sardines shows a body length from 12.5 to 22.5mm, whereas type A-I from Scombridae was divided into 2 groups of 15.05 to 20.0mm and 22.55 to 27.5mm.

The gastric contents of 100 *Sardinops m.* were examined from each sea area, and several species of Capepoda in addition to vegetable plankton and sea weed. No Nematode larvae could be detected in any of them.

Survey on Nematode Larvae from Other Marine Fish such as *Scomber japonicus*.

Five hundred and sixty fish of 22 different species, except for the above-mentioned *Sardinops m.* and *Etrumeus t.*, were surveyed for a decade (Table 8). One species each of type A-I, *Anisakis* larvae type-II (hereafter abbreviated as type A-II), *Terranova* larvae type-A (hereafter abbrebviated as type T-A). *Terranova* larvae type-C (hereafter abbreviated as type T-C) and *Contracaecum* sp. (hereafter abbreviated as *Cont.* genus), one species of *Raph.* genus and 4 species of *Thyn.* genus were detected, which made a total of 10 species of 5 genera.

Of these, type A-I were detected in 256 fish of 19 species and 109 (92.4%) of 118 mackerels showed parasitism. However, the parasitism varied in number by sea area and season, ranging from 3 to a maximum of 631.

Type A-II and type T-C were detected in fish caught in the sea areas influenced by the Kuroshio current, and more of type A-II were detected in *Scomber j.* and *Decapterus m.*, whereas two type T-C were detected in only one *Decapterus m.*. Type T-A were detected in all the fish caught on the coasts of Karatsu and Yobuko, and each one from 3 *Scomber j.* and one from 1 *Sebastiscus marmoratus* (Cuvier) were detected in a total of 4. Those in *Cont.* genus were detected in mackerel and horse mackerel. Either or both of *Thyn.* and *Raph.* genera were detected in most of the fish (21 out of 22 species, 95.5%).

Discussion

According to the 6th report by Iino in 1985 [13], there were as many as 2,252 patients with anisakiasis in the upper alimentary canal alone in the Kyushu area, and of them, all except for one with type T-A, were infected with type A-I. The author had researched a survey on Anisakidae larvae from different fish and the identification of parasites from man [14]. Acute gastric anisakiasis by ingestion of raw sardines has increased since 1985, and therefore, a survey on sardines was made selectively. The above results warrant a comparison to reports by other workers.

Table 7. The parasitic rate of the sea area and the human case by body length of type A-I

Body length of larvae	Sardines				*Scomber j.*	Human case (%)
	1. Bungo C.	2. Iki C.	3. Tsushima S.	Total (%)	Genkai (%)	
6.50–10.00	0	0	0	0	0	3 (1.1)
10.05–12.50	0	0	1	1 (1.2)	0	3 (1.1)
12.55–15.00	0	2	8	10 (11.5)	2 (3.9)	12 (4.2)
15.05–17.50	1	6	20	27 (31.0)	9 (17.3)	26 (9.1)
17.55–20.00	3	3	22	28 (32.2)	13 (25.0)	43 (15.0)
20.05–22.50	1	4	9	14 (16.1)	4 (7.7)	72 (25.2)
22.55–25.00	2	0	0	2 (2.3)	17 (32.7)	63 (22.0)
25.05–27.50	3	0	0	3 (3.5)	6 (11.5)	31 (10.8)
27.55–30.00	2	0	0	2 (2.3)	1 (1.9)	20 (7.0)
30.05–32.50	0	0	0	0	0	8 (2.8)
32.55–35.00	0	0	0	0	0	4 (1.4)
35.05–37.50	0	0	0	0	0	0
37.55–40.00	0	0	0	0	0	1 (0.4)
Total	12	15	60	87(100.)	52(100.)	286 (100.)
Average	(23.21 mm)	(17.72 mm)	(17.52 mm)	(18.34 mm)	(20.95 mm)	(22.35 mm)

Table 8. Incidence of Anisakidae larvae from marine fish caught in the near Kyushu island

Species of fish	No. of exam.	Anisakis Type-I(%)	Anisakis Type-II(%)	Terranova Type-A(%)	Terranova Type-C(%)	Contra-cacum g.	Thynnas-caris g.	Raphidas-caris g.
Scombridae								
Scomber japonicus Houttuyn	59	59 (100.)	28 (47.5)	3 (5.1)	—	+	+	+
Scomber australasicus Cuvier	41	40 (97.6)	2 (4.9)	—	—	+	+	+
Auxis thazard (Lacepede)	8	5 (62.5)	—	—	—	−	+	+
Sarda orientalis (Temminck et Schlegel)	10	5 (50.0)	1 (10.0)	—	—	+	+	+
Subtotal	118	109 (92.4)	31 (26.3)	3 (2.5)	—	+	+	+
Carangidae								
Trachurus japonicus (Temm. et Schl.)	43	19 (44.2)	—	—	—	−	+	+
Decapterus maruadsi (Temm. et Schl.)	38	28 (73.7)	—	—	—	−	+	+
Decapterus muroadsi (Temm. et Schl.)	7	5 (71.4)	—	—	—	−	+	+
Decapterus macrosoma Bleeker	98	23 (23.5)	20 (20.4)	—	1 (1.0)	+	+	+
Caranx equula (Temm. et Schl.)	16	2 (12.5)	—	—	—	−	+	+
Caranx ciliarlus (Rüppell)	12	1 (8.3)	—	—	—	−	+	+
Caranx coeruleopinnatus (Rüppell)	21	3 (14.3)	—	—	—	−	+	+
Subtotal	235	81 (34.5)	20 (8.5)	—	1 (0.4)	+	+	+
Others								
Engraulis japonica	19	—	—	—	—	−	+	+
Cypselurus heterurus doederleini (Steindachner)	41	—	—	—	—	+	+	+
Sebastiscus marmoratus (Cavier)	23	1 (4.3)	—	1 (4.3)	—	−	+	+
Cociella crocodila (Tilesias)	13	1 (7.7)	—	—	—	−	+	+
Stephanolepis cirrhifer (Temm. et Schl.)	11	1 (9.1)	—	—	—	−	+	+
Navodon modestus (Günther)	28	1 (3.6)	—	—	—	−	+	+
Navodon tessellatus (Günther)	3	—	—	—	—	−	+	+
Takifugu niphobles (Jordan et Snyder)	12	1 (8.3)	—	—	—	−	+	+
Pagrus major (Temm. et Schl.)	37	2 (5.4)	—	—	—	−	+	+
Mugil cephalus (Linnaeus)	14	—	—	—	—	−	+	−
Liza haematocheila (Temm. et Schl.)	6	—	—	—	—	−	−	−
Grand total	560	197 (35.2)	51 (9.1)	4 (0.7)	1 (0.2)	+	+	+

Survey of Anisakidae Larvae from Marine Fish   71

Reports of detection of type A-I in sardines were as follows: Yamaguti and Honda detected from *Etrumeus t.* [1,4], Honda and Kuwabara did from *Sardinops m.* [4,6], Yamaguchi, Honda, Ishida, and Hara did from *Engraulis japonica* (Houttuyn) (hereafter abbreviated as *Engraulis j.*) [2,4,7,8] and Yamaguti did from *Chirocentrus dorab* (Forskal) [1].

Reports of non-detection of larvae were as follows: Kobayashi and Kagei examined *Sardinops m.* [3,9], Katoh examined 106 [5] and Ishida did 27 from *Sardinops m.* [7], Katoh examined 77 [5] and Hara did 101 from *Etrumeus t.* [8]. Sakaguchi did 27 from *Sardinops m.*, 50 from *Engraulis j.* and 27 from *Etrumeus t.* caught in the sea near Nagasaki [10].

It is interesting to note that the present survey revealed a difference between spring and autumn in the detection of type A-I in fish of similar body length caught in the Bungo Channel. There was a considerable seasonal difference in the fish length, even in the Iki Channel, and there was a considerable difference in the parasitic rate. However, even in the same season, the parasitic rate was higher in larger fish which ingested more *Copepoda*. As a result, it appears that the difference in detection of type A-I is caused by migration of the final hosts, tides, and seasons as well as sea areas.

Kobayashi reported in 1968 that out of 354 adults, those who eat raw sardines, showed the highest positive rates of intracutaneous response to both SOM and ES antigens [15]. This could be attributed to a past infection from eating raw sardines or to the fact that sardines are a popular food of this area.

In the survey carried out in northern Kyushu the number of patients with acute anisakiasis from eating raw sardines was 31 (8.1%) between 1977 to 1986. It is interesting that anisakiasis in this district occurred frequently in 1979 and 1986, and that such cases caused by the ingestion of raw sardines has ceased since last summer. It is also interesting that people in Ooita Prefecture were first infected by eating raw mackerel, didn't eat it for a while, and had a peak later from ingestion of marinated sardines. It is feared that there may be no decrease in infection rates unless the Japanese habit of eating raw marine fish can be improved, or the final hosts are drastically reduced.

The fact that type A-II, type T-A and type T-C besides type A-I were detected in fish caught in the sea near Kyushu island, suggests a future crisis of larval parasitism. In fact the second case of the disease caused by terranovasis (type T-A) in Kyushu island has been reported in Ooita Prefecture [16]. It is advisable to pay attention to this matter, and therefore necessary to identify the parasitic body detected. It seems that the first case of type T-C was documented in fish caught in the sea near Japan.

Conclusion

Since 163 type A-I were detected in 1,429 sardines caught in the sea near Kyushu island, the possibility of type A-I infection by eating raw sardines can be presumed. However, it has turned out that the parasitic rate of fish caught, even in the same sea area, varies by seasons.

The detection of type T-A in fish caught in the sea near Kyushu island suggests a possible crisis in the future. At the same time, the detection of type A-II as

72 Y. Takao

well as type T-C must also be considered. Detected type T-C have also been reported.

References

1. Yamaguti S (1935) 10 Studies on the helminth fauna of Japan. Part. 9 Nematodes of fishes 1. Jpn J Zool 6: 337–386
2. Yamaguchi T (1966) The infection and prevention of anisakiasis. Jpn J Parasitol 15: 285–286 (in Japanese)
3. Kobayashi A, Koyama T, Kumada K, Komiya Y, Oshima T, Kagei N, Ishii T, Machida M (1966) A survey of marine fishes and squids for the presence of Anisakinae larvae. Jpn J Parasitol 15: 348–349 (in Japanese)
4. Honda T, Tsubouchi H, Noziri H (1967) On the investigations of *Anisakis* larvae in marine fishes at Nagoya-City, Nagoya-Eisei-Kenkyusho-Houkoku 14: 79–81 (in Japanese)
5. Kato T, Uminuma M, Ito K, Miura K (1968) On Anisakinae from the marine fishes at the Central Market of Japan. Shokuhin-Eisei-Kenkyu 18: 784–797 (in Japanese)
6. Kuwabara H, Takakuwa M, Shioda T, Atsumi M, Shimakawa T, Kobayashi K (1968) Investigations for the presence of *Anisakis* larvae at Mie-Prefecture. Shokuhin-Eisei-Kenkyu 18: 863–868 (in Japanese)
7. Ishida M, Higashi T, Ikegami M, Yano S, Suwa F, Ikeda Y (1969) On the investigation of *Anisakis*-like larvae at marine fishes, Nihon-Zyu-Ishikai Zasshi 22: 371–372 (in Japanese)
8. Hara I (1969) Examinations on *Anisakis*-like larvae in marine fishes from the Japan Sea. Jpn J Med Tech 18: 825–827 (in Japanese)
9. Kagei N (1969) Life cycle of Anisakinae (Nematodes). Saishin-Igaku 24: 389–400 (in Japanese)
10. Sakaguti Y, Katamine D (1971). Survey of Anisakid larvae in marine fishes caught from the East China sea and the South China sea. Tropical Medicine 13: 159–169 (in Japanese with English summary)
11. Koyama T, Kobayashi A, Kumada M, Komiya Y, Oshima T, Kagei N, Ishii T, Machida M (1969). Morphological and taxonomical studies on Anisakidae larvae found in marine fishes and squids. Jpn J Parasitol 18: 466–487 (in Japanese with English summary)
12. Hartwich G (1957) Zur Systematik der Nematoden-superfamilie Ascaridoidea, Zoolgische Jahrbucher 85: 211–252
13. Iino H (1985) Anisakiasis in Kyusyu, Japan. (Sixth survey). Gastroenterol Endosc 27: 630 (in Japanese)
14. Takao Y, Shibata O, Kudou T, Furusawa T, Kagei N (1983) Acute gastric anisakiasis. Epidemiological and morphological studies in Ooita Prefecture. Nippon-Ijishimpo 3086: 26–31 (in Japanese)
15. Kobayashi A, Kumada M, Ishizaki T, Suguro T, Koito K (1968) Skin tests with somatic and ES (Excretions and Secretions) antigens from *Anisakis* larvae. 1. Survey of normal populations on the skin sensitivity to different antigens. Jpn J Parasitol 17: 407–413 (in Japanese with English summary)
16. Takao Y, Arita T, Emoto O (1986) The second case of acute gastric terranovasis (larvae type A) in Kyushu, Japan. Rinsho to Kenkyu 63: 3636–3638 (in Japanese)
17. Ichthyological Society of Japan (1981) Dictionary of Japanese fish names and their foreign equivalents, Sanseido Co., Ltd., Tokyo, 834 pp.

Surface Ultrastructure of Anisakidae Larvae

Y. Tongu, T. Fukuda, and T. Aji

The ultrastructure of the third stage larva (L3) of Anisakidae was described using a scanning electron microscope developed by Soleim in 1974 [6], Aji et al. [1], Valter et al. [7], Smith [5], Fujino et al. [2], and Weerasooriya et al. [8]. Among them, Fujino et al. in 1984 and Weerasooriya et al. in 1986 have often referred to the fourth stage larva (L4). Special attention has been paid to the fine structure of the anterior and the posterior extremity, and the cuticular structures of the larvae. These studies are essential to identify the larva in tissue sections, larval fragments from gastric and intestinal anisakiasis patients or a worm passed through the intestine. The classification of Anisakidae larvae was determined according to the system introduced by Koyama [4].

Anisakis Larvae

The head of L3 larva of *Anisakis*-type has a triangular mouth opening (Fig. 1), a boring tooth (Fig. 1, BT), and 6 papillae (Fig. 1, P). The boring tooth (Fig. 1, BT) is situated on the ventral tip of the mouth lip. An excretory pore (Fig. 1, EP) opens out near the base of the boring tooth. It is usually difficult to locate the amphid on the head. However, Valter et al. noted the openings of the amphid at the lateral side between the head papillae in *Anisakis* sp. [7].

In the tail, *Anisakis* type I bore a small spine, namely, a mucron (Fig. 2, M). The surface of this mucron (Fig. 4) is covered with many transverse striations, while *Anisakis* type II (Fig. 5) has no mucron and only a slender tail.

Anisakis-type larva have irregular and discontinuous transverse striations (Fig. 3) with longitudinal ridges (Fig. 3, LR) seen in the spaces between these (Fig. 3, TS). The larvae are easily classified from other genera by these characteristic cuticular patterns.

Anisakis type II closely resemble *Anisakis* type I in the external appearance of the head and cuticular surface except for the tail. Regarding *Anisakis* type III, there is, as yet, no report using a scanning electron microscope.

It has been reported that the L4 larva show 3 separate-lips and a slit-like triradiate lumen of the mouth opening [2,8]. The dorsal lip is bigger than the 2 subventral ones. Each lip has 2 dentigerous ridges and a row of denticles on the inner margin of the ridges, with the total denticle number 35–45 and a different shape between the dorsal and subventral lip. The transverse striations on the

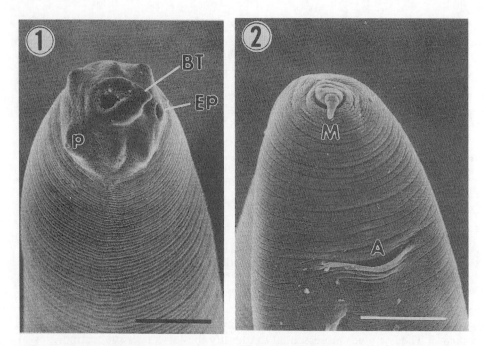

Fig. 1. Anterior extremity of *Anisakis* type I (L3). BT: boring tooth, EP: excretory pore, P: papilla, Bar = 50 μm

Fig. 2. Posterior extremity of *Anisakis* type I (L3) recovered from human. A: anus, M: mucron, Bar = 50 μm

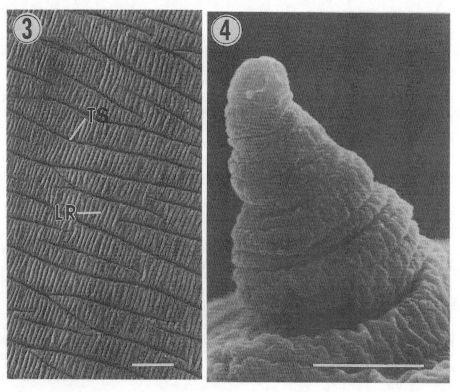

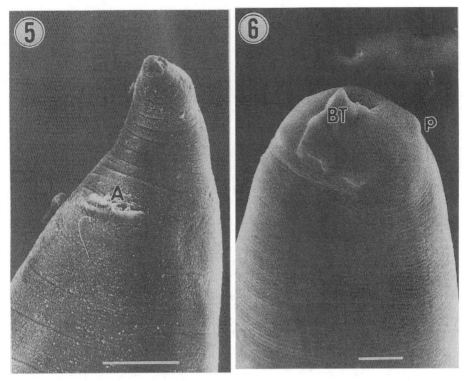

Fig. 5. Posterior extremity of *Anisakis* type II (L3). A: anus, Bar = 50 μm

Fig. 6. Anterior extremity of *Terranova* sp. (L3). BT: boring tooth, P: papilla, Bar = 10 μm

cuticle of the fourth stage larva are wide, regularly spaced and continuous, while the longitudinal ridges are regular and finer than those of L3.

Terranova Larvae

L3 larva of the *Terranova* type A (Fig. 6) have a triangular mouth opening similar to the *Anisakis*-type. A boring tooth (Fig. 6, BT) is situated on the tip of the ventral lip, with 6 papillae (Fig. 6, P) and an excretory pore seen on the head as in the case of the *Anisakis*-type. The mouth lip is not remarkable when compared with the *Anisakis*-type. A mucron covered by transverse striations is located on the tail tip of *Terranova* type A. These structural features closely resembled those of *Anisakis* type I. On the other hand, L3 larvae of *Terranova* type B lack a mucron, have a conical tail end, and the cuticle of these L3 larvae show irregular and discontinuous transverse striations.

◁─────────────────────────────────

Fig. 3. Cuticular surface of *Anisakis* type I (L3). LR: longitudinal ridge, TS: transverse striation, Bar = 10 μm

Fig. 4. A mucron of *Anisakis* type I (L3). Bar = 5 μm

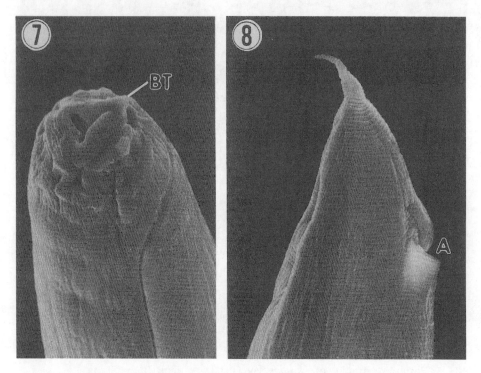

Fig. 7. Anterior extremity of *Raphidascaris* sp. (L3). BT: boring tooth, Bar = 10 μm

Fig. 8. Posterior extremity of *Raphidascaris* sp. (L3). A: anus, Bar = 10 μm

In L4 larvae, a slit-like triradiate mouth and 3 lips, equal in size and shape, have been observed [8]. Furthermore, the lip with W shape dentigerous ridges has 45 to 50 denticles on the inner margin of the ridges, with the same shape in the dorsal and subventral denticles. The transverse striations are regular and the tail of the L4 larvae has a pair of phasmids situated symmetrically as round elevations.

Raphidascaris Larvae

Although L3 larvae of *Raphidascaris* type A were smaller than the *Anisakis*-type, they have a triangular mouth opening and a boring tooth (Fig. 7, BT) displaying a good likeness to *Contracaecum* type A. The tail of *Raphidascaris* tapers off sharply to a point (Fig. 8), and resembles a mucron of *Anisakis* type I though is more slender than that of *Anisakis*. Transverse striations on the cuticle of *Raphidascaris* are irregular and discontinuous, with longitudinal ridges between the transverse striations unnoticed. In L4 larvae of *Raphidascaris*, the cuticle on the tail end is equipped with 15 to 20 spines as in the case of *Thynnascaris* type B.

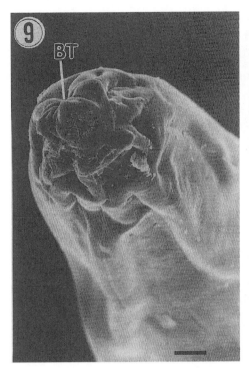 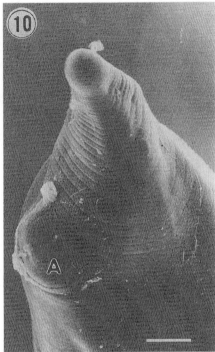

Fig. 9. Anterior extremity of *Contracaecum* type A (L3). BT: boring tooth, Bar = 10 μm

Fig. 10. Posterior extremity of *Contracaecum* type A (L3). A: anus, Bar = 10 μm

Contracaecum Larvae

L3 larva of *Contracaecum* type A (Fig. 9) were not identified with the *Anisakis*-type as to the head characteristics. Its boring tooth (Fig. 9, BT) and triangular mouth opening are very similar to those of *Anisakis*, except for the size. The transverse striations with longitudinal ridges are more regular than the *Anisakis*-type, while the tail of this larva tapers off to a point. However, the tail end was conical (Fig. 10). The cuticle has regular, patterned transverse striations.

Thynnascaris Larvae

According to Weerasooriya and Valter L3 larvae of *Thynnascaris* show a triangular mouth opening and a conical boring tooth on the anterior extremity [7,8]. Furthermore, Valter et al. (1982) discovered the papillae and amphids in L3 larva of *T. adunca*. The tip of the tail has a mucron, and the transverse striations on the cuticle are very irregular.

L4 larva of *Thynnascaris*, commonly found in fish, had separate lips (Fig. 11, L) and a slit like mouth opening. Two papillae (Fig. 11, P) were observed as

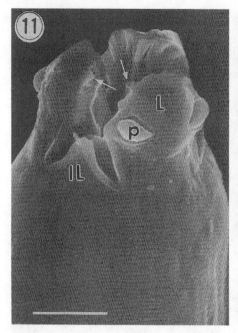 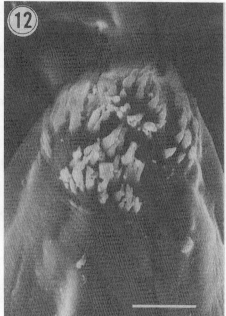

Fig. 11. Anterior extremity of *Thynnascaris* type B (L4). IL: interlabia, L: lip, P: papilla, Bar = 10 μm

Fig. 12. Posterior extremity of *Thynnascaris* type B (L4). Small spines are seen on the tail. Bar = 10 μm

round elevations on each lip. The lips have several denticles (Fig. 11, arrows) on the margin while the mouth with an interlabia (Fig. 11, IL) differed considerably from that of *Anisakis* L4, especially, in the posterior extremity, where *Thynnascaris* type B had about 100 small spines (Fig. 12) on the tail tip. Some spines branched at the tip from 2 to 4. In *Thynnascaris* type A, these spines were not found.

Mensuration of Transverse Striations

Anisakidae larvae have characteristic transverse striations (Fig. 3, TS) on the cuticle. We attempted to classify the three kinds of L3 larvae, *Anisakis* type I, *Raphidascaris* and *Contracaecum* type A, by the mean value of the distances between the transverse striations (DBTS) and the diameter of the worm trunk (DOWT) [3]. The mean DBTS and DOWT for the head, middle and tail is shown in Table 1.

The mean of DBTS differs slightly between the head, middle and tail in larval *Anisakis* type I: DBTS is wider in the middle than in the tail or head. This tendency is also observed in the other 2 species, with no significant difference between the mean for the head and tail of larval *Anisakis* type I and *Raphidascaris*. On the other hand, a significant difference ($p < 0.05$) is found between the middle and tail, and between the head and middle. In *Contracaecum* type A,

Surface Ultrastructure of Anisakidae Larvae

Table 1. Mean and confidence limits, standard deviation, and coefficient of variation of the diameter of worm trunk and the distances between the transverse striations in three larval anisakids (measurements in μm)

| Genus | Portion | DOWT | | | DBTS | | | | |
		n	mean	CL	ń	mean	CL	SD	CV
Anisakis	Cumulative	15	268.1 ±	37.73	783	5.45 ±	.125	1.784	.328
type I	Head	7	220.9 ±	47.54	376	5.00 ±	.185	1.834	.367
	Middle	6	336.7 ±	13.17	301	6.12 ±	.185	1.633	.267
	Tail	2	227.3 ±	10.71	106	5.11 ±	.268	1.389	.272
Raphidascaris	Cumulative	20	112.8 ±	9.98	996	2.92 ±	.051	.823	.281
	Head	6	99.7 ±	25.04	300	2.59 ±	.085	.749	.289
	Middle	9	125.5 ±	13.19	439	3.27 ±	.077	.826	.253
	Tail	5	105.7 ±	20.35	257	2.73 ±	.081	.662	.242
Contracaecum	Cumulative	12	73.8 ±	16.51	417	1.68 ±	.056	.580	.344
type A	Head	4	53.9 ±	32.05	110	1.38 ±	.069	.362	.263
	Middle	4	89.4 ±	34.09	149	1.98 ±	.092	.572	.289
	Tail	4	79.3 ±	25.95	153	1.62 ±	.092	.583	.359

DOWT: The diameter of worm trunk, DBTS: The distances between transverse striations, n: Number of specimens, ń: Number of DBTS measured, CL: Confidence limits ($p < 0.05$), SD: Standard deviation, CV: Coefficient of variation

significant differences ($p < 0.05$) of the mean are found between the head, middle and tail. Therefore there is a correlation between DOWT and DBTS among these 3 larval types, and in most cases a larva may be identified from the mean value of DBTS and DOWT in a clinically obtained worm fragment.

References

1. Aji T, Fukuda, T, Ho L-S, Tongu Y, Inatomi S, Motoi M, Koshimune I (1982) An intestinal anisakiasis with an ileus. Okayama Igakkai Zasshi 94: 775–782 (in Japanese with English summary)
2. Fujino T, Ooiwa T, Ishii Y (1984) Clinical, epidemiological and morphological studies on 150 cases of acute gastric anisakiasis in Fukuoka Prefecture. Jpn J Parasitol 33: 73–92 (in Japanese with English summary)
3. Fukuda T, Aji T, Tongu Y, Ishii A (1987) Classification of *Anisakidae* larvae by the distance between transverse striations (in Japanese). Jpn J Parasitol 36: Proceedings of the Regional Meetings of the Japanese Society of Parasitology (No. 1), p. 17
4. Koyama T (1974) Fishes and *Anisakidae*. Fishery Science Series 7. pp. 9–19 Koseisha Koseikaku, Tokyo, Japan (in Japanese)
5. Smith JW (1983) *Anisakis simplex* (Rudolphi 1809, det. Krabbe 1878) (Nematoda: Ascaridoidea): Morphology, and morphometry of larvae from euphausiids and fish, and a review of the life-history and ecology. J Helminthol 57: 205–224
6. Soleim Φ (1974) Scanning electron microscope observations of *Contracaecum aduncum* (Nematoda: Ascaridoidea). Norwegian J Zool 22: 171–175
7. Valter ED, Popova TI, Valovaya MA (1982) Scanning electron microscope study of four species of anisakid larva (Nematoda: Anisakidae). Helminthologia 19: 195–209
8. Weerasooriya MV, Fujino T, Ishii Y, Kagei N (1986) The value of external morphology in the identification of larval anisakid nematodes: a scanning electron microscope study. Z. Parasitenkd 72: 765–778

Restriction Endonuclease Analysis of *Anisakis* Genome

K. Sugane

Introduction

Many reports have accumulated on the human infection with the marine nematode, genus *Anisakis*. However, infection by certain other genera of marine Anisakine nematodes, including *Terranova* and *Contracaecum* have also been reported from Japan and other countries [1]–[4]. These infections have also been called anisakiasis. Many researchers have noted that the frequent presence of *Anisakis* and other *Anisakinae* larvae in the same individual host (e.g. codfish), has produced considerable taxonomic confusion [5] and that the relationships between these larvae and their adult worms are conjectural, although some indirect evidence has been provided by the analysis of isozymes or allozymes and physicochemical properties of haemoglobins [6,7] Furthermore, it should be clarified whether or not phenotypic variations in same species of *Anisakis* larvae are present.

Generally, it is necessary to collect detailed and accurate epidemiological data in endemic regions before controlling a parasitic disease. However, such work in anisakiasis is hampered by the difficulty in distinguishing the larvae of closely related genera or even species and by the lack of evidence for confirming the relationship between larvae and adult worms.

It is now apparent that the techniques of molecular biology are useful for the identification of parasites, and can provide a new approach to taxonomical study. Analysis of restriction fragment length polymorphisms (RFLPs) is an excellent method to distinguish these kinds of larvae and to clarify the relationship between larvae and their adult worms, because it can be used to detect minute differences in genomic DNA sequences among very closely related organisms.

We describe an analysis of RFLPs to distinguish *Anisakis* larvae type I, and type II as discussed by Oshima [8], and the larvae of a related genus, *Contracaecum*. The relationship between *Anisakis* larvae type I and adult worms of *Anisakis simplex* is also clarified using 25s rRNA probe.

Materials and Methods

Collection of Worms

Anisakis larvae type I were recovered from the viscera of two paratenic hosts, codfish and mackerel obtained from fish shops. Larvae were washed 4–5 times with 0.85% saline, immediately frozen in liquid nitrogen and stored at −85°C. *Contracaecum* larvae were collected from the viscera of codfish by the same method. Larval type was individually identified under the stereomicroscope according to the criteria of Koyama et al. [5]. *Anisakis* larvae type II were collected from the viscera of bonitos. *Trichinella spiralis* larvae were recovered from infected mice by the method described by Gould [9] with some modifications. Adult worms of *A. simplex* were collected form the stomach of *Globicephala macrorhyncus*.

Preparation of Genomic DNA

Genomic DNA were isolated from *Anisakis* larvae type I from codfish, and mackerel, *Anisakis* larvae type II, *Contracaecum* larvae, *T. spiralis* larvae and adult worms of *A. simplex*. Each 100mg of frozen larvae in 1ml of NET solution (0.1 M NaCl, 0.05 M EDTA, 0.1 M Tris·HCl, 1% SDS, pH 8.0) were disrupted in a Freezer/Mill pulverizer (Spex Industries Inc., USA) for 10 min. The disrupted material was repaidly transferred to a siliconized tube, incubated with occasional gentle agitation at 65°C for 60 min in proteinase K solution at 1 mg/ml. After centrifugation at 10000 rpm for 10 min at 0°C, the supernatant was collected in a sterile siliconized tube and 4.5 gm caesium chloride was dissolved in 5 ml of the supernatant by gently mixing. Then, ethidium bromide was added to the mixture at the final concentration of 600 μ g/ml and centrifuged at 42000 rpm for 36 h at 20°C in a Backman 50 Ti rotor. A single DNA band was clearly visualized under UV illumination. The DNA band was recovered and the ethidium bromide in the collected DNA solution was extracted with an equal volume of isoamyl alcohol. After dialysis against TE buffer (10 mM Tris HCl, 1 mM EDTA, pH 7.5) overnight, the DNA in aqueous phase was precipitated by two volumes of cold ethanol in the presence of 0.15 M NaCl overnight at −80°C, dried in a vacuum, and dissolved in a small volume of TE buffer.

Preparation of ^{32}P–25s rRNA

Total RNA was isolated from *Anisakis* larvae type I from codfish by the guanidinium/hot phenol method. Samples containing rRNA were electrophoresed through 1.0% agarose gel containing formaldehyde in 200 V for 2 h in MOPS buffer as described by Maniatis et al. [10]. Two bands of 25s and 17.5s rRNA can be clearly visualized after staining the gel with ethidiuml bromide (1 μg/ml) [11]. The 25s rRNA was recovered from the gel as described by McDonnell et al. [12]. The T4 polynucleotide kinase method described by Maxman and Gilbert [13] was used in the labelling of 25s rRNA with γ^{32}P-ATP (Amersham International plc, UK).

Digestion with Restriction Endonuclease and Electrophoresis

0.1 μg genomic DNA of larvae or adult worms was digested with EcoRI, HaeIII, HpaII, HhaI, HinfI and Sau3AI according to the manual of the supplier of these enzymes (Toyobo Inc., Tokyo). Restriction fragments after EcoRI digestion were electrophoretically separated on 0.8% agarose gel and those after HaeIII or HpaII digestion on 1.5% agarose gel. Fragments after HhaI, HinfI or Sau3AI digestion were separated by electrophoresis on 5% polyacrylamide gel

Restriction Endonuclease Analysis of *Anisakis* Genome 83

for clear identification of bands. λ/HindIII digest and pBR322/AluI digests were used as DNA molecular weight markers.

Southern Blot Analysis

Restriction fragments separated by agarose or polyacrylamide gel electrophoresis were transferred to a nylon membrane, Hybond-N (Amersham International plc, UK) using the method described by Southern [14] with some modification and hybridized with [32]P-25s rRNA probe according to the Amersham's manual.

Results

Detection of RFLPs in *Anisakis* Larvae Type I DNA from Different Paratenic Hosts

Variability in the lengths of digested fragments of *Anisakis* larvae type I DNA from different paratenic hosts, codfish and mackerel, was examined by Southern blot assay using [32]P-25s rRNA as a probe. In Fig. 1 and Fig. 2, lanes 1 and 2 show the fragment bands of these two kinds of DNA on different enzymes. The patterns of these two kinds of DNA fragments were exactly the same. At least three, four and six clear bands were observed in EcoRI, HaeIII and HpaII digestion, respectively (Fig. 1). Also, five, five and six bands were clearly discriminated in HhaI, HinfI and Sau3AI digestion, respectively (Fig. 2).

Differences of RELPs Among *Anisakis* Larvae Type I, *Anisakis* Larvae Type II and *Contracaecum* Larvae

Southern blot analysis of these larval genomic DNAs digested with six enzymes displayed quite different polymorphisms (Fig. 1, Fig. 2). In EcoRI digestion, *Anisakis* larvae type I, *Anisakis* larvae type II and *Contracaecum* larvae could be distinguished based on completely different fragments from each other. In terms of the other five endonucleases, the same tendencies were observed. Also, when genomic DNA from *T. spiralis* larvae were used as a control in Southern blot assay, quite different RFLPs were observed compared to those of Anisakinae larvae (Fig. 1, Fig. 2).

Comparison of RFLPs Between *Anisakis* Larvae Type I and Adult Worms of *A. simplex*

From the morphological studies, *Anisakis* larva type I is considered to be the larva of *A. simplex*. As shown in Fig. 3 and Fig. 4, the patterns of these two kinds of DNA fragments were exactly the same in the six different endonuclease digestion, respectively.

Discussion

In this study, 25s rRNA was used as a probe in the analysis of RFLPs of *Anisakis* larva type I from codfish. No differences in RFLPs between two kinds of *Ani-*

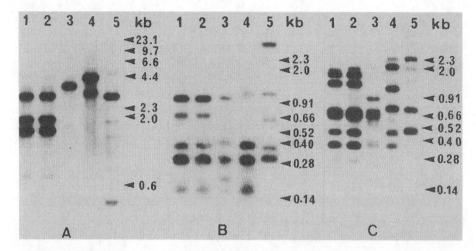

Fig. 1. Restriction fragment length polymorphisms of Anisakinae larvae. Genomic DNA was digested with EcoRI (**A**), HaeIII (**B**) and HpaII (**C**), separated on a 0.8% agarose gel for EcoRI digested fragments and 1.5% agarose gel for HaeIII and HpaII digests denatured, transferred to Hybond-N membrane and hybridized with ^{32}P-25s rRNA probe. Lane 1: *Anisakis* larvae type I from codfish; Lane 2: *Anisakis* larva type I from mackerel; Lane 3: *Anisakis* larva type II; Lane 4: *Contracaecum* larvae; Lane 5: *T. spiralis* larvae; Arrows indicate position of markers. (Sugane and Matsuura, 1989)

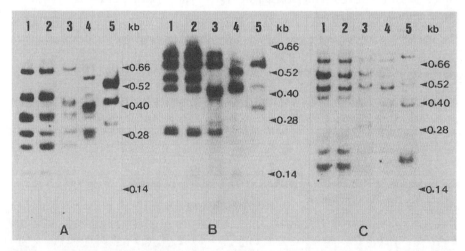

Fig. 2. Restriction fragment length polymorphisms of Anisakinae larvae. Genomic DNA digested with HhaI (**A**). HinfI (**B**) and Sau3AI (**C**) was separated by electrophoresis on a 5% polyacrylamide gel and electrotransferred to a Hybond-N membrane and hybridized with ^{32}P-25s rRNA. Lane 1. *Anisakis* larvae type I from codfish; Lane 2: *Anisakis* larva type I from mackerel; Lane 3: *Anisakis* larva type II; Lane 4: *Contracaecum* larvae; Lane 5: *T. spiralis* larvae. Arrows indicate position of markers. (Sugane and Matsuura, 1989)

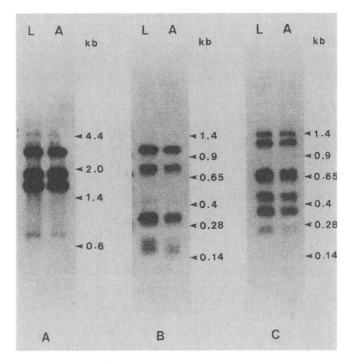

Fig. 3. Restriction fragment length polymorphisms of *Anisakis* larvae type I and adult worms of *A. simplex*. Genomic DNA was digested with EcoRI (**A**), HaeIII (**B**) and HpaII (**C**) and analysed as described in Materials and Methods. Lane L: *Anisakis* larvae type I from codfish; Lane A: Adult worms of *A. simplex*. Arrows indicate position of markers.

sakis larva type I's genomic DNA from different paratenic hosts showed that *Anisakis* larvae type I were not affected by environmental condition.

Also, the clear differences among the *Anisakis* larva type I, *Anisakis* larva type II and *Contracaecum* larvae in RFLPs of genomic DNA were shown by Southern blot assay. The species of Anisakinae larvae can be clearly distinguished from each other by their characteristic rDNA fragment patterns. The RELPs of rDNA from *T. spiralis* larvae were also examined as an example of distant relationship to Anisakinae larvae. The relationship among the four kinds of larvae clarified by RFLPs analysis agreed well with that of morphological taxonomy. This implied that the method of hybridization of 25s rRNA probe to genomic rDNA would be useful for clarifying the complicated taxonomy of the subfamily Anisakinae.

Furthermore, RFLPs of *Anisakis* larvae type I and adult worms of *A. simplex* were exactly the same. The result suggests that *Anisakis* larva type I must be the larva of *A. simplex*. When 25s rRNA from adult worms of *A. simplex* was used as a probe instead of that from *Anisakis* larvae type I, the same result was obtained.

A useful probe must been sufficiently conserved during evolution, and hybridize easily with a wide range of species. Coding sequences, e.g. rDNA, tend to

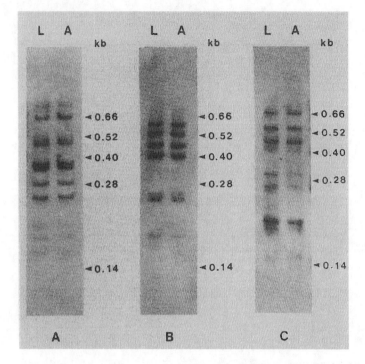

Fig. 4. Restriction fragment length polymorphisms of *Anisakis* larvae type I and adult worms of *A. simplex*. Genomic DNA was digested with HhaI (**A**), HinfI (**B**) and Sau3AI (**C**) and analysed as described in Materials and Methods. Lane L: *Anisakis* larvae type I from codfish; Lane A: adult worms of *A. simplex*. Arrows indicate position of markers.

be highly conserved in the course of evolution and the spacer sequences between the coding regions of the ribosomal cistrons tend to diverge rapidly, which accounts for the distinctive species-specific restriction fragments [15]. Thus, the RFLPs produced by the hybridization of 25s rRNA transcripted from the coding region of rDNA may possibly be able to show not only the differences between species but may also be used in estimating the genetic distances in related species.

The results in RFLPs which distinguish between *Anisakis* larvae type I and type II or *Contracaecum* larvae and identify *A. simplex* as adult worms of *Anisakis* larvae type I provided agreement with morphological studies and indicated that the 25s rRNA will prove useful in further taxonomic studies.

References

1. Shiraki T (1974) Larval nematodes of family *Anisakidae* (Nematoda) in the northern sea of Japan as a causative agent of eosinophilic phlegmone or granuloma in the human gastrointestinal tract. Acta Medica et Biologica 22: 57–98
2. Suzuki H, Ohnuma H, Karasawa Y (1972) *Terrranova* (Nematoda: *Anisakidae*) in-

Restriction Endonuclease Analysis of *Anisakis* Genome

fection in man I. Clinical features of five cases of *Terranova* larva infection. Parasitology 21: 252–256

3. Kates S, Wright KA, Wright R (1973) A case of human infection with the cod nematoda *Phocanema* sp. Am J Trop Med Hyg 22: 606–608
4. Little M, Most H (1973) Anisakid larva from the throat of a woman in New York. Am J Trop Med Hyg 22: 609–612
5. Koyama T, Kobayashi A, Kumada M, Komiya Y, Oshima T, Kagei N, Ishii T, Machida M (1969) Morphological and taxonomical studies on *Anisakidae* larvae found in marine fishes and squids. Jpn J Parasitol 18: 466–487
6. Orecchia P, Paggi L, Mattiucci S, Smith JW, Nascetti G, Bullini L (1986) Electrophoretic identification of larvae and adults of *Anisakis* (Ascaridida: Anisakidae). Helminthol 60: 331–339
7. Agatsuma T (1982) Electrophoretic studies on glucosephosphate isomerase phosphoglucomutase in two types of *Anisakis* larvae. Int J Parasitol 12: 35–39
8. Oshima T (1972) *Anisakis* and anisakiasis in Japan and adjacent area. In: Progress of Medical Parasitology in Japan Morishita, Komiyay, Matsubayashi (eds) Vol. IV, pp. 301–393, Meguro Parasitological Museum, Tokyo
9. Gould SE (1970) In: Trichinosis in man and animals, Gould ED (ed) pp. 190–221. Charles C. Thomas Publisher: Springfield, U.S.A.
10. Maniatis T, Fritsch EF, Sambrook J (1982) Molecular cloning. A larboratory manual pp. 194–203. Cold Spring Harbor Laboratory, U.S.A.
11. Sugane K, Matsuura T (1989) Restriction fragment length polymorphisms of *Anisakinae* larvae. J Helminthol 63: 269–274
12. McDonnell MW, Simon MN, Studier FW (1977) Analysis of restriction fragments of T7 DNA and determination of molecular weights by electrophoresis in neutral and alkaline gels. J Mol Biol 110: 119–128
13. Maxman AM, Gilbert W (1980) Sequencing end-labeled DNA with Base-specific chemical cleavages. Methods in Enzymology 65: 499–506
14. Southern EM (1975) Detection of specific sequences among DNA fragments separated by gel electrophoresis. J Mol Biol 98: 503–517
15. Cameron ML, Levy P, Nutman T, Vanamala CR, Narayanan PR, Rajan TV (1988) Use of restriction fragment length polymorphisms (RFLPs) to distinguish between nematodes of pathogenic significance. Parasitol 96: 381–390

Clinical Features of Intestinal Anisakiasis

H. Ishikura

Anisakiasis is a parasitic disease caused by eating raw seafood containing *Anisakis* larvae. The larvae emerge and separate from the muscle tissue of the fish in the oral cavity, the esophagus, or the stomach, and the disease occurs when they penetrate the wall of the digestive tract. The relationship between *Anisakis* larvae and the human body is complex and unknown. Larvae which cannot penetrate the stomach wall move into the intestinal cavity, and parasite-host relationship divides them into larvae which penetrate the intestinal wall and larvae which are discharged through the anus. The larvae which penetrate the intestinal wall are further divided into those which either stop in the wall, or those which perforate through.

It is assumed that when *Anisakis* larvae are active and the environment in the intestinal cavity is suitable for their movement, the larvae perforate the intestinal wall and penetrate into the abdominal cavity in a very short time. There are reports of a mild form of anisakiasis in the abdominal cavity with no display of signs or subjective symptoms that only requires out-patient treatment.

The diagnosis of intestinal anisakiasis is made from pathological changes to the intestinal wall, when intestinal excision show larvae at the place of infection, or when the tissue at the point of excision apparently indicates the presence of larvae. Recently cases with perforation of the intestinal wall have increased, and when this is accompained by bacterial infection, the perforated tissue in the intestinal wall undergoes histological morbid changes with symptoms of acute abdominal upset. The following describes the clinical symptoms and laboratory results of these cases.

General Symptomatology

In the nation-wide parasitological survey of anisakiasis conducted by the author in 1967, 278 cases were located: 196 cases (70.5%) were gastric, 77 (27.0%) [6] were intestinal anisakiasis, and 4 were extra-gastrointestinal anisakiasis (mild form) and one was unknown. The main symptoms of the cases of intestinal anisakiasis, including the 77 cases diagnosed by the author are detailed in Table 1.

Of more than 216 cases of anisakiasis in one geographical area, 87 displayed symptoms of acute ileus, necessitating laparotomy, an additional 10 cases also received laparotomy. Intestinal excision took place in 46 cases, and *Anisakis* larvae were found in 19 cases. Intestinal anisakiasis was diagnosed in the remain-

90 H. Ishikura

Table 1. Subjective complaints in patients with intestinal anisakiasis

Complaint	Number of cases		
	(15)[a] X-ray's diagnostics	(77)[b] Laparotomy done	(77)[c] Nation-wide examination
Nausea	6	54	19
Vomiting	4	54	22
Abdominal bulging	2	47	3
Abdominal induration	3	20	7
Meteorism	—	—	11
Fatigue	—	—	1
Location of subjective pain			
Epigastric	4	3	7
Upper abdomen	(whole abdomen 1)		
Umbilical	3	24	
Lower abdomen	1	20	
Right lower quadrant	5	26	
Left lower quadrant	1	2	
Unknown	2	2	
Evacuation of the bowels			
Constipation	1	24	
Diarrhea	5	20	
Blood in stool	3	4	
Mucus in stool		1	
Unknown		(normal 34)	
No complaint			3
Found by operation for another disease			2
Post-mortem dissection			1

[a] Ishikura H. (1965): Jpn. J. Clin. Radio. 10: 576.
[b] Ishikura H. et al. (1965): Surg. Treat. 13: 144.
[c] Ishikura H. (1968): Hokkaido J. Med. Sci. 4–6: 83.

ing cases from histopathological findings. the remaining 119 cases were treated with conservative internal therapy (evacuation of the intestinal tract by Miller-Abbott tube and pharmacotherapy). Among these, 15 cases that were diagnosed as intestinal anisakiasis by X-ray showed very slow progress with conservative treatment, and 5 cases were subjected to surgery after suddenly worsening symptoms [10]. The main complaints of the author's 92 cases are listed in Table 1.

In the majority of intestinal anisakiasis cases, the clinical diagnosis shows rapidly developing symptoms such as intestinal colic; or when initially mild cases are observed they gradually develop complications like peritonitis. Symptoms which start to appear at the time of the initial diagnosis are critical (Table 2). The clinical diagnosis is made from an evaluation of subjective, objective, and general symptoms as well as the results of tests.

Clinical Features of Intestinal Anisakiasis

Table 2. Interval between the onset and the first medical examination (107 cases)

Interval between the onset and the first medical examination	Number of cases			
	The worm was identified[a]	Intestinal resection done (included 5 cases of worm found)[b]	Laparotomy done (not resected foci)[b]	X-ray diagnostic cases (including 5 cases of operation performed)[c]
within 2 hours			1	
3			1	
6		1		
12		1	1	
(within 24 hours)		(2)	(3)	
1 day	10	19	15	1
2 days	2	9	6	3
3		2	3	4
4		1	3	1
5	2	1	1	2
8			2	
10		3	1	
15				1
25	1	1		
over 1 month				
15		1	1	
unknown	1	4		3
Total	16	43	33	15

Annotation: from the papers of [a]Ishikura H. et al. (1968): Arch. Jpn. Chir. 36: 663. [b]Ishikura H. et al. (1965): Surg. Treat. 13: 144. [c]Ishikura H. (1965): Jpn. J Clin. Radio. 10: 576.

Subjective Complaints

Abdominal Pain

There are numerous cases of assymptomatic intestinal anisakiasis as is also the case with abdominal anisakiasis. Symptoms, when present, depend on whether *Anisakis* larvae have invaded the intestinal wall and entered the abdominal cavity or remain in the intestinal wall. When the intestinal wall is perforated, it does not become morbid with pain only arising from physical perforation. There are even cases where the pain disappears so quickly that patients do not seek treatment. It is always the subjective symptoms that make patients report for out-patient treatment, and the most common complaint of such out-patients is abdominal pain.

92 H. Ishikura

Anisakis larvae may invade any part of the digestive tract, and the location of abdominal pain varies. In cases diagnosed by the author (Table 1), 91% were in the right hypogastrium, or umbilical region [2]. It is important to note that the location is different from appendicitis, and it does not appear only in one place.

Nausea and Vomiting

Nausea and vomiting are positive symptoms of an acute inflammatory digestive tract disease. Both occur with anisakiasis, with 40–70% of the author's cases and 25 % of the nation-wide survey reporting nausea; 27–70% of the author's cases and 29% of the national sample reporting vomiting. The apparent differences in the incidence of the author's cases and the nation-wide survey arise from the author distinguishing cases with severe symptoms while the nation-wide survey deals with averages, and the cases that have been included are different.

Abdominal Bulging and Induration

Of the 77 cases requiring laparotomy, 61% had abdominal bulging and 26% of the patients felt induration.

Meteorism

The statistics show no records of meteorism, but experience shows it to be common. Symptoms of meteorism are also detected objectively with X-rays. The symptoms are related to evacuation of the bowels.

Evacuation of the Bowels

There are numerous reports of constipation with intestinal anisakiasis. This is because surgery is attempted when the symptoms indicate intestinal colic with strong acute abdominal pain.

Before dealing further with this, it is necessary to consider the condition of patients suffering from anisakiasis. A primary or later infection may be complicated by a secondary bacterial infection through intestinal perforation. Histopathological experiments show that firstly a foreign body reaction occurs and the tissue reaction is localized with no appreciable exudative inflammation. Even when fresh *Anisakis* larvae penetrate into the intestinal wall, the pain assoicated with this intrusion will not cause meteorism but there may be some diarrhea. Even with strong pain from larval penetration into the abdominal cavity, the pain is shortlived with rapid relief and gives rise to meteorism. The stool is generally normal. There is extensive eosinophilic cell infiltration with exudative phlegmon in the intestinal wall and a resulting edematous thickening of the intestinal wall restricts the passage. The resulting ascites and removal of food residue exudate leads to constipation; the food-remain in the thickened parts and the opening of the intestine feels like a sausage. For these reasons, although constipation is not a diagnostic symptom of anisakiasis, it is helpful in providing information on the extent of the disease.

Clinical Features of Intestinal Anisakiasis

Table 1 shows a few cases with blood or mucus in the stool. This arises when the intestinal wall is ulcerated from acute bacterial peritonitis due to perforation of the intestinal wall by the *Anisakis* larvae.

Objective Symptoms

Like other acute intestinal diseases with peritoneal symptoms, there is little information on clinical observation and diagnosis utilizing percussion or palpation.

Coated Tongue

Experience has shown that tongue coating with intestinal anisakiasis is generally white while a dark-brown coating associated with acute peritonitis and the advanced stages of acute appendicitis can be seen. As shown in Table 3, the 77 cases diagnosed by the author is divided into 27.2% without a coated tongue, 39% lightly coated, 11.6% with medium coating, 16.9% heavily coated, and 5.2% undetermined (4 cases).

Abdominal Bulging

Abdominal bulging can be divided into cases where the volume of the intestinal tract increases due to gas accumulation and cases where abdominal volume increases due to accumulation of ascites.

There is generally no gas accumulation in the intestine with the first infection, occurrings during later infections when the thickening of the intestinal wall narrows and blocks the passage and when the larvae have penetrated the wall and bacterial infection has caused peristaltic paralysis due to acute peritonitis. When there is a lot of gas, percussion gives a tympanic resonance, while in the case of ascites the sound is dull. Many cases suffer from both conditions, and to differentiate between these, X-ray and ultrasonic diagnosis may be used. These will be detailed separately. The presence of ascites and its properties is a critical element in the diagnosis and treatment of intestinal anisakiasis with ultrafine laparoscopy or puncture used to determine the presence of eosinophilic cells or bacteria in the ascites. Ascites was found in all the twenty cases where larvae were found in the abdominal wall [3,7] with the volume of ascites about 10 ml ~ 500 ml. In another 77 cases reported by the authors, a considerable volume of lemon yellow ascites was determined within 24 hours of the attack. Within 48

Table 3. Coated tongue of intestinal anisakiasis (in 77 cases)

	Number of cases	%
None	21	27.2
Slight	30	39.0
Middle	9	11.6
Severe	13	16.9
Unknown	4	5.2

94   H. Ishikura

hours, this edema became transparent or plasma-like, within 72 hours the volume was reduced with very little remaining after 5 days.

In the 65 cases from the Kanazawa area reported by Naka et al. [13], 64 displayed accumulations of ascites. In 23 cases this was plasma-like and in the remaining 41 cases serum-like. Naka et al. distinguished semitransparent, tubid and opaque, and a pus-like color as·suppurative peritonitis, (this case may have had a bacterial infection with perforation by the larvae).

Muscular Defense

The muscular defense with intestinal anisakiasis is slight when compared with allergic reactions like acute appendicitis and acute ileus not caused by parasites, or other purulent bacterial infections. Of 123 cases, the majority (65.8%) showed no muscular defense, especially in cases with perforation and bacterial peritonitis (Table 4).

Localization of the Objective Painpoint

Anisakis larvae may enter the intestinal wall anywhere between the duodenum and rectum, and the illness is not localized to any particular place. The subjectively felt pain and the objectively determined painpoint also do not always coincide. The objectively determined painpoint in the 87 cases diagnosed by the author are as follows: epigastric 1, umbilical 31 (35.6%), right lower quadrant 1, McBurney's point 26 (29.9%), upper abdomen 6 (6.9%), and one undetermined. The pain occurs most frequently (54%) in the right lower quadrant (including McBurney's point) and the umbilical region (35.6%). Table 5 shows the relationship between the subjectively felt pain and the objectively determined painpoint. The subjectively and objectively determined painpoint coincide in 13 cases (35.6%) and nearly coincide in 24 cases (27.6%), showing that the symptoms are generally felt in the vicinity of the illness. A further 30% of both the objective and subjective determinations were in the lumbar region. The place of the disease for these 87 cases with laparotomy is as detailed in Table 6. It must be noted that 64.4% are within 50cm of the oral site of the Bauhin's valve.

Table 4. Muscular defense of intestinal anisakiasis (123 cases)

Degree of muscular defense	Method of diagnosis (author's cases)			By the paper of another author
	By larva itself	By histopathologic findings	By intraperitoneal macroscopic findings	
None (−)	12	29	21	19
Slight (+)	4	10	9	4
Middle (++)	2	3	2	1
Severe (+++)	1	0	1	1
Unknown		2		2
Total	19	44	33	27

In all 123 cases: (−) 81 (65.3%), (+) 27 (22.0%), (++) 8 (6.5%), (+++) 3 (2.4%) and unknown 4 (3.3%).

Clinical Features of Intestinal Anisakiasis

Table 5. Relationship between the subjective abdominal pain and the objective pain point of intestinal anisakiasis

Subjective abdominal pain		Objective pain point	
Epigastric	3	umbilical	3
Upper abdomen	2	umbilical	2
Umbilical	26	umbilical	15
		right lower quadrant	3
		McBurney's point	7
		lower abdomen	1
Lower abdomen	20	lower abdomen	6
		right lower quadrant	5
		left lower quadrant	1
		umbilical	5
		McBurney's point	3
Right lower quadrant	31	right lower quadrant	12
		McBurney's point	10
		umbilical	8
		epigastric	1
Left lower quadrant	2	left lower quadrant	1
		right lower quadrant	1
Right hypochondric	1	McBurney's point	1
Unknown	2	right lower quadrant	1
		unknown	1
Total	87		87

Table 6. Location of pathological process of intestinal anisakiasis

Location			No. of cases
Jejunum			7
Ileum	terminal		17
	10cm		2
	20cm	64.4%	10
	30cm		15
	40cm		4
Jejunoileum	50cm		8
(oral distance from the Bauhin's valve)			
Ileocaecum			7
Caecum			5
Sigmoid colon			1
Skip areas			1
Intraperitoneal			10
Total			87

Interviewing the Patient

Intestinal anisakiasis occurs when parasite larvae living in marine organisms are transferred to humans. When humans have not eaten raw fish or squid that act as paratenic hosts for the parasitic larvae, infection will not occur. At the initial examination it is therefore critical to inquire whether fresh seafood has been eaten, and if so what kinds of marine organisms. It is also necessary to know what marine organisms are landed at what times in the general area where the patient resides. Further information includes details of the transport of paratenic hosts from the coast to markets, and a thorough knowledge of changes in the dietary habits of the inhabitants of the area. Recently there has been an increase in the variety of marine organisms that are eaten fresh in Japan. In addition to the seafood eaten nationally, somespecies are only eaten locally. Sculpins, *Osmerus eperlanus mordax* and Alaska pollack (*Theragra chalcogramma*), for example, are only eaten fresh in northern Japan.

Diagnosis with X-ray, ultrasonography, and endoscopy are also of importance in the clinical diagnosis.

Results of Laboratory Examination

There are few clear and unambiguous clinical signs of intestinal anisakiasis. It can be divided into a mild and a fulminant form: The mild form shows eosinophilic granuloma forming tumors in the intestinal walls, and movement in the constricted intestine. It is difficult to differentiate from other tumor-like protuberances. The fulminant form often has symptoms of acute ileus and it is difficult to perform detailed tests. Treatment centers on alleviating the symptoms of intestinal colic with an acute lack of clinical data for deciding to perform surgery.

Though there are few clear symptoms of intestinal anisakiasis, Table 7 lists the results of some biochemical tests utilised in the past 20 cases. There is seroimmunological research and investigations into the relationship of intestinal anisakiasis to allergic reactions, and this will be reported in detail elsewhere.

The following summarizes the test results for symptoms in the author's cases shown in Table 7.

1. Fever. Generally there is no fever. When the temperature exceeds 38 °C it can be assumed that the larvae have perforated the wall with resulting bacterial peritonitis.

2. Increases in leucocyte count. The typical increase associated with other bacterial infections is not shown, however there is a surprising increase without a rise in the body temperature.

3. High eosinophilic cell count. The count is not high in the initial stage of the illness. There is a peak two weeks after the onset of the illness and then after the third week there is a gradual decrease. However, a case with 42% at the first examination has been recorded. The eosinophilic cells are either active in the intestinal wall tissue or the cell number in the blood does not increase in the first week after the onset.

4. Change in erythrocyte count. Nearly normal in the first week, followed by a slight decrease; in the mild form it then returns to the normal level.

Table 7. Result of clinical laboratory examination on intestinal anisakiasis

Case No.	Age and Sex of patient	Tempera- ture	Leucocyte	Eosino- phil	Hb (sahli)	Ht	Erytho. Sed. (1 hour)	GOT	GPT	Author
1.	28 ♂	37.7°C	11,000	0 %	13.0g/d		10mm			Furukawa A. (1974) [14]
2.	60 ♂	36.6	8,800	2	13.8	12.0%	55	44	8	Sasaki Kaoru et al. (1985) [15]
3.	37 ♀	36.0	13,100							Hayasaka H. et al. (1970) [4]
4.	32 ♀		6,100	1	(63%)					Inoue K. et al. (1974) [16]
5.	43 ♂		8,600	0	(73%)					Inoue K. et al. (1974) [16]
6.	58 ♂		8,200		17.6	54.3		normal		Maruyama A. et al. (1982) [17]
7.	73 ♂		9,400	4	11.1	33.6	56			Maruyama A. et al. (1982) [17]
8.	37 ♂		12,900	0		50.0		30		Fukada S. et al. (1984) [18]
9.	73 ♀		15,800			52.3		24		Fukada S. et al. (1984) [18]
10.	33 ♂		14,000	0			54	20		Fukada S. et al. (1984) [18]
11.	24 ♂		8,050	3	(78%)					Yoshimura H. et al. (1966) [19]
12.	36 ♂	38.7	14,000		12.2			normal		Yoshimura H. et al. (1979) [20]
13.	32 ♀	36.7	18,100		14.9	44.0				Sasaki M. et al. (1978) [21]
14.	28 ♂		6,300	6	12.1	38.0		17	15	Ishikura H. (1968) [6]
15.	52 ♀	normal	6,900	4	16.2					Sasaki H. et al. (1982) [22]
16.	39 ♂	36.8	10,200		14.2			normal		Hiraoka T. et al. (1980) [23]
17.	60 ♂	36.7	8,700	2	(104%)	52.0		15	11	Furukawa M. et al. (1972) [24]
18.	54 ♂	37.2	11,700	2	16.6	50.0		18	11	Fukushima H. et al. (1978) [25]
19.	61 ♂	36.2	8,600	4	14.2		33	21	15	Shirakabe K. et al. (1984) [26]
20.	38 ♂		7,800		(103%)	48.4				Iwata M. et al. (1969) [27]

98   H. Ishikura

5. Pigmentation index. The arithmetic average is 82.2%. Within four days 95.2%, and within 10 days decreasing to 64.7%.

6. Erythrocyte sedimentation rate. Medium acceleration in the first week.

7. Prothrombin rise. There is one case which showed 32 sec. within the first 24 hours, ordinarily the value is normal early in the attack with a slightly increasing tendency later.

8. Hypoproteinemia. Most cases underwent emergency surgery and so few underwent this test. The 30 cases where the test was performed showed normal values.

9. Latent vitamin B deficiency. With progression of the intestinal anisakiasis, there is constriction of the intestine and an accumulation of ascites leading to vomiting and anorexia which causes dehydration and vitamin B deficiency with symptoms of cheilitis, glossitis and xerosis cutis. This affects the ileum and so vitamin B12 absorption is possibly upset, although there are no reports of tests to verify this.

10. Liver damage. Chronic cases are extremely rare, and while there are reports of cases with hepatic demage, the chronic cases in Table 7 show that both GOT and GPT are practically normal.

11. Ascites. The accumulation of ascites is a critical symptom as reported in detail already. Despite its complexity, puncturing is important to determine the existence of ascites and its composition. More than 30% of the cells in the ascites have increased eosinophilic cell content. This occurs not only in ascites, but also in exudative pleurisy where the hydrothorax show dramatic increases in eosinophilic cells [29].

There is a strong need for bacterial cultivation, and when bacteria are determined, to diagnose perforation of the intestinal wall by anisakiasis larvae, and to initiate chemotherapy.

Conclusion

The mild form of intestinal anisakiasis does not display the characteristic clinical symptoms of intestinal anisakiasis, with tumors in the intestinal wall forming localized swelling and constriction of the cavity making diagnosis very difficult. To reach a diagnosis the presence of larvel bodies forming nuclei of tumors (antigen) need to be observed. Surgery to obtain such proof and to avoid a misdiagnosis is not a mistaken approach.

The fulminant form rapidly develops symptoms of intestinal colic making it necessary to decide to perform surgery within a short time. Such cases arise within two or three days after the appearance of symptoms and patients nearly always remember what fresh marine organisms, or paratenic larval hosts they have eaten. This explains the extreme importance of interviewing patients. Even with the lack of unique clinical symptoms, by employing X-ray, ultrasonic tests, working to relieve the acute ileus by the Miller-Abbott tube, or in performing an immunodiagnosis, there is an increasing number of possibilities for avoiding unnecessary surgery. By stressing observation of the progression of the illness, it becomes possible to raise the ratio of correct diagnoses of intestinal anisakiasis.

References

1. Ishikura H, Hayasaka H, Kikuchi Y (1967) Acute regional ileitis at Iwanai in Hokkaido,–with special reference to intestinal anisakiasis. Sapporo Med J 4: 183–196
2. Ishikura H, Kikuchi Y (1967) Larva migrans due to the *Anisakis simplex* Larva. J Jpn Med Assoc 57: 1649–1655 (in Japanese)
3. Ishikura H, Kikuchi Y, Hayasaka H (1967) Pathological and clinical observation on intestinal anisakiasis. Arch Jpn Chir 36: 663–679 (in Japanese)
4. Hayasaka H, Ishikura H, Mizugaki H, Asaishi K, Iakagi R, Iwano H (1969) A case of anisakiasis caused by two *Anisakis* Larvae penetration. Hokkaido J Surg 14: 141–146 (in Japanese)
5. Hayasaka H, Ishikura H, Miyagi H, Ueno T, Utsumi A, Sato Y (1967) On clinical studies in early stadium of intestinal anisakiasis. Hokkaido J Surg 12: 155–161 (in Japanese)
6. Ishikura H (1968) Clinical and immunopathological studies on anisakiasis. Hokkaido J Med Sci 43: 83–99 (in Japanese)
7. Ishikura H (1969) Occurrence of anisakiasis and its presentation. Saishin Igaku 24: 357–365 (in Japanese)
8. Ishikura H, Kikuchi K, Ishikura H (1983) Enteritis acuta caused by *Anisakis* larvae. Stomach and Intestine 18: 393–397 (in Japanese)
9. Hara K, Yokoyama T (1985) A clinical study on possible anisakiasis intestinalis causing acute intestinal obstruction. J Jpn Soc Clin Surg 46: 416–421 (in Japanese)
10. Ishikura H (1965): Radiologic festures of intestinal anisakiasis. Jpn J Clin Radiol 10: 576–588 (in Japanese)
11. Matsui T, Iida M, Murakami M, Kimura Y, Fujishima M, Yao T, Tsuji M (1985) Intestinal anisakiasis: Clinical and radiologic features. Radiology 157: 299–302
12. Matsui T, Iida M, Fujishima M, Naritomi O, Sugiyama K, Yao T, Murakami M, Sakai T, Kimura Y, Tsuji M (1985) Radiological study of the intestinal anisakiasis. Jpn J Clin Radiol 30: 741–747 (in Japanese)
13. Naka T, Aikawa K, Shinno I, Kuranishi H (1969) Experience with acute nonspecific regional enteristis. Clin Surg 24: 129–133 (in Japanese)
14. Furukawa A (1974) Anisakiasis: Its history and a case of acute ileitis, attributable to a living larva of *Anisakis* in the peritoneal cavity. J Jpn Soc Clin Surg 35: 63–69 (in Japanese)
15. Sasaki K, Sasaki N, Nagamine Y (1984) A case of intestinal anisakiasis with skip legion and mesenteric granuloma formation. J Jpn Soc Clin Surg 45: 1183–1187 (in Japanese)
16. Inoue Z, Shimizu N, Yoshida Y, Fujii T, Adachi H (1974) Clinical studies on 6 cases of intestinal anisakiasis: particularly 2 cases of intestinal anisakiasis with skip lesion. Clin Surg 29: 808–814 (in Japanese)
17. Maruyama A, Inaba K, Osanai H, Suzuki S, Fujita T (1981) Two cases of intestinal anisakiasis: Skip lesion and perforation. Geka Shinryo 23: 517–519 (in Japanese)
18. Fukada S, Hachisuga K, Yamaguchi A, et al. (1984) Three cases of anisakiasis causing acute intestinal abstruction. Clin Surg 39: 707–711 (in Japanese)
19. Yoshimura H, Kaneta J, Suzuki T, et al. (1966) A case of acute abdomen by the penetrated *Anisakis*-like larva through the intestinal wall. Surg Treat 15: 626–630 (in Japanese)
20. Yoshimura H, Kondo K, Akao N, Ohnishi Y, Watanabe K, Shinno B, Aikawa K (1979) Two cases of eosinophilic granulomas formed in the large omentum and mesentery by the penetrated *Anisakis* larva through the gastrointestinal tract. Stomach and intestine 14: 519–522 (in Japanese)
21. Sasaki M, Aoki Y, Syoji M, Matsumoto K, Okamoto S, Katsumi M (1978) A case of intestinal perforation due to the *Anisakis* larvae. J Jpn Soc Clin Surg 39: 61–65 (in Japanese)

22. Sasaki H, Watanabe H, Suzuki Y, Koyama T (1982) A case of *Anisakis* infection in the second portion of the duodenum in which a worm was isolated 17 days after onset of symptoms. Gastroenterol Endosc 24: 667–671 (in Japanese)
23. Hiraoka T, Ishihara A. Nosaka K, Katoh Y, Iwamoto T, Hiraaki K (1980) A case of anisakiasis causing acute ileus. J Hiroshima Med Sci 33: 1319–1323 (in Japanese)
24. Furukawa M, Kawawaki S, Furumoto I, Misawa K (1973) A case of intestinal anisakiasis. Surg Treat 14: 1647–1650 (in Japanese)
25. Fukushima H, Yuge S, Yamakawa R, Adachi T, Kudoh T (1975) A case of intestinal anisakiasis attributable to a living worm. J Jpn Soc Clin Surg. 36: 721–725 (in Japanese)
26. Shirakabe K, Sato M, Kamachi H, Kodama Y, Inuzuka S (1984) A case report of colonic anisakiasis diagnosed preoperatively as cancer of the transverse colon. Med Bull Fukuoka Univ 11: 309–311 (in Japanese)
27. Iwata K, Nishimura T, Takemura T, Urano E, Oda T (1968) Clinicopathological studies on anisakiasis in Wakayama prefecture. Wakayama Med Rep 19: 59–67 (in Japanese)
28. Ishikura H, Tanaka M, Goto T, Aizawa M, Kanemoto T, Hagihara I, Kikuchi K, Tsuji Y, Takahashi T (1965) Studies on regional ileitis (No.2): Clinical observation of 87 cases which occurred at Iwanai district in Hokkaido. Surg Treat 13: 144–154 (in Japanese)
29. Kobatashi A, Tsuji M, Dwight LW (1985) Provable pulmonary anisakiasis accompanying pleural effusion. Am J Med Hyg 34: 310–313

Radiographic Features of Intestinal Anisakiasis

T. Matsui, M. Iida, M. Fujishima, and T. Yao

Introduction

Intestinal anisakiasis was formerly considered to be a rare occurrence in Japan [1,2], with only a few case reports diagnosed by a preoperative radiological study [3–6]. We obtained clinical, radiologic and immunologic evidence of anisakiasis [5] and suggested that the specific radiological picture was edema and/or stenosis of the bowel. The degree of edema or stenosis differed due to the wide spectrum of clinical presentation. However, we concluded that radiological evaluation might be helpful in establishing the diagnosis.

Materials and Methods

From 1983 to 1987, we treated 30 patients with acute intestinal anisakiasis— 7 women and 23 men, aged 24–62 years; average age, 44.5 years—Table 1). Mackerel had been eaten by all except for two who had eaten squid. Abdominal pain was a major symptom and developed 5–48 hours after the patients had eaten raw mackerel. Pain was present in the epigastrium as well as in the lower portion of the abdomen.

All 30 had undergone combined upper gastrointestinal (GI) and follow-through small-bowel studies, while barium enema examination was done in 4

Table 1. Clinical features of intestinal anisakiasis

	No. of cases
Age (year)	43
Sex (M:F)	23:7
Ingested fish	
mackerel	28
squid	2
Incubation period	19 (h)
Ileus	13/30
Leucocytosis ($>8000mm^3$)	25/30
Eosinophilia	0/21
Positive CRP	18/21
Accelerated ESR ($>15mm/h$)	6/20

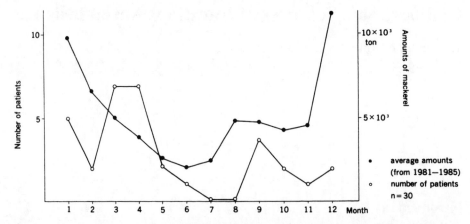

Fig. 1. Total occurrence of anisakiasis in each month from 1984 to 1987 and average amount of mackerel handled per month at the Fukuoka fish wholesale trade market

patients. Radiological examinations were performed when bowel sounds were audible, despite small amounts of fluid levels found on the plain radiographs. In all patients the upper GI series disclosed no abnormalities in the stomach or duodenum.

Anisakis infections are characterized by a good response of immunoglobulins, and though the ascarids have a marked degree of antigenic cross-reactivity, a sensitive and reliable immunodiagnostic test for anisakiasis is now available. Tsuji [7] used immunoelectrophoresis to study homologous and heterologous antibody-antigen reactions from various helminths and stated that specific bands were obtained for larval *Anisakis*, and that larval and adult antigens of *Anisakis* are different. Using this method, specific antibody to *Anisakis* larvae were detected in blood samples obtained 1 to 70 days after the onset in all 30 cases.

Causative Fish and Seasonal Occurrence

In our series, mackerel was the most frequent culprit (Table 1). The occurrence of acute intestinal anisakiasis in each month was investigated for four years with the disease occurring most frequently in March and April (Fig. 1). The amounts of mackerel handled at the Fukuoka wholesale trade market in each month were also obtained, since these figures are representative of the amounts of mackerel consumed by Fukuoka city residents. There is a good correlation between the seasonal occurrence of the disease and seasonal consumption of the related fish, with this seasonal occurrence corresponding to that found in Kyushu island, confirmed by Iino's large series [8].

Radiologic Features

Characteristic radiographic features are marked edematous changes of the bowel wall, thickening and blunting of the Kerckring fold, and irregular narrow-

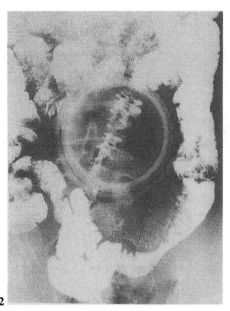 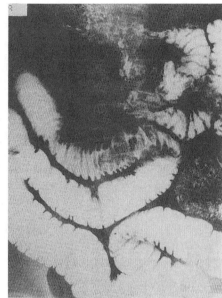

Fig.2. Follow-through small-bowel study reveals a coarse thickening of the ileum with mucosal edema (without preceding ileus)

Fig.3. Jejunal involvement with thickened mucosa and proximal dilatation (with preceding ileus).

ing of the bowel lumen [4–6]. In 1965 Ishikura [3] demonstrated radiographic findings of an acute regional enteritis, namely intestinal anisakiasis, but the radiography presented was not consistent with that in our series.

The most common site of involvement was the ileum, 20/30, (Fig. 2), followed by the jejunum, 6/30, (Fig. 3) and the colon, 4/30, (Fig. 4) (Table 2).

The small-bowel studies showed irregular narrowing with thickening of the bowel wall and blunting of the folds, the "picket-fence appearance", (Fig. 5). The length of the narrowed bowel ranged from 15 to 90 cm, with diseased segments as long as 40 cm common (Table 2), and even longer lesions were present in 9 patients (Fig. 6).

Table 2. Radiological findings of intestinal anisakiasis

	No. of cases
Site of involvement	
jejunum	6
ileum	20
colon	4
Length of involvement (cm)	40
Out-line of worm	5

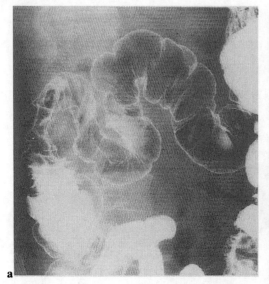
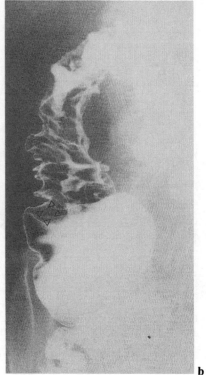

Fig.4. A double-contrast barium enema examination discloses an extremely swollen colonic segment in the hepatic flexure with a reduced lumen (**a**) and a thread-like filling defect (**b** arrow) (without preceding ileus)

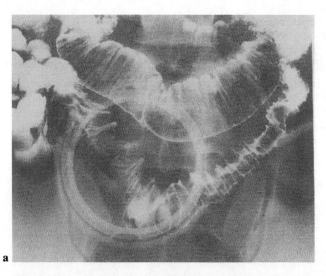

Fig. 5. Compression radiograph shows irregular mucosal thickening of the terminal ileum ("picket-fence appearance") of a severe degree (**a** with preceding ileus) and mild degree as long as 15 cm (**b** without preceding ileus)

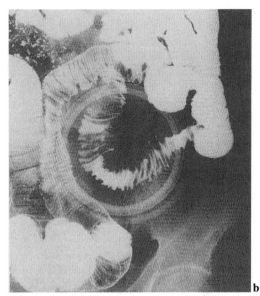

Fig. 5

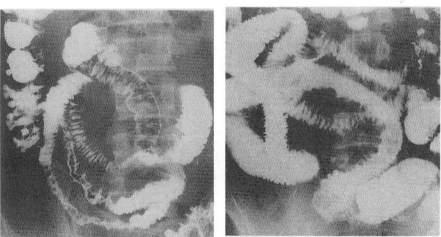

Fig. 6. A 90 cm involvement of the ileal segment (with preceding ileus)

Fig. 7. Compression radiograph reveals a narrowed segment and dilated proximal bowel (without preceding ileus)

Various degrees of dilatation of the bowel proximal to the narrowed lesion were frequently seen (Fig. 7). When ileus developed, the dilatation was more severe (Figure 8). Ulceration was not evident, although the folds were edematous. A thread-like filling defect (Figs. 4 and 9) in the bowel, suggesting a worm itself, was visualized in 5 patients. The outline of the worm was 1mm in diameter and 15 to 30 mm in length, and was visualized at the center of the diseased segment

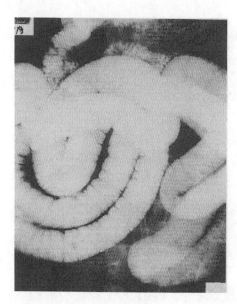

Fig. 8. Barium study discloses dilated jejunal loops filled with bowel fluid and undigested food (with preceding ileus). From [5] with permission

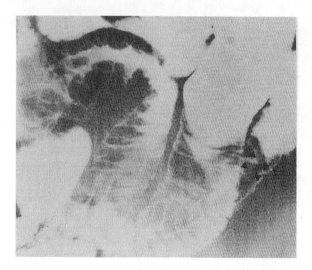

Fig. 9. Follow-through small-bowel radiograph shows mucosal edema and a thread-like filling defect (air contrast radiograph without intention)

where edema was most severe, in the same way as the worm out-line in the stomach (9). Compression or air contrast radiograph done without intention of a double-contrast study was useful to delineate the worm out-line. There are only two reports which showed the worm outline in the intestine radiologically [5,6].

Differential Diagnosis

Differential diagnosis of intestinal anisakiasis includes acute appendicitis, neoplasia, intussusception, diverticulitis, ileus, food poisoning, and Crohn's disease. Eating raw fish before the onset is an important factor in its diagnosis. Abdominal pain is not sharply demarcated as in acute appendicitis, and laboratory findings suggest only nonspecific acute inflammatory changes. Therefore, the radiologic evaluation, as well as the immunologic examination is important for the diagnosis of intestinal anisakiasis.

The pathognomonic evidence is to delineate the larva itself in the diseased bowel segment [4,5] as in gastric anisakiasis [9]. However it is difficult to identify *Anisakis* larvae without bowel surgery, but we found evidence of the worm itself in the bowel, in 17 % of the radiographs. If the worm is invisible, radiographic features of anisakiasis resemble those of regionalenteritis, ischemic ileitis, or intestinal submucosal hemorrhage. When there is a history of raw mackerel intake and the clinical symptoms, the radiologic diagnosis is not difficult.

Treatment and Clinical Course

Symptoms and signs ameliorate spontaneously without any accompanying complication during 1-2 weeks after the onset. There were no abnormalities of the bowel evident on repeated radiologic examinations performed in 17 of our 30 cases 1-2 weeks (average, 11 days) after the onset and none of the cases required surgical intervention.

Conclusion

In conclusion, we obtained clinical and radiologic evidence of anisakiasis and suggested that the specific radiologic picture was edema and/or stenosis of the bowel. When there is a history of raw mackerel intake with the typical clinical symptoms, the radiologic diagnosis is not difficult, and might be essential in establishing the diagnosis.

References

1. Oshima T (1972) *Anisakis* and anisakiasis in Japan and adjacent area. Morishita K, Komiya Y, Matsubashi H (eds) Prog Med Parasitol in Japan. Meguro Parasitol Museum 4: 301–393
2. Van Thiel P H (1980) The present state of anisakiasis and its causative worms. Trop Geographic Med 28: 75–85
3. Ishikura H (1965) Radiography of the acute regional enteritis. Clin Radiol 10: 576–588 (in Japanese)
4. Richman R, Lewicki A (1973) Right ileocolitis secondary to anisakiasis. A J R 119: 329–331
5. Matsui T, Iida M, Murakami M, Kimura Y, Fujishima M, Yao T, Tsuji M (1985) Intestinal anisakiasis: clinical and radiological features. Radiology 157: 299–302

6. Higashi M, Tanaka K, Kitada T, Nakatake K, Tsuji M (1988) Anisakiasis confirmed by radiography of the large intestine. Gastrointest Radiol 13: 85–86
7. Tsuji M (1975) Comparative studies on the antigenic structure of several helminths by immunoelectrophoresis. Jpn J Parasitol 24: 227–236 (in Japanese)
8. Iino H (1984) Anisakiasis in Kyushu. Proceedings of 27th Annual Meeting of the Japanese Association of Gastro-intestinal Endoscopy: 230 (in Japanese)
9. Nakata H, Takeda K, Nakatake K (1980) Radiological diagnosis of acute gastric anisakiasis. Radiology 135: 49–53

Diagnosis of Intestinal Anisakiasis by Ultrasonography

T. YAMAMOTO and K. MINAMI

Introduction

The diagnosis of gastro-intestinal disease by ultrasonography has been considered to be difficult because of the presence of digestive tract gas and has therefore been used only in selective cases. However, with improvements in equipment and techniques, it can also be used in the diagnosis of gastro-intestinal disease. In recent years there have been increasing reports of aniaskiasis, but most of these are of the gastric type with few reports on intestinal anisakiasis. In this article ultrasonography of intestinal anisakiasis is described.

Subjects and Methods

Seventeen cases with intestinal anisakiasis diagnosed from March 1986 to December 1987 are described. They were divided into 2 groups: 7 cases were affected in the jejunum, 10 in the ileum while there were no cases found in the large intestine. All subjects had eaten raw fish and then chiefly complained of peri-umbilical pain. Intestinal anisakiasis was suspected because of ileus shadows or small intestinal gas showen by simple abdominal X-rays. Stenosis by edematous swelling of the small intestine (particular to this disease) was discovered by radiography using contrast material. In these cases ultrasonography was performed prior to radiography of the small intestine.

Ultrasonographical Characteristics of the Normal Intestine

Small Intestine

The small intestine normally shows almost no gas or intestinal juice and in most cases cannot be detected with ultrasonography. Therefore, in the presence of Kerckring's folds (characteristic to the small intestine) or the detection of intestinal juice stasis, an obstructive intestinal disease should be considered. However, if recently developed equipment is used, the small intestine can normally be detected as a thin linear high echoic image. Identification of the terminal ileum in which a high incidence of disease occurs is especially important.

Large Intestine

The ultrasonic image of the large intestine under normal circumstances consists of a sonolucent echo zone showing the intestinal wall and intestinal contents [1]. Kuramoto et.al found that in the excised intact large intestine, a 5 layered structure was arranged in the following order: high, low, high, low, high echo zone [2], while Sudo et al. has shown that the normal width of large intestinal wall is less than 4mm, compared to 5mm or more when thickened [3]. The transverse and sigmoid colon do not run straight and therefore are difficult to detect, but the ascending and descending colons are easily revealed by the detection of the characteristic haustra. Even in an empty stomach, there are often feces remaining in the large intestine and frequently the feces show echo images similar to those of tumors. Furthermore, the presence of large intestinal gas make detection of the intestinal wall difficult. Therefore an extensive examination should be performed after cleansing of the intestinal tracts using a warm water enema.

Ultrasonographic Characteristics of Intestinal Anisakiasis

The ultrasonographic characteristics of diseased intestine are classified into 4 different findings: dilatation of the intestine, thickening of the intestinal wall, image of masses and peripheral ascites [4]. In our 17 cases, the above-described findings were noted in 16 patients: 12 showed dilatation of the intestine, 11 showed thickening of the intestinal wall, 12 showed peripheral ascites (Table 1). There were no cases showing an image of a large mass. The most important finding is the thickness of the intestinal wall, though other obstructive intestinal diseases cannot be ruled out only by the findings of dilatation or ascites. The intestinal wall thickness is noted as a uniform low echogram, similar to that seen in the stomach, however a layered structure can be detected even in the thickened part of the intestine, and this thickened layer equals the submucosa. This finding is in agreement with edematous swollen lesions found by contrast radiography. We have no experience with large intestinal cases, but Yabunaka et.al have reported ultrasonic examination of 2 cases of large intestinal anisakiasis and described the same wall thickness features as seen in our cases [5]. Therefore it is possible that the ultrasonographic characteristics of anisakiasis in the small intestine may be similar to those in the large intestine.

Case Reports

Case 1: 25 Year old male (jejunal case)
Chief complaint: Upper-umbilical pain

Table 1. Ultrasonic findings of intestinal anisakiasis

Positive findings	16/ 17 cases	(94%)
Dilatation	12/ 17 cases	(71%)
Wall thickness	11/ 17 cases	(65%)
Mass image	0/ 17 cases	(0%)
Ascites	12/ 17 cases	(71%)

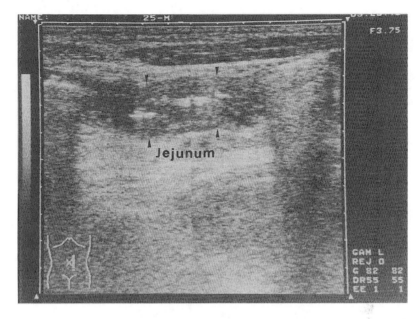

Fig. 1. Ultrasonography of a case affecting the jejunum. The arrow points out the thickness of the jejunal wall and dilatation to the oral side

On the night of February 21, 1987, the subject ate some pickled mackerel. Eight hours later, he experienced severe upper-umbilical pain necessitating a hospital visit.

Abdominal X-ray findings: Marked small intestinal gas and air-fluid levels were observed.

Abdominal ultrasonic findings: Severe wall thickness of about 10cm in length was revealed in the left umbilical area in which the jejunum was found (Fig. 1). The thickness reached a maximum of 10mm, and dilatation in the oral side of the lesion and a small amount of ascites in the lower left abdominal area were seen. From the above findings, small intestinal anisakiasis was suspected and radiography of the small intestine with contrast material was performed.

Small intestinal X-ray findings with contrast material: A severe localized stenosis of about 10cm in length was seen in the upper jejunum. The affected area showed an edematous swelling and a generalized uniform thickening, a serrated shape, and no erosions or ulcers (Fig.2).

Clinical course: After in-patient therapy the ileus was so improved by the next day, that the patient was released.

Case 2: 52 Year old female (ileal case)
Chief complaint: Peri-umbilical pain
At dinner on March 16, 1987, the subject ate raw horse mackerel. Twelve hours later, she visited hospital with peri-umbilical pain.

Abdominal X-ray findings: The ileus was much the same as in case 1.

Abdominal ultrasonic finding: The small intestine was greatly dilatated over an extensive area. The wall was thickened in a part of the right lower abdominal

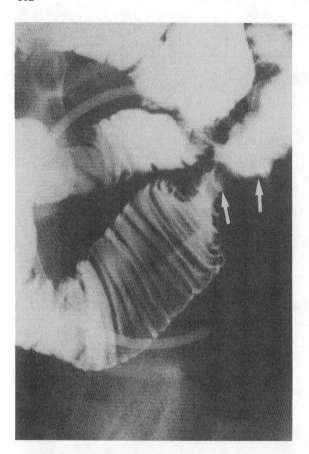

Fig. 2. Small intestinal X-ray of the case affecting the jejunum. The arrow points out an edematous stenosis of 10cm in length of the upper jejunum

Fig. 3. Ultrasonography of a case affecting the ileum. The arrow points out the thickness of the ileal wall and peripheral ascites can be seen

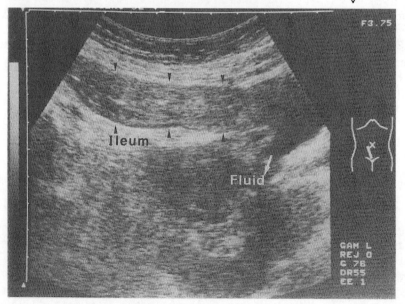

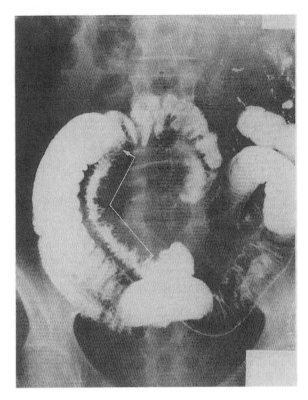

Fig. 4. Small intestinal X-ray of the case affecting the ileum. The arrow points to an edematous stenosis of about 20cm in length at the end of the ileum and to the oral side, dilatation with some remains of food can be seen

ileum, and a moderate amount of ascites were seen in the Douglous pouch (Fig. 3). Because of the above, small intestinal anisakiasis was suspected and radiography with contrast material was performed.

Small intestinal X-ray findings with contrast material: In the distal portion of the ileum, there was a severe localized edematous swelling of about 20cm in length like that in case 1, and at the oral side of the lesion, intestinal dilatation with foods and fluids remained markedly increased (Fig. 4).

Clinical course: After in-patient therapy, the symptoms improved rapidly, with the patient released the next day.

Differential Diagnosis with Other Intestinal Diseases Using Ultrasonography

Intestinal Obstruction

If dilatated intestinal tracts are detected in which stasis and to-and-fro movements of intestinal contents are seen, the diagnosis of intestinal obstruction is easily obtained, and in most cases, ascites are also present [6]. There are some

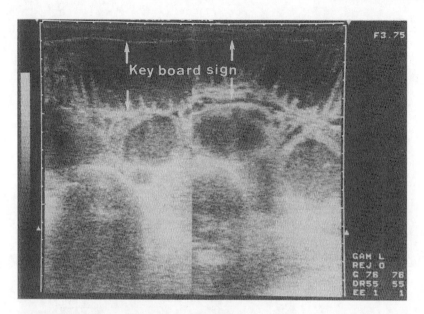

Fig. 5. Ultrasonography of a case affecting the adhesive ileus. The marked dilatation of small intestine so called "Key-board sign' and ascites pooling between the dilatated intestines are noted

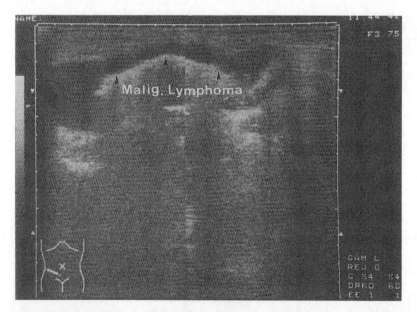

Fig. 6. Ultrasonography of malignant lymphoma of the small intestine. When compared to the wall thickness of intestinal anisakiasis, this case obviously shows a low echoradiography

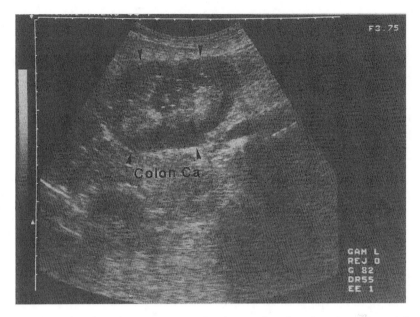

Fig. 7. Ultrasonography of a colon cancer. As a first impression there is a circumferential low echo with central high echo that can be confused with the kidney (Pseudo-Kidney sign). This sign is not seen in intestinal anisakiasis

cases of intestinal obstruction due to intestinal anisakiasis, but usually symptoms are mild and disappear within several days. With mild intestinal dilatation and detection of the wall thickness and if there is a history of raw fish intake, intestinal anisakiasis should be considered and the clinical course should be observed conservatively. Figure 5 shows the ultrasonic findings of an adhesive ileus case.

Intestinal Malignant Lymphoma

The ultrasonic findings of intestinal malignant lymphoma is marked wall thickness with a uniform low echo of the margin and central high echo (Pseudo-Kidney sign) [7]. This sign is actually an image of a mass which can be seen even in a localized disease such as large intestinal cancer, and so the presence of this sign can be used to easily differentiate intestinal anisakiasis from this disease. However malignant lymphoma often shows a uniform low echogram and does not show this sign until its in the advanced stage. In this respect, malignant lymphoma must be differentiated from intestinal anisakiasis, but differential diagnosis is not difficult as local lymph node swelling is sometimes seen in malignant lymphoma and the wall thickness is obviously low echoic compared to that of intestinal anisakiasis. In Fig. 6 and Fig. 7, ultrasonic findings of malignant lymphoma of small intestine and colon cancer are shown.

Terminal Ileitis

The ileocecum is highly affected by this disease. Yuasa et.al have reported on cases with terminal ileitis who had acute digestive tract symptoms and showed

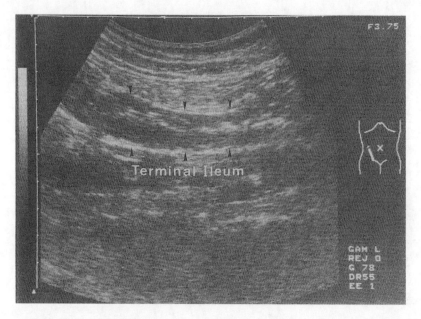

Fig. 8. Ultrasonography of terminal ileitis. In addition to this wall thickness, the local lymph node swelling can be seen in this case (not shown in the figure). But with these findings alone, it is almost impossible to differentiate from intestinal anisakiasis

edematous thickening of the terminal ileum by ultrasonography. According to that study, the most common cause is bacterial enteritis, but there are many cases of negative feces culture, so that the viral or allergic mechanisms such as anisakiasis etc. must be considered. Ultrasonographically edematous thickening of the terminal ileum, surrounding lymph node swelling, enlargement of Peyer's patches and mesenterial thickening etc. have all been observed [8]. Figure 8 shows the wall thickness of terminal ileitis. In this case, since the feces culture was negative and there was no history of raw fish intake, the cause is unknown, and it was almost impossible to associate this ultrasonic finding only with intestinal anisakiasis.

Appendicitis

In ultrasonography of appendicitis, it is most important to detect the enlarged appendix. An appendix enlarged by inflammation can be detected with a uniform low echoic image, but it should be mentioned that we occasionally find it difficult to differentiate the enlarged appendix with the thickened wall of the terminal ileitis.

Other Intestinal Diseases

Other than those mentioned above, there are many intestinal diseases which show wall thickness ultrasonographically, making differential diagnosis at times difficult. However, the ultrasonic image should differ according to the layer of the intestinal wall which is mainly affected. For example, ulcerative colitis, drug-induced colitis, radioactive enteritis, etc. have their main lesions in the mucosa or submucosa. The original layered structure can be seen preserved under careful examinations, and if irregularity of the mucosal layer is marked, it can be detected as an irregularity of the central high echoic band. On the other hand, Crohn's disease, intestinal tuberuculosis, Behçet syndrome affecting G-I tract and advanced cancer etc. affect all levels, destroying the intestinal layered structure and the inner echo of the thickened wall is rough, with irregularity of the mucosal layer. Since the main lesion of intestinal anisakiasis is the thickened submucosa with a minimal mucosal change, its characteristics show a uniform wall thickness with an intact layered structure.

Conclusion

Until now intestinal anisakiasis appeared to be a relatively rare disease, difficult to discover, but it has now become possible to identify easily by the use of ultrasonography which is extremely useful. The image shows a uniform wall thickness with an intact layered structure. If eating habits and past medical history are carefully considered, a differential diagnosis from other intestinal diseases should be relatively easy.

References

1. Kawamoto C, Watanabe H, Yamanaka T, Kimura K (1985) Ultrasonographic diagnosis of colonic diseases. Clinical trial of 7.5MHz probe (abstract in English). Proceedings of the 46th Meeting of the Japan Society of Ultrasonics in Japan: 893
2. Kuramoto H, Otani Y, Yamao T, Oka S, Kinjo M, Omiya H, Takahashi T, Hiki Y, Fujiu T (1986) A clinical study of ultrasonographic examination on the colo-rectal cancer (1st report) (abstract in English). Proceedings of the 49th Meeting of the Japan Society of Ultrasonics in Japan: 657
3. Suto T, Kunikane M, Moriyama Y, Tushima K, Kondoh H, Yoshida Y (1985) Ultrasonic findings using water enema for colonic diseases with thickening of the colonic wall (abstract in English). Proceedings of the 47th Meeting of the Japan Society of Ultrasonics in Japan: 707
4. Yuasa H. Hirooka T, Itákura K, Yamamoto H, Okamura Y, Fukui H, Ide M, Kurohara S (1983) Ultrasonic examination of Intestine.—about Ileum lesion—(abstract in English). Proceedings of the 43th Meeting of the Japan Society of Ultrasonics in Japan: 725
5. Yabunaka K, Yuasa H, Hirooka T, Ohchi H, Uetaka F, Kishimoto A, Ide M, Saito M, Kiyohara S (1987) Two cases of anisakiasis of the large intestine by the sonographic examination (abstract in English). Proceedings of the 51th Meeting of the Japan Society of Ultrasonics in Japan: 471
6. Ogata M, Hashimoto T, Kuroki T, Tomita S (1987) Ultrasonographic diagnosis of strangulation ileus (abstract in English). Proceedings of the 50th Meeting of the Japan Society of Ultrasonics in Japan: 125
7. Ohashi I, Suzuki T, Yasumoto M, Shibuya H, Horiuchi J, Suzuki S, Yoshimatsu S (1986) Sonographic finding of small intestinal involvement of malignant lymphoma (abstract in English). Proceedings of the 49th Meeting of the Japan Society of Ultrasonics in Japan: 659
8. Yuasa H, Hirooka T, Itakura K, Yamamoto H, Ohchi H, Nishihara H, Yoza S, Ide M, Kurohara S (1986) Terminal Ileitis (abstract in English). Proceedings of the 48th Meeting of the Japan Society of Ultrasonics in Japan: 525

Differential Diagnosis of Intestinal Anisakiasis

H. Ishikura

Introduction

Anisakiasis an infectious disease, requires anisakid larvae, the infecting agent, to be determined in the patient for an accurate diagnosis. Unlike gastric, oral and esophageal anisakiasis, a positive determination of larvae is very difficult for intestinal and abdominal anisakiasis.

Some of the difficulty is shown Table 1. Larvae were not established in any of the cases with the mild form where the clinical diagnosis before surgery was intestinal anisakiasis, or in the national total where the post surgery or histological diagnosis was also intestinal anisakiasis [11–13]. In the fulminant form only four cases were clearly intestinal anisakiasis, 30 cases very likely so, and in 56 cases there was some suspicion; the 56 cases that were mistakenly diagnosed as acute appendicitis are the most numerous. These cases were all diagnosed before 1974 but even with improved examination methods larvae are not often found. This is even true of cases where there is a strong suspicion of intestinal anisakiasis, or in those suspicious cases that, however, are treated with conservative therapy.

Parasitic ailments are often determined after discovery of eggs, which the vast majority produce; however with larva migrans the eggs are not discharged from the human body, adding to the difficulty of establishing a diagnosis. However, treatment is only possible when an ailment is clinically diagnosed, therefore for intestinal anisakiasis a number of approaches are possible when attempting to establish a diagnosis.

Approaches to Diagnosing Intestinal Anisakiasis

Introduction of the source of infection to the body. Anisakid larvae are always introduced to the human body by the intake of an uncooked (raw) paratenic host, showing the need to know what marine organisms act as such hosts. It is important therefore to know what marine organisms in the seas around Japan act as hosts and the time of the year these organisms are caught; also to know what seafood is usually eaten and how they are transported from the port of landing. It is of utmost importance to learn from the patients what marine organisms were ingested prior to the appearance of symptoms. This would amount to an epidemiological approach.

Table 1. Clinical preoperative diagnose of intestinal anisakiasis

	No. of cases by nation-wide examination (1) in 1968.[a] (Ishikura)	Nation-wide examination (2) in 1974.[b] (Iwano et al.)	Author's cases in 1965.[c]
Fulminant Form			
Anisakiasis int.	2	2	17
Regional ileitis	12	1	24
Acute abdomen	2	2	28
Appendicitis	22	6	3
Acute ileus	9	19	4
Postop. adhesion	4	1	
Invagination		1	
Peritonitis acute		1	
Mild Form			
Eosino. granuloma	1		
Appendicitis chronica	1		
Tumor of intestine	4		
Ileum tuberculosis	1	6	
Salpingitis	1		
Diverticulm of intestine	1	2	
Pylorus stenosis	1		
Cholelithiasis	1		
Cancer of intestine	1	1	
Polyp of duodenum	1		
Fistelformation of caecum			1
Chance upon the operation of another disease	1		

[a] Ishikura H: Hokkaido J Med Sci 43: 83 ~ 99 (1968)
[b] Iwano H, Ishikura H. et al.: Geka Shinryo 16: 1336 ~ 1342 (1974)
[c] Ishikura H et al.: Surg Treat 13: 144 ~ 154 (1965)

Objective and subjective clinical symptoms. Abdominal ailments are associated with a number of universal symptoms such as abdominal pain, vomiting, pain-point, defence musculaire, temperature increase, and increasing leucocyte number. Simple observation is not enough to determine the ailment, and must include and not only experience with actual cases but also test results. This shows the need for a statistical approach based on the clinical conditions.

The biochemical and histopathological state of the ailment. One characteristic of the symptoms of larval movement is the chemotactic factor ECF-P in the parasite [14], and the concept of the larvae being a foreign antigenie stimulus to the human body. This means the first and later infections are different with the clinical symptoms also differing.

With intestinal anisakiasis, particularly when it is not the first infection, there

Differential Diagnosis of Intestinal Anisakiasis

is an acute danger that an intestinal colic-like state will develop early. This may necessitate an immediate decision of whether to perform surgery or not. In such cases a speedy diagnosis is necessary, made possible by a discrimination of the symptoms described in this section, and also an understanding of the acute responses, considerations that are based on the peculiarities of the host response to the parasite. The human body is not the final host of the larvae with the larvae remaining alive and infiltrating the abdominal cavity to form cysts, thus passing through the human as through a paratenic host. However, the human body becomes the dead-end-host where extinction occurs. This must be kept in mind to understand the mechanism of the illness, including automatic morphological changes in the abdominal wall and its thickening and constriction. The accumulation of abdominal dropsy and localized changes in the abdominal wall by exudative phlegmon in later infections are the result of the Schultz–Dale reaction and the Arthus phenomenon. When the larvae perforate the intestinal wall and reach the abdominal cavity peritonitis perforative occurs, together with bacterial infection of the abdominal cavity. Adhesion in the vicinity of the perforations causes abdominal colic, and the progression of the ailment must be kept clearly in mind when evaluating the clinical symptoms.

Auxiliary diagnosis. With present capabilities it is more difficult to observe larvae on X-ray's of intestinal than of gastric anisakiasis, however when larvae are determined it is very helpful. Ultrasonic images allow the observation of localized hydremic hypertropics in the abdominal wall. For a sero-immunological diagnosis, the most accurate and distinguishing method, monoclonal antibodies can be produced. Though it must be assumed that the healthy majority of Japanese already have antibodies. Therefore, a diagnosis by this method requires at least two weeks and repeated serodiagnosis, making a determination of the need for surgery difficult to reach.

Necessary Symptoms for Differential Diagnosis

Evacuation of the bowels. Acute intestinal colic leads to stoppage of the stool, and often to constipation, however, this is also mistakenly thought to occur with intestinal anisakiasis. It is critical to remain aware of this with the changes caused by the illness. When anisakid larvae penetrate into the intestinal wall the Schulz–Dale reaction exacerbates intestinal peristalsis and often induces diarrhea resulting in normal stool movement. Localized Arthus phenomena in the intestinal wall and the bodies immune response lead to exudative morbidity, so that after passing lymph large amounts of abdominal fluid accumulate in the intestinal cavity. Localized morbidity then induces constriction and the food at the opening is dehydrated and coagulates in small lumps, leading to constipation. Next the mucus membrane becomes ulcerated leading to diarrhea with a mucous stool, and ulcer bleeding results in hemafecia often leading to peritonitis perforativa with bacterial infection. Knowledge of these mechanisms makes an evaluation of the progression of the ailment possible. In the 87 cases where laparotomy was performed, 34 had normal stool (41%), 20 diarrhea (24.1%), 24 constipation (28.9%), one mucous in the stool (1.2%), and 4 blood in the stool (4.8%).

Abdominal bulging. In acute cases there are other symptoms in the early stages. This may be gas in the abdomen, accumulation of abdominal dropsy, or a combination of the two, distinguished by a dull or tympanic sound given off by tapping, and shown clearly by X-ray. When the abdomen is swollen, it is softer and less painful than with other acute illnesses of the stomach, and less gas accumulates than with colic.

Abdominal pain and the painpoint. Cases with violent and continuous spontaneous abdominal pain are common, but there are also cases with either continuous dull pain arising from the larvae remaining in the intestinal wall or violent temporary pain from perforation. Indirect pain is a symptom of intestinal constriction and interruption, while continuous violent pain often accompanies bacterial peritontitis. The position of the spontaneous pain and the painpoint do not necessarily coincide, with the painpoint (induration) often moving.
Defence musculaire. This symptom is generally not pronounced, but with extensive perforation, the muscular defence becomes stronger similar to that seen with abdominal colic.

Four Main Characteristics of Intestinal Anisakiasis

To enable a differentiation of intestinal anisakiasis from other acute abdominal complaints the author has continued to point to four clinical symptoms (since 1968).

1. Inquiries establish that before the attack the patient has consumed raw marine organisms that act as paratenic hosts for anisakid larvae.

2. Temperature, increases in leucocytes, and defence musculaire symptoms differ from other acute abdominal ailments like acute appendicitis, acute abdominal colic, etc.

3. Painpoint (place of perceived tenderness). In the case of acute appendicitis it is nearly always in one place in the right hypogastrium, and with acute abdominal colic it is also generally in one place or affects the whole stomach. In intestinal anisakiasis it is different for different cases, and it moves. The soft induration at the painpoint also moves.

4. X-rays show peculiarities. Few cases of intestinal anisakiasis suffer from much gas in the abdomen, but X-rays often show a mirror–like shape similar to acute abdominal colic. However with intestinal anisakiasis the general condition is better and other clinical symptoms are also lighter than with colic. Localized shadows show swellings in the affected parts, with indentations from the constricted part towards the mouth of the intestine. A barium shadow shows swollen blocked areas indicating dehydrated granules of food in the intestinal cavity (further details in a later section).

With these four points it is still necessary for further analysis to differentiate intestinal anisakiasis from other ailments. Table 2 shows the temperature, leucocyte count, and eosinophilic cell count for patients with intestinal anisakiasis from different geographical areas (Iwanai in Hokkaido, Ishikawa and Fukui Prefecture, and Northern Kyushu). The left column for Ishikawa Prefecture are cases where the symptoms necessitated surgery, and the right column shows

Differential Diagnosis of Intestinal Anisakiasis

Table 2. Clinical features of intestinal anisakiasis from several different districts

Kind of symptom	Cases of Iwanai[a] District in Hokkaido	Cases of Ishikawa Pefecture[b]	Cases of Ishikawa Prefecture[c]	Cases of Fukuoka Prefecture[d]
Temperature (Celsius scale)				
normal	47	13	17	Not described
37.0°~37.5°	28	16	} 4	
37.6°~38.0°	4	17		
38.0°~	5	18		
unknown	4	1	5	
Leukocytosis				
leukopenia	1	1	8	1
under 8000	8	9	6	40
8000~10000	15	12	7	2
10000~12000	16	12	4	5
12000~14000	9	8		
14000~	30	16		
unknown	8	7	1	1
Eosinophilia				
under 4%	19			10
4~9 %	3		9	
10~20%				
20~40%	4			
unknown	63	65	4	2

[a] Ishikura H et al.: Surg Treat 13: 144~154 (1965)
[b] Naka P et al.: Clin Surg 24: 129~133 (1969)
[c] Hara K et al.: J Jpn Clin Surg Sac 46: 416~421 (1985)
[d] Matsui T et al.: Jpn Clin Radiol 30: 741~747 (1985)

cases with suspicion of intestinal anisakiasis that were treated conservatively. The cases from Fukuoka Prefecture had been diagnosed as having intestinal anisakiasis from X-ray observations. The cases from Iwanai, Hokkaido and the left column for Ishikawa represent relatively serious cases, and it may be assumed that the right column for Ishikawa and Fukuoka represent mainly mild cases. The temperature, leucocytosis, defence musculaire, and the interval between the onset and the first medical examination lead to the following observations.

Of the 87 cases from the Iwanai area, 5 had fever above 38°C, three of these within 24 hours of the appearance of symptoms and two around the 8th to 10th day. The leucocyte counts for the three early cases were 8,400, 12,800, and 14,000 and for the late fevers 8,400 and 12,200. The muscular defence for all three early fevers was medium, and the two late cases had one with and one without strong muscular defence reations. Surgery revealed relatively strong localized morbidity in both late cases. Two other cases required intestinal excision, one with fever within 24 hours, and one with fever on the 10th day. In the two cases with strong fever and localized morbidity requiring intestinal excision no larvae were found in the intestinal wall. All of the 15 cases with intestinal excision had only slight fevers, below 37.3°C, and of these only three cases were over 37°C. Two were diagnosed within 24 hours of the appearance of symptoms and had leucocyte counts of 12,200 and 20,400, while the third case was diagnosed within 48 hours and the leucocyte count was 15,600. All cases were without muscular defence reactions.

There were 5 cases with leucocyte counts above 20,000 among the authors 88 cases requiring intestinal excision and, these all had temperatures below 37.3°C with the majority diagnosed shortly after the apearance of symptoms, one in 3 hours (leucocyte count 28,410), 2 within 12 hours (25,000 and 37,200), and one within 24 hours (20,200), and only one on the 4th day after symptoms started (leucocyte count 21,400).

One case had larvae in the perforated intestinal tract, one bacterial infection in the intestinal wall, and in one case there was bacterial infection in the intestinal cavity.

The following relates to the 65 cases reported by Naka et al [9]. Among 38 cases diagnosed at the same hospital (after the cases listed in Table 2), *Anisakis simplex* larvae were found in 11 of the excised sample, and a further 8 were determined to suffer from anisakiasis by histological test [15]. All 65 cases had abdominal dropsy, which was generally aseptic. *E. coli*, staphylococcus, an anaerobic bacteria have been cultured from ascites (7 cases), fibrous fur (23 cases), and mesentery (4 cases).

These results show that Naka's cases had a much higher incidence of abdominal bacterial peritonitis complicating the larval perforation of the intestine than the Iwanai cases. It is not clear whether there is some geographical factor in the mechanism of the larval infection, though there are reports of experimental results showing interspecies differences in the infestiousness of paratenic hosts. Comparing the statistics from cases in Iwanai and Ishikawa (Kanazawa), 75 cases (86.2%) from Iwanai and 9 cases (44.6%) from Kanazawa had none or slight fever; there were only 5 cases (5.7%) with fever above 38.0°C in Iwanai, but 29 (44.6%) of the 65 cases from Kanazawa were in the 38-39°C range, show-

Differential Diagnosis of Intestinal Anisakiasis 125

ing the need to consider baterial infection in the latter cases. Leucocyte counts above 14,000 were determined in 30 (34.5%) of the 87 Iwanai cases, which was very different from the 16 (24.6%) of 65 cases from Kanazawa. This is in part because the increase in leucocytes is relatively strong, even when the temperature remains normal or slight, and is useful in distinguishing intestinal anisakiasis from other acute abdomen, where fever is strong and the leucocyte increase is much less.

The eosinophil cell count was not done for most of the cases in Table 2, but it has been reported that 7 out of 22 cases under conservative therapy for suspicion of anisakiasis eosinophilic cell fractions were more than 5%, reaching a peak in the second week of the ailment and decreasing after the third week [9]. All of Matsui et al cases in Table 2 had normal values [8].

Conclusion

Intestinal anisakiasis, as gastric anisakiasis can be classified as either mild or a fulminant. A diagnosis of the mild form is difficult even when it has been clinically determined that there is tumorous hyperplastic inflammation in the intestine. A diagnosis becomes possible when there are repeated relapsing and releaving symptoms, and sero-immunological tests show concomitant increases and decreases in the eosinophilic cell count and immunoglobulins specific for *Anisakis* larva.

The fulminant form quickly develops ileus symptoms and as the acute abdominal symptoms require a quick determination of the necessity of performing a laparotomy, it is necessary to be able to distinguish it from other inflammatory ailments.

Intestinal anisakiasis is the result of infection caused by anisakid larvae and the ingestion of raw marine organisms that act as paratenic hosts must be established. This is achieved by interviewing the patient, and is the first step towards a diagnosis. Further investigation of the symptoms then establishes the progression of the accumulated abdominal fluid. The abdomen is distended, with resonance found on percussion. It is critical to obtain samples of the abdominal fluid by laparoscope or puncturing, and to determine the eosinophilic cell infiltration and bacteria (culture). Increased eosinophilic cell count in the early stage makes a diagnosis of intestinal anisakiasis 80% certain.

A combination of two or more of the clinical symptoms in Table 3 will also allow a diagnosis. That is, when there is slight fever but the increase in leucocyte count is stronger than that in other inflammatory diseases, when there is no bacterial infection and the muscular defence is negative or slight, the abdomen is distended but relatively soft, the painpoint is not in one place, indurations move around, or when X-ray and ultrasonography shows places with localized swelling and constrictions. These symptoms are lighter than in other kinds of intestinal colic. When evaluating the contents of the intestine from the afflicted area to the opening with a Miller-Abbott tube, the symptoms generally improve quickly and it is possible to perform immunodiagnosis to establish the final diagnosis.

By utlising knowledge of the disease progression, and with some experience it is not difficult to establish a correct diagnosis. However, when developments are

Table 3. Comparison of clinical characteristics between intestinal anisakiasis and other acute abdomens

Clinical features	Intestinal Anisakiasis	Acute ileus	Appendicitis
Temperature	±	+++	++
Nausea and vomitting	+	+++	++
Evacuation of the bowels	±	Constipate	−
Abdominal pain	+	+++	++
Abdominal swelling (1) gas stagnant	+	+++	±
Abdominal swelling (2) ascites stagnant	+++	+	−
Defence musculaire	−	+++	++
Leucocytosis	+++	+++	++
Subjective pain point	Irregular	Whole abdomen	right lower abdomen
Objective pressure point	Unsettled	Whole abdomen	Mc. Burney

− : none, + : slight, ++ : middle, +++ : severe.

slow there is occasionally fever, the leucocyte count keeps increasing, vomiting does not stop, and when bacteria have been determined in the abdominal fluid, it is necessary to prepare for the possibility that larvae have penetrated into the abdominal cavity.

References

1. Nanbu T, Tani K, Fujiwara T, Kinoshita T, Sada M (1983) The clinical and roentgenological features of 27 patients with "acute edematous ileitis". Stomach and Intestine 18: 373–379 (in Japanese)
2. Nishiki S, Konishi K, Samejima H, Toume I (1985) Clinical investigation on 27 cases of acute edematous enteritis. Jpn J Gastroentero 82: 2005 (in Japanese)
3. Takamiya H, Izumi H, Asakawa S (1986) Investigation of 17 cases of intestinal anisakiasis using roentogenological diagnostic method. Jpn J Gastroenterol 83: 280 (in Japanese)
4. Naritomi O, Karai K, Gamachi T, Yao T (1985) A case report of ileitis caused by Anisakis larvae. Jpn J Gastroenterol 82: 2005 (in Japanese)
5. Matsuoka Y (1966) Studies on peripheral blood picture and serum protein in experimental anisakiasis. Shikoku Acta Med 22: 556–580 (in Japanese)
6. Hara K, Yokoyama T (1985) A clinical study on possible anisakiasis intestinalis causing acute intestinal obstruction. J Jpn Soc Clin Surg 46: 416–421 (in Japanese)
7. Ishikura H, Tanaka M, Goto T, Aizawa M, Kanemoto T, Hagihara I, Kikuchi K, Tsuji Y, Takahashi T (1965) Studies on regional ileitis No.2. Clinical observation of 87 cases which occurred at Iwanai district in Hokkaido. Surg Treat 13: 144–154 (in Japanese).
8. Matsui T, Iida M, Fujishima M, Naritomi O, Sugiyama K, Yao T, Murakami M, Sakai T, Kimura Y, Tsuji M (1985) Radiological study of intestinal anisakiasis. Jpn J Clin Radiol 30: 741–747 (in Japanese)
9. Naka T, Aikawa K, Shinno T, Kuranishi H (1969) Experiences with acute nonspecific regional enteritis. Clin Surg 24: 129–133 (in Japanese)
10. Ishikura H (1965) Radiologic features of intestinal anisakiasis. Jpn J Clin Radiol 10: 576–588 (in Japanese)

Differential Diagnosis of Intestinal Anisakiasis

11. Ishikura H (1968) Clinical and Immunopathological studies on anisakiasis. Hokkaido J Med Sci 43: 83–99 (in Japanese)
12. Ishikura H (1969) Occurrence of anisakiasis and its presentation Saishin Igaku 24: 357–367 (in Japanese)
13. Hayasaka H, Ishikura H, Mizugaki H, Utsumi A, Saeki H, Asaishi K, Takagi R, Iwano H (1969) Studies on anisakiasis 22 especially conservative treatment of intestinal anisakiasis. Jpn J Parasitol 18: Suppl 720 (in Japanese)
14. Torisu M, Iwasaki K, Tanaka J, Iino H, Yoshida T (1983) *Anisakis* and eosinophil: pathogenesis and biologic significance of eosinophilic phlegmon in human anisakiasis. Immunobiology of the eosinophil 343–367. Elsevier Biomedical New York Amsterdam Oxford
15. Shiraki T, Suzuki T, Otsuru M, Naka T, Kubota H, Ishikura H (1969) Nineteen cases of intestinal anisakiasis found in Kanazawa City over 8 years. Jpn J Parasit 18: 652 (in Japanese)

Pathology of Intestinal Anisakiasis

Y. Kikuchi, H. Ishikura, and K. Kikuchi

Introduction

Anisakiasis (AN) is classified as gastric, intestinal and extra-gastrointestinal, which all share common features. The major pathological change in anisakiasis is an eosinophilic cell infiltration, a chemotactic effect and immunological reaction caused by the *Anisakis* larval antigens. However, there are some clinical differences among these types depending on the affected organ.

AN is subdivided into a mild or fulminant form, and a fulminant form of intestinal anisakiasis (IA) is diagnosed after unlike gastric anisakiasis (GA), cannot be diagnosed endoscopically, and is diagnosed only by identifying removed larva or, microscopic examination of resected specimen.

A mild form of IA is found more rarely than the fulminant form, and is often misdiagnosed as a tumor, chronic appendicitis and other intestinal inflammations, because clinical symptoms are very slight and slowly progressing.

In GA, clinical symptoms disappear in a few hours after endoscopic removal of the antigen (larva). On the other hand, in IA, removal of larvae itself is difficult if not done by surgical intestinal resection. Furthermore, the allergic reaction of the intestine takes a severe seroexudative form leading to thickening of the intestinal wall, which in turn prolongs the obstruction of intestinal lumen, compared to GA.

Histopathologically, IA shows more severe and typical acute eosinophilic cell infiltration and phlegmonous inflammation than GA. When the specific symptoms persist for several days, it is often found that larva cannot be identified. In 63% of resected intestine of histologically highly suspected IA cases, the larva was not found [1]. As for the above fact, the author has often criticized unsuitable histopathological examination.

Recently, however, an increasing number of cases of intestinal perforations by worms have been reported. The perforating orfice can be found on the intestinal serosa, and causing a persistence of abdominal symptoms due to bacterial contamination. So macroscopic inspection at the time of laparotomy is important in the case of IA.

In this section histopathological findings are described in macroscopic and microscopic terms separately.

Macroscopic Findings in the Peritoneal Cavity

IA can be diagnosed by careful observation with surgical treatment performed when the symptoms of acute ileus appear or when the diagnosis is uncertain and thus proved by laparotomy. However, most of the case of IA are cured by conservative treatment. Macroscopic findings refer to the surgical findings of the peritoneal cavity or serosal changes of the intestine.

Fulminant Form

Changes of peritoneum. The peritoneum shows a different appearance from that found with other intestinal diseases and is thin and transparent containing ascites and floating intestine in the abdominal cavity. These findings are so typical that anyone can be diagnosed as having anisakiasis if their peritoneum has this appearence.

Ascites. As much as 300~500 ml of ascites were found in all 19 cases reported by Ishikura [1], though a few cases without any ascites have been reported for those in the very early stages. The ascites has a serum like transparent or yellowish translucent color differing from that of other peritonitis (ileus or appendicitis perforative acuta), that are thick yellow or cloudy brown. Aspirated ascites should be carefully examined for larva which may have migrated through the intestinal wall [2], as well as lymphatic cells and neutrophils. Eosinophils are also typical in this disease, accounting for as many as 30% of the infiltrating cells. Bacteria can be found in some cases [3].

Greater omentum. Mild edema, hyperemia and thickening are noticed, but necrosis is not found, unlike suppurative inflammation. Adhesions are fibrous and easily dissected. A soft tumor may be found at the site of adhesions and larva may be present in this tumor. There is always lesion at the site of adhesion between the omentum and the intestine, and all portions of the intestinal wall should be inspected because the multiple lesion, like skip lesions are not that rare [5,12]. Several cases with the main lesion at the terminal ileum, one lesion at the upper jejunum with omentuam adhesion and the third lesion at sigmoid colon have been reported, with small tumors containing relatively fresh larva in different sites from the peritoneal wall and the serosa of abdominal organs being found [12].

Appearance of Intestine. Inflammatory changes are strictly localized but vague reddening is the only findings in the primary infection. Generally, severe local edema leads to obstruction and proxymal dilation (found on rentogenography) can be noticed (Fig. 1). Food residue is dehydrated in the intestinal lumen and palpated as small lumps, leading to obstructive change causing ileus like an acute abdomen.

Lesion of the Intestinal Serosa (Fig. 2). Inflammation is localized; the dilatation of lymphatic ducts, petechiae, hyperemia, edema, cloudy swelling, sometimes necrosis and fibrin clots are observed (Table 1). Sometimes larvae that have penetrated the serosa can be found moving on the surface of serosa.

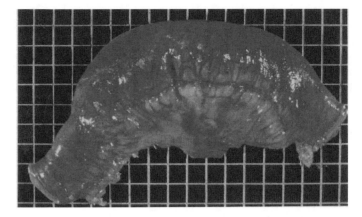

Fig. 1. Inflammatory changes are strictly localized in the lesion and severe local edema leads to obstruction of the intestine and proximal dilatation

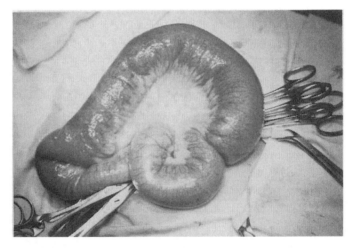

Fig. 2. Localized inflammation which shows petechiae, hyperemia, edema, cloudy swelling of serosa and mesenterium

Mesenterium. Local mesenterium is diffusely edematous in most cases.

Lymph nodes. Local mesenteric lymph nodes are swollen, sometimes bigger than the size of a thumb-tip, and sometimes hidden in the swollen mesenterium.

Mild Form

This type of IA shows no or mild symptoms compared to the fulmimant form in which acute and ileus–like symptoms often necessitate surgical treatment. Many cases of this form have been found accidentally on laparotomy for other diseases

Table 1. Macroscopic findings in the abdominal cavity of intestinal anisakiasis (Fulminant form)

Case number	Name of patient	Age and sex	Bleeding of serosa	Muddiness of serosa	Edema of serosa	Necrosis of serosa	Stenosis of wall	Swelling of lymph node	Necrosis of lymph node	Ascites	Location: oral site from Bauhin's vulve
1	KA	43♂	+++	+++	+	+	+++	++	++	+++	45cm
2	HA	30♂	++	++	++	−	+	+++	−	++	20
3	MN	17♀	++	++	++	−	−	++	−	+	50
4	NT	39♂	+	++	++	−	++	++	++	++	TM
5	FM	10♀	++	++	++	±	+	+++	−	+++	20
6	SK	36♀	++	++	++	−	+	±	−	+++	150
7	KO	17♂	++	+	++	−	+++	++	−	++	J
8	OH	19♂	+++	+	++	−	±	+	−	++	10
9	FM	34♂	++	+	++	−	−	+++	−	+++	20
10	UY	24♂	++	+++	+++	+	++	−	−	+++	TM
11	KY	27♀	++	+	++	+	−	++	−	+	60
12	MS	18♂	+++	+	±	−	+	±	−	+++	30
13	KH	21♂	++	++	±	−	±	+	−	+	70
14	SK	22♂	++	++	+++	++	++	+++	−	+++	30
15	AM	35♀	++	++	++	−	±	++	−	+++	70
16	HN	19♂	++	+	++	−	±	++	−	++	70

TM: terminal ileum, J: jejunum

or during an autopsy [1]. It is mostly a primary infection, and the pain caused by mechanical irritation by the migrating larva is usually torelated with the patient either not presenting to the physician or it cannot be diagnosed by the physician. Palliative treatment can cure the pain but the persisting small abdominal tumor man increase in size. Obstruction then causes chronic abdominal symptoms, which are misdiagnosed as benign or malignant tumors. Finally, diagnosis must be made by microscopic examination of the resected specimen.

Acute intra-abdominal changes such as ascites or localized serosal changes that are found in the fulminant form are rarely found in the mild illness. Tumors on the intestinal wall, mesenterium, greater omentum, peritoneum and other organs or located adhesions can only be noticed by careful inspection.

Reinfection takes place if one eats raw fish after a primary infection, with an immunological reaction complicated by acute symptoms causing a complex disease. The following experimental findings help to understand this phenomenon. When larva are introduced into the subcutaneous tissue of rats, and reaction of the host and larva in both the primary infection and reinfection are examined, it is found that edematous change in the host is mild in the primary phase but an abscess is formed around the larva [4]. Fibrosis and granulomatous changes appear from the 7th day, foreign body giant cells on the fifth week, and suppurative granulation on the eleventh week. On the other hand, in reinfection, severe

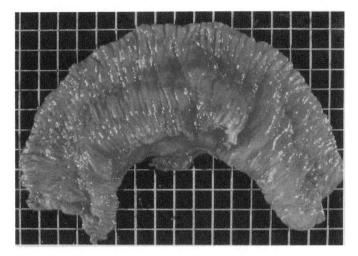

Fig. 3. Inside of localized imflammatory lesion shows intense edema of mucous membrane with many petechiae. No larve can be seen

edema appears at first, then abscess (suppurative inflammation) from the first to fourth day, fibrinous swelling from the 5th day, granulation tissue on the first week and giant cells in the third week. This means granulomatious change is more rapid in the case of reinfection.

Larvae can remain alive for three to seven days in the primary infection, but die after three to five days in a sensitized rat, with disintegration of larva also faster in reinfection. Degeneration of the excretory organ is especially fast with larva hyalinized in seven to fourteen days in some cases. A figure of 40~50% (some variation depending on the species) of orally administered larvae are excreted anally, with others remaining in the body of rats [16]. Larvae penetrate from the gastrointestinal wall into the peritoneal cavity rather than stay in the gastric wall, and are thought to form parasitic granulomas which are then absorbed in a few days.

It has been noted that more larvae than expected penetrate the intestinal wall into the peritoneal cavity even in humans [17]. Cases of gastrointestinal penetration have been reported increasingly in recent years, strongly suggesting that many patients with primary infection show no symptoms but have a parasitic granuloma in their abdominal cavity. Those found by laparotomy for complication make up only a small population, therefore, when reinfection happens in the patients with a primary infectious granuloma, the time between raw fish ingestion and surgery necessitated by acute abdominal symptoms does not correlate with the host histological reaction and the degree of typical larva degeneration (Kojima et al. [15]). Such cases and typical mild form cases are listed in Table 2.

Case Report of Reinfection

Case 1 Sasaki et al. [15].
Sudden onset of severe abdominal pain around the umbilicus, tenderness at the same site, abdominal distension, accelerated bowel movement, air-fluid levels

Table 2. Macroscopic intraabdominal findings of mild form of intestinal anisakiasis

No. of patients	Age and sex	Eating raw fishes	Foci of the subjective pain	Touch the tumor or not	Interval between the onset and operation	Characteristic features of the abdominal cavity	Change of serosa	Location of the tumor (oral distance from the Bauhlin's vulva)	Adhesion	Ascites	Swelling of lymph node	Degenerations grade of *Anisakis* larva	Type of the histopathologic change (mild form)	Reporter
1	60♂	?	Um	−	1D	Skip legion (jejunum, ileum and Messenteum)	Ileumphlegnon jejunum perfolation Messenteum-tumor	Me	−	++	−	+++	AG	Sasaki K. et al. (1984)[5]
2	23♀	?	Lc	−	1D	Ascites, Stenosis	Swelling coated fibrinous	−	−	++	+	+	A	Oouchi S. et al. (1971)[6]
3	16♀	?	Lc	?	3Y2D	Tumor	Hyperaemie Swelling	20 cm	−	−	+	+++	AG	Oouchi S. et al. (1971)[6]
4	43♀	?	Riq	?	7D	non	non	Me	−	+	++	−	A	Nishimura T. et al. (1974)[7]
5	36♀	?	lc	+	10D	Hard Tumor	non	Ti	?	?	+	+++	AG	Hotta T. et al. (1968)[8]
6	28♂	?	?	?	20D	Tumor	non	Je	?	?	?	C	A	Iwata M. et al. (1968)[9]
7	28♂	?	?	?	21D	?	?	Ti	−	?	?	+	AN	Ishikura H. et al. (1968)[10]
8	29♂	++	Um	?	23D	Tumor Adhesion	Bleeding Swelling	Sq	+++	−	?	+++	AG	Ooshio T. et al. (1973)[11]
9	43♂	?	Mo	−	25D	Stenosis of intestinal wall	Bleeding Coated fibrinous	45	−	++	++	+++	A	Ishikura H. et al. (1967)[12]
10	15♂	+	Lc	−	1M	Stenosis	Claudy Swelling	40	−	?	?	+	A	Kikuchi S. et al. (1968)[13]
1i	61♂	Mac	La	+	1M	Tumor	Tumor Swelling	Ct	++	−	?	+++	A	Schirakabe K. et al. (1984)[14]
12	28♂	?	Lc	?	1.5M	Stenosis Hyperemie ?	Tumor Swelling	Ti	−	−	++	−	AG	Oouchi S. et al. (1971)[6]
13	36♀	?	Lc	+	2M	?	Swelling	Ti	?	?	?	C	AG	Kajima K. et al. (1966)[15]
14	7♂	?	Ua	+	7M	Tumor	?	Je	−	?	?	+	AG	Ishikura H. et al. (1968)[16]
15	18♂	?	?	?	3Y		non	Je	−	?	?	+	AG	Ishikura H. et al. (1968)[16]

1. Eating raw fishes
   Mac: mackerel
2. Foci of the subjective pain
   Um: umbilical   Ma: middle abdomen
   Lc : ileocecal   La : lower abdomen
   Riq: right lower quadrant   Ua: upper abdomen
3. Interval between onset and operation
   D: day   M: month   Y: year
4. Location of the tumor
   (oral distang from the Bauhin's vulva).

Me: mesentery
Je : jejunum
Sq : sygmoid

5. Degenerations grade of *Anisakis* larvae
   C: cuticle
6. Type of the histopathologic change (mild form)
   A : (2nd stadium) abscess formation type
   AN: abscess formation with necrosis type
   AG: (3rd stadium) abscess-granuloma formation type

Ti : terminal ileum
Tc : transverl colon

Pathology of Intestinal Anisakiasis 135

on X-ray film, nausea and vomiting were all experienced. One day after onset, a laparotomy was performed.

In the peritoneal cavity, there was 200 ml of yellow ascites with localized acute exudative inflammation and obstruction by the intestinal contents such as edema and spotted bleeding in ileum 60 cm proxymal to the Bauhin's valve, intestinal distension in this site, similar skip lesion in the jejunum 100 cm proximal to the former one, and mesenteric lymph node swelling. The jejunal lesion and lymph node lesions showed changes of the fulminant form, but the larva in the ileum was hyalinized. In this case, hyalinized larva, associated with suppurative granuloma of anisakiasis, was thought to be the primary infection. The primary infection had not caused any symptoms, but sensitized the patient strongly, leading to severe symptoms at the reinfection.

Case 2 Oouchi et al. [6].
Severe pain in the ileocecal region and vomitting led to a diagnosis of acute appendicitis with surgery performed on the day of onset. A small-sized tumor was resected in the ileum 40 cm proximal to Bauhin's valve, and serosal reddening and thickening was found in another site. The resected tumor was eosinophilic granuloma (abscess-granuloma formation type), and thought to be the primary infection. If further examination was performed in the incised portion, larvae might be found.

Case 9 Ishikura et al. [12].
Dull pain in the middle of the abdominal wall was noticed 25 days before surgery, worsening upon walking, but then temporarily disappeared. Surgery was performed because the diagnosis for the persisting pain was uncertain. A small volume of cites, severe edema, severe thickening and hyperemia in the ileum 45 cm proximal to Bauhin's valve, fibrin clot, abscess with serosal necrosis in 2 other regions, obstructive change with dilated proximal intestine and local lymph node swelling were all observed. At the site of the fibrin clot, adhesion of the omentum to the intestine was noted. Considering the macroscopic findings, and the clinical course of 25 days, the case does not appear to be of the fulminant type, whereas the intra-abdominal findings, were of the fulminant type. This discrepancy was resolved by microscopic findings. Larvae were degenerated and hyalinized, surrounded by a neutrophilic abscess with necrosis suggesting bacterial contamination. Serosal necrosis and omental and intestinal adhesion around the fibrin clot also suggested bacterial contamination.

Case 15 Ishikura et al. [16].
Right lower quadrant pain did not disappear for 3 years after appendectomy and the patient was operated upon again for post-appendectomy adhesion. A hard tumor of finger-tip size was found in the midportion of the jejunum and was resected. Pathologically it was an abscess-granuloma formation type, with the other larva shell found surrounded by a large eosinophilic abscess with necrosis showing 2 layers. The outer layer showed periodic change suggesting that a long time had passed since the infection. Considering this histopathological finding and the fact that the symptoms did not disappear after appendectomy, a more precise examination of other parts of the intestine should have been done when the appendectomy was performed.

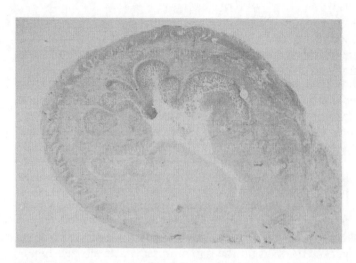

Fig. 4. Transverse section of ileum which shows narrowing inside because of intensive edema. (X4, H.E.)

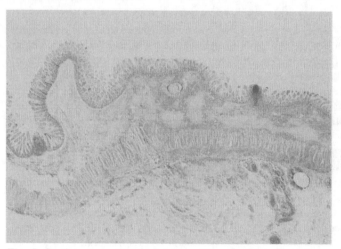

Fig. 5. In the mucosa and submucosa there is intensive edema. It shows homogeneous thin colored area with dilated veins congested with blood. A cut surface of *Anisakis* larva is found. (X20, H.E.)

Histological Findings

Clinically, the anisakiasis lesion has been described in a fulminant and mild form [19], and the histological findings will also be described by this classification.

Pathology of Intestinal Anisakiasis

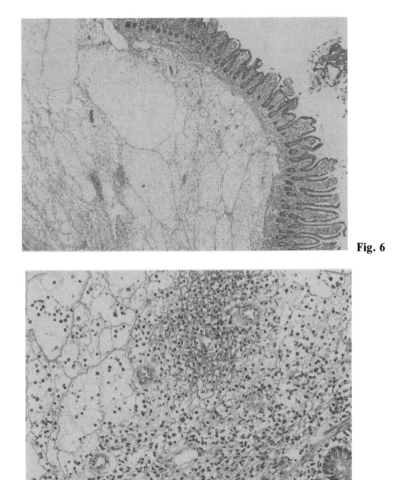

Fig. 6

Fig. 7

Figs. 6 and 7. High magnification of submucosal edema with fibrin, petechiae and infiltration of inflammatory eosinophils and neutrophils. Fig. 6 (X40, H.E.), Fig. 7 (X200, H.E.)

Fulminant Form

The thickness of intestinal wall in this form is 3-5 times thicker than the normal intestinal wall (Fig. 4,5). This phenomenon is caused by intensive edema and cell infiltration especially in the submucosal through serosal layer, including mainly massive eosinophils, neutrophils, monocytes and lymphocytes (Fig. 6,7). The cut surfaces of *Anisakis* larva are found most frequently in the submucosal layer, with the most intensive fulminant change also observed in this submucosal layer (Fig. 8–10). Even though *Anisakis* larva may not be found in one area of phlegmonous wall, occasionally they might be found several centimeters close by, and sometimes two or several cut larval surfaces can be seen by reason of coil-

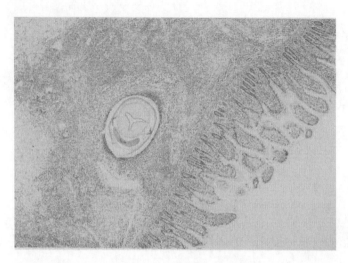

Fig. 8. Cut surfaces of typical *Anisakis* larva in the submucosal layer. (X40, H.E.)

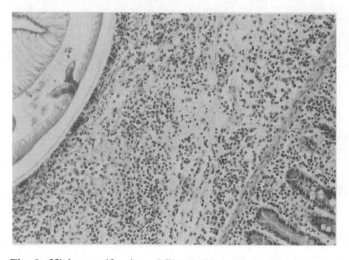

Fig. 9. High magnification of Fig. 8. Around the larva is intensive infiltration of eosinophils, lymphocytes and neutrophils with interstitial edema. (X100, H.E.)

shaped migration of larva or migration by more than one larva (Fig. 11). The probability of discovering larval cut surfaces might depend on the number of tissue blocks. Even though *Anisakis* larvae are not found in these areas, it is possibly due to larva escaping out of the intestinal wall. The most intensive histological changes are observed around *Anisakis* larva which indicate tissue necrosis and severe cell infiltration including eosinophils. The larva is usually intact and clearly visible in this form since it might take only 48 hours after larval migration. Also intensive edema with inflammatory exudate is shown accompanying exudated fibrin, and small hemorrhagic lesions are observed in this

Pathology of Intestinal Anisakiasis

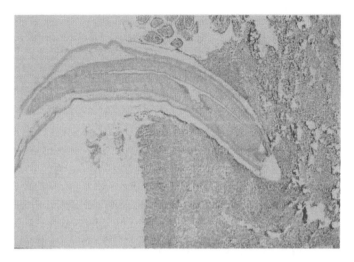

Fig. 10. Sagittal cut surface of larva invading submucosal layer from mucosal surface. (X40, H.E.)

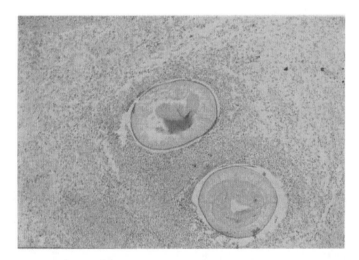

Fig. 11. Two cut surfaces of larva in the submucosal area. This larva might migrate with a coil-shaped action into the tissue. (X50, H.E.)

layer. In the mucosal layer there are no findings of ulceration or necrosis at all but lymphoid follicles are found in most cases. The muscular layer shows weaker inflammatory changes than the submucosal layer, without edema and fibrin exudation and little cell infiltration seen in this layer. Sometimes ganglion cells of Auerbach neuronal plexus are swollen, degenerated or infiltrated by reactive cells. The serosal layer may have massive cell infiltration, weak edema and fibrin exudation continuing into the muscular and submucosal layers, and the most remarkable hemorrhages are observed in the serosal layer since many capillaries belong to this area anatomically. In several cases the subserosal area has been swollen with fibrosis especially at perivascular areas. Regional mesenterium of these phlegmonous intestine shows weak inflammation including exudation and cell infiltration. Finally, these pathological findings are similar to an Arthus–type allergic reaction, that is a secondary reaction by the *Anisakis* larval antigens [20,21,23].

Mild Form

This form corresponds to findings of chronic inflammation compared to the fulminant form which indicates acute inflammation. If the fulminant form is an Arthus–type allergy by *Anisakis* antigens following secondary infection, the mild form appears to be caused by prolongation of this allergic reaction due to longstanding larval antigen from the primary infection or even chronic foreign body inflammation with bacterial contamination by primary infection of *Anisakis* larva. The low incidence depends on the mild symptoms in this form, with no resection of the infected lesions necessary. Anisakiasis has been classified into 4 stages, **1st stadium—phlegmonous type**. According to Kojima's classification the 1st phlegmonous stage corresponds closely to the fulminant form by Suzuki [19].

2nd stadium—abscess formation type. Most cases arise from complication of bacterial infection with abscesses marked by many eosinophils, neutrophils, histiocytes, and lymphocytes around the slightly degenerating larva or its debris. In some cases the degenerating larva is surrounded by massive necrotic tissue at the inner layer with infiltration of eosinophils into the larva (Fig. 12). A small amount of granulomatous tissue surrounding the abscess is infiltrated by inflammatory cells, with accompanying edema and fibrin exudation. Kojima called this type of reaction an "excervation" reaction (Fig. 13) [15] resulting from exposure to parasitic antigen,—especially excreted material (ES antigen) or visceral antigens—which might react as secondary antigens to the host, previously immunized with a primary infection of *Anisakis* larva.

3rd Stadium—abscess-granuloma formation type. Most cases of this type are found incidentally when intestinal diseases such as ileus, submucosal tumors and chronic enteritis are operated upon. When abscess formation is prolonged and diminished these lesions indicate growth of fibroblast and granuloma. At the center of this abscess-granuloma tissue, intensive degenerating larva are observed which may not be identified as *Anisakis* larva at all. There is a less intensive reacting cell infiltration, than found with abscess-formation (stage 2) type. The degenerating larval-like materials are invaded by neutrophils and eosinophils, and sometimes surrounded by foreign body giant cells. Lymphocyte infiltration may be dominant instead of eosinophils in this lesion.

4th Stadium—granuloma formation type. This is the end stage of anisakiasis, seen very rarely since almost all of these cases are operated and resected before reaching this end stage, though it can be observed in gastric anisakiasis [22,24]. Even if intestinal granuloma formation is found, it cannot be identified as granuloma caused by anisakiasis because of no *Anisakis* larva itself and few eosinophiles.

Pathology of Intestinal Anisakiasis

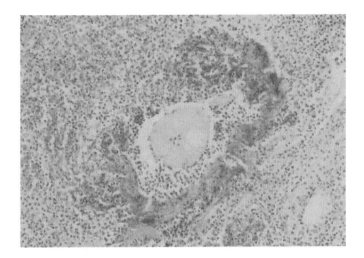

Fig. 12. Degenerating larva is surrounded by massive necrotic tissue and the inner layer of larva is infiltrated by eosinophils and neutrophils. (X40, H.E.)

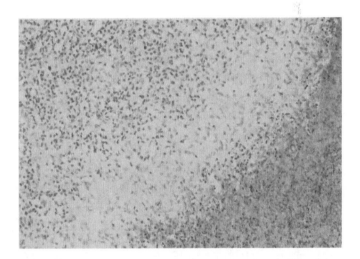

Fig. 13. Higher magnification of necrotic granulation surrounding destructed larva. This type of necrosis means "excervation" reaction by destructed larval antigens. (X100, H.E.)

Destruction of larva might progress systematically. According to duration from infection suggesting that the grade of larval destruction could conversely estimate the period of infection. However these pathological stages of anisakiasis are not strictly separated but form a continuum, making such estimation difficult.

Discussion

Intestinal anisakiasis can be divided into a fulminant and mild form, which have different pathogenesis. The fulminant form is initiated by a secondary allergic reaction. If larva stay in the intestinal wall, granulation occurs around it with periodic change occurring which may show pathological findings identical to the mild form. But there are occasions in which larvae are not found at all and yet are histologically identical. In such cases there may have been some technical failure in preparing the histological specimen, or the larva which had once migrated into the intestinal wall come out on to the mucosal surface, with only the head stuck into the intestinal wall. This is called the jumping phenomenon [18]. Larvae that have migrated into the intestinal wall may also disappear into the abdominal cavity or intestinal lumen, but the ES antigen left in the intestinal wall can cause a secondary allergic reaction, without any granuloma formation. In such a case, inflammatory changes take place rapidly and the larva cannot be found, with intestinal resection not necessary. Therefore, when surgeon operates upon the fulminant form, macroscopic findings facilitate the decision of whether or not intestinal resection should be performed. Macroscopic findings are thought to be more important than histological findings for surgeons.

The mild form, in primary infection, causes only minor symptoms, and is therefore only rarely diagnosed when the patient is operated upon for other diseases causing persistent abdominal pain and ileus. In such cases obstruction by mild inflammatory edema and hyperemia are found.

Reinfection causes acute abdominal symptoms and surgery may be performed. If a surgeon is confused with the findings of reinfection and does not carry out a thorough examination, the primary parasitic granuloma may remain in the abdominal cavity.

Even though intestinal anisakiasis shows more intensive histological findings than gastric anisakiasis, they are caused by the same fundamental pathological process [24].

References

1. Ishikura H (1968) Clinical and immunopathological studies on anisakiasis. Hokkaido J Med Sci 43: 83–99 (in Japanese)
2. Furukawa A (1974) Anisakiasis, its history and a case of acute ileitis, attributable to a living larva of *Anisakis* in peritoneal cavity. J Jpn Soc Clin Surg 35: 63–69 (in Japanese)
3. Naka T, Aikawa K, Niino T, Kuranishi (1969) Experiences with acute nonspecific regional enteritis. Clinical Surgery 24: 129–133 (in Japanese)
4. Saeki H, Mizugaki H, Ishikura H, Hayasaka H (1972) Immunological studies on anisakiasis (2) Participation of immune response in host-tissue reaction and destruction of paracite bodies. Hokkaido J Med Sci 47: 541–550 (in Japanese)
5. Sasaki K, Sasaki T, Nagamine Y (1984) A case report of intestinal anisakiasis with skip lesion and mesenteric granuloma formation. J Jpn Soc Clin Surg 45: 1183–1187 (in Japanese)
6. Oouchi K, Sugiyama Y, Abo Y, Ito Y, Izai S, Abe K, Okudera S (1971) Regional Ileitis. Surgical Treatment 13: 843–853 (in Japanese)

Pathology of Intestinal Anisakiasis

7. Nishimura T, Tanaka, Ito Y, Sugihara Y, Morishita K, Watanabe S, Watanabe S (1974) Report of three cases of human anisakiasis. Larva, each recovered from different organs of men and their morphological studies. J Kobe Medical College 2: 124–139 (in Japanese)
8. Hotta T, Okano T, Konishi Y (1967) A case of ileocoecal granuloma with eosinophitic infiltration. Clinical Surgery 22: 1467–1469 (in Japanese)
9. Iwata K, Nishimura T, Takemura T, Urano E, Oda T (1968) Studies on anisakiasis in Wakayama prefecture especially its clinicopathologic consideration. J Wakayama Med Soc 19: 59–72 (in Japanese)
10. Ishikura H, Kikuchi Y, Hayasaka H, Miyagi H, Ueno T (1968) Studies on anisakiasis in Hokkaido Japan. J Jpn Soc Clin Surg 29: 49–60 (in Japanese)
11. Oshio T, Nishii H, Harada R, Usaya N, Ogawa K (1973) A case report of cured Anisakiasis in sigmoid colon. Surgical Treatment 15: 207–210 (in Japanese)
12. Ishikura H, Kikuchi Y, Hayasaka H (1967) Pathological and clinical observation on intestinal anisakiasis. Arch Jpn Chir 36: 663–679 (in Japanese)
13. Kikuchi S, Kosugi K, Hirabayashi H, Hayashi, Uno H, Yanagishita, Harada A, Tanaka T, Kamiya K, Ino H (1968) A case report of intestinal anisakiasis. J Yokohama Med Sci 20: 286–288 (in Japanese)
14. Schirakabe K, Sato M, Kamachi H, Kodama Y, Inuzuka S (1984) A case report of colonic anisakiasis diagnosed preoperatively as cancer of the transverse colon. Med Bull Fukuoka Univ 11: 309–311 (in Japanese)
15. Kojima K, Koyanagi T, Schiraki K (1966) Pathological studies of anisakiasis (parasitic abscess formation in gastro intestinal tracts) Jpn J Clin Med 24: 134–143 (in Japanese)
16. Okumura T (1967) Experimental studies on the anisakiasis. J Osaka City Med Center 16: 465–502 (in Japanese)
17. Suzuki T, Ishikura H (1974) Studies on the etiologic mechanism, it's symptom and diagnosis of anisakiasis. Fishes and *Anisakis* 58–72 (in Japanese)
18. Karasawa Y, Kawakami Y, Hirafuku I, Hoshi K, Koyama T (1983) Studies on anisakiasis and terranovasis of the digestive tract. Jpn Med J 3079: 30–34 (in Japanese)
19. Suzuki T (1968) Studies on the immunological diagnosis of anisakiasis. Antigenic analysis of *Anisakis* larvae by means of electrophoresis. Jpn J Parasitol 17: 213–220 (in Japanese)
20. Kikuchi Y, Ueda T, Yoshiki T, Aizawa M, Ishikura H (1967) Experimental immunopathological studies of intestinal anisakiasis. Igaku No Ayumi 62: 731–736 (in Japanese)
21. Saeki H (1975) Studies on cell-mediated immunity in experimental anisakiasis. J Sapporo Medical College 44: 309–322 (in Japanese)
22. Shiraki T (1969) On the pathological diagnosis of gastrointestinal larva migrans (on anisakiasis). Saishinigaku 378–389 (in Japanese)
23. Smith J W, Wootten R (1978) *Anisakis* and anisakiasis. Adv in Parasitol Vol. 16. Bake J R, Muller R (eds) Academic Press, London and New York, pp. 93–163
24. Kukuchi Y, Ishikura H, Kikuchi K, Hayasaka H (1989). Pathology of gastric anisakiasis. Gastric Anisakiasis in Japan. Ishikura H, Namiki M (eds), Springer, London, Heidelberg and New York, pp. 117–127.

Clinical Patho-Parasitology of Extra-Gastrointestinal Anisakiasis

H. Yoshimura

Previous investigations have demonstrated that *Anisakis* larva orally administered to experimental animals can easily penetrate through the gastrointestinal tract and reach the abdominal cavity a few days after ingestion of the larva [1–4]. Since the first case of extra-gastrointestinal anisakiasis was reported in Holland [5], 16 other cases have been documented in other countries, though the majority were from Japan [6–15] (Table 1). The locations of *Anisakis* larvae in the tissues were abdominal cavity (3), large omentum or mesentery (6), subcutaneous tissues (4), pleural cavity (1) and others (3). All except three cases, harbored a larva in the involved tissues, and five patients were examined pathoparasitologically by means of immunodiagnoses (Table 1).

Presentation of the Cases

Case 1 (No. 8 in Table 1). A 22 year-old man complained of abdominal pain, vomitting and tarry or bloody stool for a period of 8 days. The day before the onset of the disease, he consumed raw mackerel and bluefin tuna *(Thunnus thynnus)* and the symptoms began to appear at midnight. Leucocyte count was 9,000, eosinophil rate was 2%, and the stool was strongly positive for occult blood. A surgical operation was performed on the ninth day of the illness, and at laparotomy, a $2.2 \times 1.3 \times 1.6$ cm sized tumor was found on the large omentum near the greater curvature of the stomach, suggesting a mestastatic focus of a malignant neoplasm (Fig. 1). However, examination of a section revealed a disintegrated thread-like nematode in the tumor tissues (Fig. 2). Histopathologically, no malignant cell or tissue was recognized while a nematode larva was observed in the eosinophilic granulations, with marked edema and fibroblastie proliferation noted, *Parasite*: The transverse sections of a nematode, approximately 0.46×0.25 mm in diameter were seen in the serial sections of the affected tissues. The polymyarian-type muscle cell layer under the smooth cuticle, muscular esophagus, renette cell and particularly Y-shaped lateral cords were considerably well preserved, therefore the parasite was identified as an *Anisakis simplex* larva (Fig. 3). Latex agglutination using *Anisakis simplex* larvae antigen was strongly positive with a $1:2^{10}$ titer, while the Ouchterlony' test was also positive (Table 2).

Case 2 (No. 9 in Table 1). A 78 year-old woman complained of epigastric colic and vomitting that continued for one week. The leucocyte count was 13,400,

Table 1. Case reports of extra-Gastrointestinal anisakiasis

No.	Age	Sex	Residence	Location of Anisakis larva	Reporters (Year)
1	13	F	Holland	Abdominal cavity	van Thiel & van Houten (1967)
2	28	M	Japan (Tokyo)	Abdominal cavity	Furukawa et al. (1974)
3	43	F	Japan (Osaka)	Mesentery	Nishimura et al. (1974)
4	67	M	Japan (Kashiwara)	Mucous membrane of oral cavity	Nishimura et al. (1974)
5	58	F	Japan (Toyonaka)	Mucous membrane of pharynx	Nishimura et al. (1974)
6	30	M	Japan (Kanazawa)	Subcutaneous tissue (abdominal wall)	Kagei & Sakaguchi (1977)
7	32	F	Japan (Wakayama)	Large omentum	Sasaki et al. (1978)
8[a]	22	M	Japan (Kanazawa)	Large omentum	Yoshimura et al. (1978)
9[a]	78	F	Japan (Maizuru)	Large omentum	Yoshimura et al. (1978)
10[a]	36	M	Japan (Kanazawa)	Abdominal cavity[b]	Yoshimura et al. (1979)
11[a]	42	F	Japan (Ishikawa)	Subcutaneous tissue (abdominal wall)	Yoshimura et al. (1980)
12[a]	3	M	Japan (Toyama)	Suhcutaneous tissue (inguinal)	Yoshimura et al. (1980)
13	54	M	Japan (Iwate)	Lymph node (mesentery)	Monma et al. (1985)
14	11	M	Japan (Iwate)	Large omentum	Monma et al. (1985)
15	23	F	Japan (Iwate)	Subperitoneum (parietal)	Monma et al. (1985)
16	37	M	U.S.A.	Pleural cavity[b]	Kobayashi et al. (1985)
17	unknown	F	France (Paris)	Subcutaneous tissue	Godeau et al. (1986)

[a] Nos. 8, 9, 10, 11 and 12 (*Case* 1–5 described in this paper) were examined in our laboratory.
[b] *Anisakis* larva was not found, but suspected.

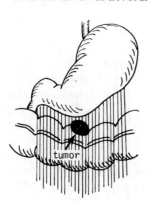

Fig. 1. Location of the granulomatous tumor as seen in the large omentum

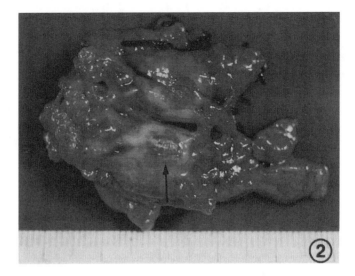

Fig. 2. A disintegrated *Anisakis* larva (divided into two parts) found on the cutting surface of the large omentum

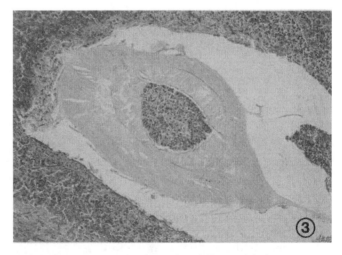

Fig. 3. Transverse section of the larva surrounded by eosinophilic granulation

eosinophil was 6%, and the stool was positive for occult blood. On X-ray examination a shadow defect suggesting gastric cancer was located at the antrum of the greater curvature of the stomach. Symptoms of gastric anisakiasis started to appear 8 hours after eating raw spanish mackerel *(Scomberomorus niphonius)* sashimi. After gastric endoscopy, a laparotomy was done on the eighth day of the disease (Fig. 4). A localized tumor measuring 8 × 4 cm in diameter was located near the pylorus of the stomach, and two enlarged, hard nodules sug-

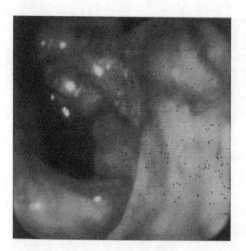

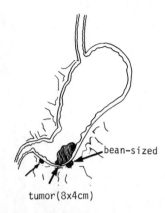

Fig. 4. Gastroendoscopic finding suspecting an ulcer or cancer of the stomach

Fig. 5. A tumor-like palpable mass (8 × 4 cm) was located at the antrum of the greater curvature of the stomach. Two nodules are also seen on the large omentum (arrows)

gesting cancerous metastatic lumps or granulomas were located on the large omentum of the stomach (Fig. 5). On macroscopic observation of the resected stomach, the erosive and ulcerated large focus was seen near the pylorus and a small punched out hole penetrating through the stomach wall was present (Fig. 6). Histopathological diagnosis of this lesion was given as a subacute gastric ulcer and perforation possibly due to penetration by the parasite. No malignant proliferation was seen, but abundant eosinophils were observed in the stomach wall, with the two removed nodules also characterized by granulations containing massive eosinophils. The transverse sections of the nematode larva revealed the characteristic feature of *Anisakis* measuring 0.39× 0.22 mm in diameter (Fig. 7). Latex agglutination and Ouchterlony' tests were positive (Table 2).

Case 3 (No. 10 in Table 1). A 36 year-old man was admitted to hospital due to severe abdominal pain resembling that of an acute ileus with tarry or bloody stool for a period of 5 days. Four weeks before onset of the disease, he ate raw mackerel sashimi. Slight fever, leucocytes numbering 14,000, red cells 410 × 10^4 and no anomalies of liver or urinal tests were seen. The abdomen was distended and typanic, and acute appendicitis was suspected before the performance of laparotomy.

On macroscopic observation, the terminal ileum was thickened, edematous and a reddish mesentery near by the focus had a hard red bean-sized nodule. When the terminal ileum was longitudinally opened, a small pore which was a probable canaliculi due to its penetration of *Anisakis* larva was seen (Fig. 8). Microscopically, the mucosal layer of the intestine revealed marked catarrhal inflammation with massive eosinophils and edema, and an exudative or phlegmonous reaction was seen in the submucosa to the serosa. No parasite was found in the sections of the intestinal wall, while the small mesentery nodule was composed of fibrous or collagenous connective tissue, presumably scar, and no para-

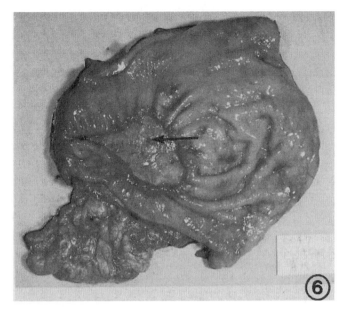

Fig. 6. Inner wall of the stomach resected. Erosive and ulcerated focus with a size of approximately 8 × 4 cm was seen near the pylorus. A small punched hole (arrow) penetrating through the focus was found

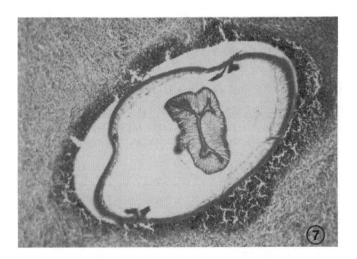

Fig. 7. Typical feature of *Anisakis* larva transversely sectioned in the eosinophilic phlegmon of the nodule

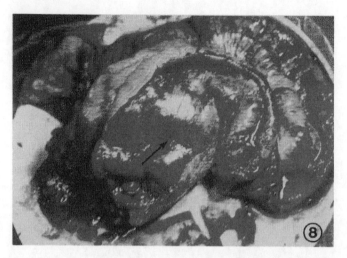

Fig. 8. Macroscopic finding of the focus of the terminal ileum surgically resected. At the center of the focus a small pore which probably indicates perforation or penetration into the abdominal cavity was seen (arrow)

Table 2. Results of immunological tests on five cases of extra-gastrointestinal anisakiasis

				Latex antigen			Anisakis antigen	
No.	Age	Sex	Location of Anisakis larva	Anisakis	Pseudo-terranova	Ascaris	Ouchterlony	IEP
6[a]	30	M	Abdominal wall	2^{10}	2^6	N.D.	N.D.	N.D.
8	22	M	Large omentum	2^{10}	N.D.	N.D.	+	N.D.
9	78	F	Large omentum	2^9	2^1	2^2	+	N.D.
10	36	M	Abdominal cavity?	2^5	N.D.	N.D.	+	N.D.
11	42	F	Abdominal wall	2^{10}	2^2	2^4	+	+

Numbers were referred to as those in Table 1.
N.D.: not done   F: female   M: male   IEP: immunoelectrophoresis
[a] Clinical findings of No. 6 were reported by Kagei and Sakaguchi(1977).

site was seen in the tissues. Latex-agglutination test was positive (1:2^5) and Ouchterlony' test revealed three precipitin bands (Table 2).

Case 4 (No. 11 in Table 1). A women aged 42 years presented with a 4.0 × 3.0 × 8 cm sized nodule, palpable in the subcutaneous tissues of the median line under the navel of the abdominal wall. The tumor was surgically removed and macroscopically had dermoid-like features, while histopathology showed a transverse section of *Anisakis* larva in an eosinophilic abscess (Fig. 9). The patient had eaten raw mackerel and squid 3 months prior to the operation. Ouchterlony' test and immunoelectrophoresis were both positive (Fig. 10), as well as the latex agglutination (1:2^{10}), but cross reactivity revealed for the *Ascaris* antigen (1:2^4) (Fig. 11).

Clinical Patho-Parasitology of Extra-Gastrointestinal Anisakiasis 151

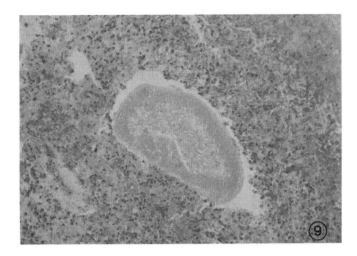

Fig. 9. Transverse section of a degenerated larva seen in the eosinophilic abscess

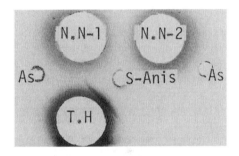

Fig. 10. Ouchterlony test: This patient's serum was positive for *Anisakis* larva antigen, but negative for *Ascaris* antigen. (N.N-1 and N.N-2 were healthy)

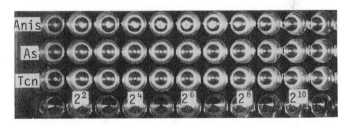

Fig. 11. Latex agglutination: The patient's sera (Case 11) showed a positive reaction with antibody titer 1:2^{10} against *Anisakis* antigen, 1:2^4 for *Ascaris* and negative for *Toxocara* antigens

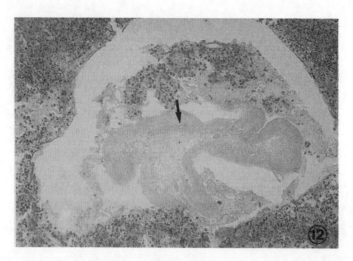

Fig. 12. A disintegrated worm in the sectioned tissue showing an eosinophilic abscess. A renette cell can be faintly observed (arrow)

Case 5 (No. 12 in Table 1). A 3 year-old boy received surgical treatment to remove a tumor located in the left inguinal subcutaneous tissue which was palpabale two months after eating sashimi such as cod, squid and yellowfish. The tumor gradually increased in size. Macroscopically, a hard tumor was sharply demarcated from the adjacent tissues and had a yellowish-white appearance at the cut surface. Histopathological features were characterized by massive eosinophils associated with neutrophils and edema, and the tumor harbored several longitudinal-transverse sections of the nematode, presumably *Anisakis* larva measuring 0.99 − 0.27 × 0.29 − 0.13 mm in diameter. A renette cell was faintly seen in the body cavity of the parasite (Fig. 12). No immunodiagnositc test was done.

Discussion

There have been more than a few cases with sudden and severe abdominal pain due to deeply invasive or penetrating *Anisakis* larva into the mucosal layer of the gastro-intestinal canal, though the larva did not reach the abdominal cavity [18–23]. Actually, the diagnosis of extra-gastrointestinal anisakiasis can be hard to ascertain because there are many differentiation difficulties in differentiating it not only from acute or subacute anisakiasis, but also from other illnesses such as ileus, appendicitis, neoplasm and so forth. In the case with tumor-like granulomas in the abdominal cavity or subcutaneous tissues, the period of time from ingestion of the larva to appearance of clinical symptoms is not always clear, with some occurring with the acute type and others with the chroinc type. In consideration of the above, the necessity of immunodiagnostic investigation for this disease must be emphasized. The use of the radioallergosorbent test (RAST) as a sensitive and specific method has been recommended [24]. As shown in Table 2, we applied latex-agglutination and Ouchterlony' tests for the

Clinical Patho-Parasitology of Extra-Gastrointestinal Anisakiasis 153

extra-gastrointestinal infections, finding all of the five sera examined were latex-agglutination-positive and four of those sera were Ouchterlony-positive against *Anisakis simplex* larval antigens. Some cases of anisakiasis often revealed cross-reactivity against *Toxocara* or *Ascaris* adult antigens [19,25,6]. Result of the latex-agglutination and Ouchterlony' tests, however, seemed to be tentatively useful as an aid for preoperative immunodiagnosis of extra-gastrointestinal anisakiasis. Kobayashi *et al.* reported a case with probable pulmonary anisakiasis examined by Ouchterlony' test and immunoelectrophoresis which showed specific precipitin bands for *Anisakis simplex* larval antigens [16], though cross reactivity was seen for *Toxocara canis* and *Taenia saginata* antigens.

In Japan, consumption of sashimi or sushi using raw sea fish and squid are quite common. Therefore, the status of subclinical infection or sensitization with *Anisakis simplex* larvae antigen may likely occur [26–28]. In addition, Japanese people may be exposed at all times with antigens of various nematodes such as *Toxocara*, *Ascaris* or *Dirofilaria immitis*. Further studies on pathogenesis, pathoparasitology and immunodiagnosis for extra-gastrointestinal anisakiasis should be performed.

References

1. Yoshimura H (1966) Migration of *Anisakis*-like larva, causing eosinophilic granuloma in the alimentary tract of man. Minophagen Med Review 11: 105–114 (in Japanese)
2. Asami K, Inoshita Y (1967) Experimental anisakiasis in guinea pigs; Factors influencing infection of larvae in the host. Jpn J Parasitol 16: 415–422
3. Oyanagi T (1967) Experimental studies on the visceral migrans of gastrointestinal walls due to *Anisakis* larvae. Jpn J Parasitol 16: 470–493 (in Japanese with English abstract)
4. Ruitenberg EJ (1970) Anisakiasis: Pathogenesis, serodiagnosis and prevention PhD thesis, Rijks University, Utrecht, pp. 33–45
5. Van Thiel PH, Van Houten H (1967) The localization of the herringworm *Anisakis marina* in and outside the human gastrointestinal wall. Trop Geogr Med 19: 56–62
6. Yoshimura H, Akao N, Kondo K, Ohnishi Y, Funaoka Y, Yamane K (1980) Two cases of extra-gastrointestinal infection with *Anisakis* larvae and their immunodiagnoses. Jpn J Clinical Pathol 28: 708–712 (in Japanese)
7. Furukawa A (1974) Anisakiasis, its history and a case of acute ileitis, attributable to a living larva of *Anisakis* in the peritoneal cavity. J Jpn Soc Clin Surgery 35: 63–69 (in Japanese)
8. Nishimura T, Tanaka E, Ito Y, Sugihara Y, Morishita K, Watanabe S, Watanabe S (1974) Report of three cases of human anisakiasis: Larvae, each recovered from the different organs of men, and their morphological studies. J Hyogo College of Med 2: 124–139 (in Japanese with English abstract)
9. Sasaki S, Aoki Y, Shoji M Matsumoto K, Okamura S, Katsumi M (1978) A case of the intestinal perforation due to *Anisakis* larva. J Jpn Soc Clin Surg 39: 61–65 (in Japanese)
10. Kagei N, Sakaguchi Y (1977) Interesting cases due to *Anisakis* larva. Nihon Igi Shinpo 2786: 32–34 (in Japanese)
11. Matsuki N, Ariga T, Tsuchihara K, Furukawa N, Kozaka S (1979) A case of abdominal wall mass due to anisakiasis. J Clin Surgery 34: 1169–1171 (in Japanese)
12. Yoshimura H, Kondo K, Akao N, Ohnishi Y, Watanabe K, Shinno B, Aikawa K (1979) Two cases of eosinophilic granulomas formed in the large omentum and mesentery by the penetrated *Anisakis* larva through the gastrointestinal tract. Stomach and Intestine 14: 519–522 (in Japanese with English abstract)

13. Yoshimura H, Akao N, Kondo K, Ohnishi Y (1979) Clinicopathological studies on larval anisakiasis, with special reference to the report of extra-gastrointestinal anisakiasis. Jpn J Parasitol 28: 347–354
14. Yoshimura H, Akao N, Kondo K, Ohnishi Y (1980) Two cases of subcutaneous involvement due to *Anisakis* larva. Jpn J Parasitol 29 (Suppl): 52 (in Japanese)
15. Momma N, Iwasaki T, Satodate R, Ito I (1985) Three cases of parasitic granulomas due to *Anisakis* parasitic in the lymph node, large omentum and parietal subperitoneal tissues. Iwate Med J 37: 919 (in Japanese)
16. Kobayashi A, Tsuji M, Wilbur D (1985) Probable pulmonary anisakiasis accompanying pleural effusion. Am J Trop Med Hyg 34: 310–313
17. Codeau P, Danis M, Bouchareine A, Nozais J (1986) An unusual case of aedema: *Anisakis*. Helminthol Abstract 55: 297–298
18. Yoshimura H, Kaneda J, Suzuki T, Takaso T, Mikoshiba Y (1966) A case of acute abdomen due to probable penetration of *Anisakis*-like larva into intestinal wall. Surgical Treat 15: 626–630 (in Japanese)
19. Yokogawa M, Yoshimura H (1967) Clinicopathological studies on larval anisakiasis in Japan. Am J Trop Med Hyg 16: 723–728
20. Ishikura H, Kikuchi Y, Hayasaka H (1967) Pathological and clinical observation on intestinal anisakiasis. Arch Jpn Chir 36: 663–679 (in Japanese with English abstract)
21. Maruyama A, Inaba, Aiuchi Y, Suzuki S, Fujita T (1981) Two cases of intestinal anisakiasis—Skip lesion and perforation. Surgical Diag and Treat 23: 517–523 (in Japanese)
22. Sasaki K, Kamita N, Yamaguchi Y (1982) Four cases of anisakiasis, especially a case of intestinal perforation cause by *Anisakis* larvae. J Jpn Soc Clin Surg 43: 1374–1380 (in Japanese)
23. Tsukamoto H, Koizumi W, Atari E, Okudaira M, Yoshizawa S, Maekawa K, Mieno H, Hamashima H, Ishikawa J, Takahashi T, Hiki Y, Aso K (1987) A case of gastric anisakiasis, causing gastric perforation. Jpn J Gastroenterol 84: 104–107 (in Japanese)
24. Desowitz RS, Raybourne RB, Ishikura H, Kliks MM (1985) The radioallergosorbent test (RAST) for the serological diagnosis of human anisakiasis. Transact Roy Soc Trop Med Hyg 79: 256–259
25. Yoshimura H, Kondo K, Ohnishi Y, Akao N, Tsubota N (1978) Summary of human anisakiasis during past three years in our laboratory—with special reference to clinicopathology and immunodiagnoses. Nihon Igi Shinpo 2837: 29–32 (in Japanese)
26. Kobayashi A, Kumada M, Ishizaki T, Suguro T, Koito K (1968) Skin tests with somatic and ES (excretions and secretions) antigens from *Anisakis* larvae. II. The difference of antigenicity between the two antigens. Jpn J Parasitol 17: 414–418 (in Japanese with English abstract)
27. Suzuki T, Shiraki T, Sekino T, Otsuru M, Ishikura H (1970) Studies on the immunological diagnosis of anisakiasis. III. Intradermal test with purified antigen. Jpn J Parasitol 19: 1–9 (in Japanese with English abstract)
28. Suzuki T, Ishida K, Asaishi K, Nishino C (1976) Studies on the immunodiagnosis of anisakiasis. 6. Analysis of criteria on intradermai and indirect hemagglutination tests by means of radioimmunoassay. Jpn J Parasitol 25: 17–23 (in Japanese with English abstract)

Immunodiagnosis for Intestinal Anisakiasis

M. Tsuji

Introduction

Endoscopical examination provides a definite diagnosis for gastric anisakiasis but without bowel surgery to identify *Anisakis* larve it is very difficult to diagnose intestinal anisakiasis. Eating raw fish within a few days of the onset of disease is an important factor, while laboratory findings may only suggest nonspecific acute inflammatory changes. Therefore, immuno-serological examination is very important for the clinical diagnosis of intestinal anisakiasis.

In the past few years, several serological studies have been performed for the diagnosis of intestinal anisakiasis, such as complement fixation test, indirect hemagglutination test, Ouchterlony test, immunoelectrophoresis and indirect immunofluorescence. Results of these tests have all indicated that positive serological tests for anisakiasis are closely connected with the surviving worms in patients.

The practical value of sero-diagnosis for helminthic diseases was compared for several techniques and the results summarized (Table 1). Among infections due

Table 1. Comparison of results of sero-diagnosis for helminthic diseases

	CFT	IHA	IFT	IEP	
Anisakiasis	85	85	95	95	
Ascariasis	0	0	20	20	
Ancylostomiasis	0	0	15	5	
Toxocariasis	90	85	85	90	
Filariasis (with *D. immitis* Ag.)	75	85	85	85	
Schistosomiasis	90	90	92	95	(cop 98)
Paragonimiasis	95	90	95	98	
Fascioliasis	98	95	98	98	
Clonorchiasis	45	30	50	50	
Metagonimiasis	5	5	15	5	
Taeniasis	20	15	25	20	
Echinococcosis	90	85	98	95	
Diphyllobothriasis	20	15	25	20	
Sparganosis	90	85	98	95	

CFT: Complement fixation test, IHA: Indirect haemagglutination test, IFT: Indirect immunofluorescence test, IEP: Immunoelectrophoresis, COP: Circumoval precipitin test

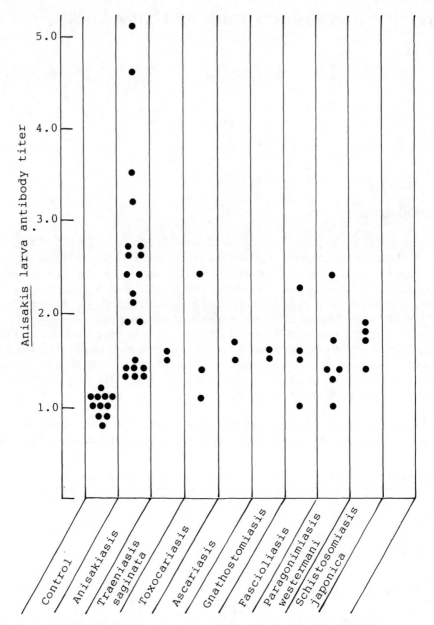

Fig. 1. *Anisakis* larva antibody titer in sera from patients with helminthiasis

to tissue parasites such as anisakiasis, toxocariasis, filariasis, schistosomiasis, paragonimiasis, fascioliasis, echinococcosis and sparganosis, a good response is shown by immunological techniques. On the contrary, serological tests for infections due to digestive duct parasites, ascariasis, ancylostomiasis, clonorchiasis, metagonimiasis, taeniasis and diphyllobothriasis shown very poor results [1].

Immunodiagnosis for Intestinal Anisakiasis   157

However, in these helminthic diseases the eggs are very easy to detect by stool examination.

Recently enzyme-linked immunosorbent assay for the detection of the anisakiasis antibody in the patients sera was used [2]. *Anisakis* larvae antigens were prepared from 0.1% saline extracts of *Anisakis* larvae which were collected from the mackerel's peritoneal cavity. An enzyme-linked immunosorbent assay (ELISA) has been developed for detecting *Anisakis* larvae antibody with *Anisakis* larvae antigen. In this assay, peroxidase-labeled goat anti-human IgG serum was used as a conjugate and 5-aminosalicylic acid was used as a substrate. The optimal concentration of antigen was found to be 20 μg/ml and the optimal dilution of peroxidase-labeled goat anti-human IgG serum was 1:800. Of the 14 sera from patients 5 days post–infection with *Anisakis*, 11 showed positive results by ELISA. Of 7 *Anisakis* larvae positive sera from patients with anisakiasis, one serum was found to show a positive result by ELISA. Of the other 23 sera from patients with helminthiasis, only 3 sera showed positive results (Fig. 1).

However, in the cases of primary infection, the first positive reactions in all serological tests were recognized 10 to 30 days after infection [3], and should therefore have follow-up examinations. In the re-infection cases, the first positive reactions were recognized 6 to 24 hours after re-infection. In follow-up examinations antibody titers increased, with maximum titers shown at 3 to 10 weeks post–infection. These titers showed a tendency to decrease and finally became negative within 18 months.

On the problem of cross reactivity, the strongest reactions were observed between the antigen and its homologous anti-sera in all tests, and the antigens of close species should be diagnosed for differentiation. The detection of a specific band of *Anisakis* by immunoelectrophoresis is also very useful for the diagnosis.

Usunally, a surgical operation is not necessary in most patients with intestinal anisakiasis because of its good prognosis with conservative treatment. Therefore, immunoserological examinations as well as radiologic evaluation, a history of raw fish intake and the clinical symptoms are all important for the diagnosis of intestinal anisakiasis. The serological tests are very useful parameters for the diagnosis, and should be conducted simultaneously using several techniques.

References

1. Tsuji M (1986) Sero-diagnosis for parasitic diseases. Kagaku Ryoho no Ryoiki 2 (3): 381–386 (in Japanese)
2. Tohgi N (1983) Detection of antibody of *Anisakis* larvae by enzyme-linked immunosorbent assay with *Anisakis* larvae antigen. Hiroshima Daigaku Igaku Zasshi 31 (6), 936–970 (in Japanese)
3. Tsuji M (1989) General remarks, Serological and immunological studies on gastric anisakiasis, Gastric Anisakiasis in Japan, Springer, Tokyo, pp. 89–95

Skin (Intradermal) Testing Using Several Kinds of *Anisakis* Larva Antigens

H. Ishikura, Y. Kikuchi, O. Toyokawa, H. Hayasaka, and K. Kikuchi

Introduction

In 1962 the first case of intestinal anisakiasis was reported by van Thiel et al. in the Netherlands and 2 years later nationwide studies on this disease started in Japan. The majority of Japanese eat raw marine fish and squid, so this study was very important and has progressed rapidly. The initial stages of study mainly involved immunological experiments for pathogenesis and diagnosis. Skin tests were studied quickly and isolated rapidly in that period.

Skin tests for parasitic diseases had already been extensively for several species of parasite, and also in mass medical screening. The skin test for *Anisakis* looked for an immediate reaction, as did the tests for other parasitic disease, and was called a reaginic reaction. In this reaction antigen are injected intradermally, the antibody (reagin) then fix into the specimen's cell and when combined, are released. This inevitably causes flare (angiectasia) and swelling, due to changes in cell membrance permeability, asthenia, angioatelectasia, and liquid exudation at the side of the host's body. This reagin was shown to be IgE by Ishizaka in (1967).

As the analysis of specific antigen was not so developed then, it was difficult to specify the individual name of the disease by total IgE measurement alone, leading to confusion with other allergens. Today, the specific monoclonal antibody of *Anisakis simplex* larva has been isolated by Takahashi S. et al in 1986, and the seroimmunological diagnosis using the specific antibody by micro-ELISA method has been accomplished successfully. This test is more precise than skin test. And then, the skin test performed at present.

Studies of skin (intradermal) testing for anisakiasis started in the Gifu area [1–3] then continued in other parts of Japan [4–15,17,20–22] are discribed in this paper.

Antigens Used for Skin Test (ST test)

It has often been pointed out that *Anisakis* larvae have complicated antigenicity. These many antigen groups present seroimmunohistopathological lesions, such as swelling, exudation and eosinophilic cell infiltration into the tissue as well as clinical symtoms such as nausea, vomiting, abdominal pain and leucocytosis.

160

However, purified antigen excluding many other common Ascaridoidea antigens have been used in experiments to reproduce specific anisakiasis pathogenicy and in the seroimmunological or immunohistopathogical diagnosis of the anisakiasis patient.

In one study intact antigens of both *Anisakis* and adult *Ascaris* were electrophoresed by the starch-gel electrophoretic method, finding that the water-soluble protein components were very similar in both [8], and the electrophoretic patterns of *Anisakis* larval antigens were complicated. The gel was separated into 9 fractions as indicated by Aminoblack 10B. This component was extracted, antigenetic specificity was tested with immune house rabbit's blood serum by the Ouchterlony method, which showed a fair specificity in the 6th fraction [1]. Since them efforts have been made to purify specific antigens [10].

Recently monoclonal antibody has been prepared, which will make the extraction of specific antigens increasingly possible, the details of which will be introduced in a separate section. We describe here the respective antigens which were used for the skin test (ST) in different studies.

Kinds of Intact Antigens Used for Skin Test (ST)

Saline soluble antigen. Morishita T. et al. (1965) and Taniguchi A. (1966) prepared antigens by first washing raw *Anisakis* larvae, collected from horse mackerel, and *Scomber japonicus*, which were available on the market in Gifu city, with physiological saline, adding an adequate amount of distilled water to them, before homogenizing well. They were then vacuum-freeze-dried, and diluted 100 times with pH 7.2 physiological saline. They were left for 2 hours at 37.0°C and extracted after 48 hours at 5.0°C, followed by centrifuging at 12,000 rpm for 60 minutes at 0.0°C, thus making a clear supernatant fluid. Then 0.2% phenol was added to increase the volume 100 times. Raw antigens used by Hayasaka et al. and Ishikura were also prepared in the same way after washing *Anisakis larvae* (which was picked out of the peritoneal cavity of *Pleurogrammus* sp. or *Theragra chalcogramma*) well with physiological saline and adding antibiotics (penicillin or Streptomycin).

V.B.S. antigen. This raw antigen was prepared by Suzuki et al. and was same as that used by Hayasaka and Ishikura et al. This was prepared by freeze-depressor-drying raw larvae from *Scomber japonicus* and pulverizing at low temperature and then adding a small amount of physiological saline. This was then centrifuged at 8.500 rpm for 30 minutes. After drying and weighing, they added pH 7.4 veronal buffered saline weighing 100 times their weight, then cold-extracting with agitation for 24–48 hours at 4.0°C, and centrifugating at 13,000 rpm for 30 minutes. The supernatant was then increased by a factor of 100 with physiological saline plus marzonin.

Somatic antigen extracted with Unger's solution. This antigen was prepared by Kobayashi et al. in 1968. One hundred pieces of *Anisakis simplex* larvae from *Gadus macrocephalus* were nipped, freeze-thawed ten or more times repeatedly, and freeze-dried again after the parasitic body was destroyed. At this stage, the weight was 150 mg, and were kept in a cool dark place. Before use, they were ground in a mortar, then delipidized for eight hours by aethyleter in Soxlet device at normal temperature. After Unger's solution, 50 times as much as dry weight was added, it was extracted for 48 hours at 4.0°C, and centrifugated at 15,000 rpm for 30 minutes. And then the supernatant liquid was dialysed and sterilized to make SOM antigen's standard solution, adjusting the amount of protein to 30 μg per 1 ml by ultra-violet ray.

Excretary-secretary antigen (ES-antigen). This is a raw antigen which has been widely used. Third stage larvae are bred in physiological saline for 3–4 days at 37.0°C. they molt to 4th-stage larvae, discharging a large volume of molting fluid from the excretary opening, which is the antigen. One hundred and fifty pieces of *Anisakis simplex* larvae from *Gadus macrocephalus* were bred in 0.85% physiological saline at 37.0°C with breeding fluid renewed every day and collected 4 days later, freeze-dried (dry weight 10 mg) after dialysis with running water. When used, they were lysed with 5cc Aq. distilata, treated with NaCl to regulate osmotic pressure, and filtrated by a Seitz filter to adjust the protein concentration (30 μg/ml).

Freeze-dried powder antigen for oral administration. This antigen is not for intradermal injection but was experimentally used for oral administration to immune animals by Ishikura et al in 1968. In this case, powder, equivalent to 20 larvae, was administered to house rabbits in capsule once a day.

Other antigens are saline insoluble fractions for testing of delayed subcutaneous immunolo-reactions.

Hemoglobin antigen Suzuki. Raw antigens extracted from *Anisakis* larvae were put in DEAR-cellulose chromatography, lysed continuous NaCl gradient, and isolated with 5 fractions. Starch-gel and disk electrophoresis methods were then carried out, followed by gel infiltration with Sephadex D200 in order to eliminate the minor component of the 3rd and 4th fractions in N6. As the N6 had the nature of delayed solution, it was purified in this method and consequently concentrated into chromoprotein hemoglobin antigen.

Kikuchi also carried out ST using several antigens, comparing the strength of the reaction. He found that the reactions were stronger in the order of ES, SOM and VBS with the same protein level's antigen and that histological lesions were also more conspicuous in the same order. The intensity of these skin reactions was not necessarily parallel to that of serum antibody titer by the Boyden method.

Since cross reactions with other parasitose or host allergic reactions to other diseases are strong, it is necessary to purify the raw antigens. This was done with isolated hemoglobin antigens by Suzuki and used for ST, described in the following section. In addition, cuticle antigens, have been prepared though these have not been used for ST [10].

Results of Skin Testing for Anisakiasis in Japan

Acute symptoms of anisakiasis overwhelmingly manifest intestinally, clinically presenting as an acute abdomen which resembles ileus. Therefore there have been many opportunities to undertake histopathologic examination of the resected intestine. Symptoms of anisakiasis result from immunological reactions, besides eosinophil chemotactic factors. Since Japanese have a habit of eating raw fish, it was presumed that people who looked healthy and symptomless could have been already immunized by *Anisakis* larval antigens, leading to re-

162 H. Ishikura et al.

search on ST of healthy people, which will be described by another author in a separate section.

Animal Experiments

Skin testing using raw larvae and saline soluble or insoluble fractions of antigen intradermally or subcutaneously were examined by Kikuchi in 1967 [25]. The primary subcutaneous infection of raw larvae led to a foreign body reaction accompanied by eosinophilic infiltration caused by a chemical mediator released from the larvae. Secondly, eosinophilic granuloma were formed by gradual release of granuloma formation factors from the degenerative bodies of surrounded parasites. With reinfection, parasitic collapse progressed rapidly, causing acute exduadative inflammation around the granuloma accompanied by eosinophilia. When the *Anisakis* fractional antigen was subcutaneously injected into immune rabbits, the supernatant showed immediate reaction whereas the deposit showed a delayed reaction, suggesting that cellular immunity as well as reaginic reactions (IgE type) was also involved. Injection of fractional antigen into the intestinal wall of sensitized rabbits indicated eosinophilic, fibrinous and acute lesions, similar to what many human cases experienced, and which was recognized as allergic reaction.

Passive cutaneus anaphylaxis (PCA) mainly using immune guinea pigs showed that the intensity of intradermal reactions were in the order of ES, SOM and VBS [16–17]. When cross matching with *Toxocara canis* it was reported that no correlation between serum antibody titer and the intradermal Boyden reaction could be found [19].

ST on Human Anisakiasis

Not many patients have had ST for human anisakiasis. From separate researchers there have been: one cases of gastric anisakiasis [1,3], 3 cases of intestinal disease [12–13], five gastric patients [4], 11 gastric and 20 intestinal [6] and 37 gastric anisakiasis patients (of which 16 were pseudoferranouasis) [21] have been reported seventy two patients out of 86 were positive, providing a very high positive percentage rate of 83.7%, but the elapsed time between the onset and the test must be taken into consideration (Table 1). According to Suzuki all the negative patients had been infected several years previously (2–9 years), and as this disease was considered to be pathologically involved in allergy, that the antibody might disappear after many years. Also, people who constantly ate raw fish mgiht be reinfected so people showing negative immune reactions are either not infected or their antibody has diappeared, whereas positive patients are either presently ifnected, or have been in the past.

Conclusion

Skin testing, carried out with various raw antigens and hemoglobin antigens made differentiation between *Ascaris* and *Anisakis* possible, although no immunological differentiation between *Anisakis* and *Pseudoterranova* larvae could

Table 1. Intradermal test with Anisakiasis antigen

Kind of antigen	Concentration	No. of patients	Positive rate	Author	
Saline extract	1:10000	1 (G)	100 %	Morishita et al, (1965)	Taniguchi (1966)
Saline extract VBS extract	1:10000	3 (I)	100 %	Hayasaka et al, (1968)	Ishikura (1968)
Som. antigen		5	0 %		
(Ungers solution) ES antigen	Protein 30μg/ml	5 (G)	80 %	Kobayashi et al. (1968)	
Hemoglobin antigen	Protein nitrogen 4μg/ml	35 (G.8) (G.M.7) (I.20)	(100 %) (42.7 %) (80 %)	Suzuki et al. (1968)	
Hemoglobin antigen	Protein nitrogen 4μg/ml	37 (G2.1) (G.P.16)	(100 %) (100 %)	Asaishi et al. (1975)	

G: Gastric anisakiasis, I: Intestinal anisakiasis, M: Mild form, P: Pseudoterranovasis

be obtained. However, monocolonal antibody by Takahashi et al. can discriminate strictly between *Anisakis* and *Pseudoterranova* larvae, though *Anisakis simplex* larvae specific antigen derived from monoclonal antibody is not used as ST antigen, because the immune test (e.g. ELISA method) can be used which is less painful to patients than ST.

References

1. Morishita T, Kobayashi M, Sakata R, Goto M, Yamada I, Sakakibara H, Mishima S, Furuhashi T, Hiraoka Y, Yamada M (1965) On skin tests of anisakiasis. Jpn J Parasitol 14: 230–232 (in Japanese)
2. Taniguchi M (1965) Immunological study on anisakiasis. Jpn J Parasitol 14: 619 (in Japanese)
3. Taniguchi M (1966) Studies on *Anisakis* (1). On its antigenicity. Jpn J Parasitol 15: 502–506 (in Japanese)
4. Kobayashi A, Kumada M, Ishizaka T (1968) Skin test with somatic and ES (excretions and secretions) antigens from *Anisakis* larvae. I Survey of normal populations on skin sensitivity to different antigens Jpn J Parasitol 17: 407–413 (in Japanese)
5. Kobayashi A, Kumada M, Ishizaki T, Suguro T, Koito K (1968) Skin test with somatic and ES (excretions and secretion) antigens from *Anisakis* larvae. II The difference of antigenicity between the two antigens. Jpn J Parasitol 17: 414–418 (in Japanese)
6. Kobayashi A (1969) Skin test of anisakiasis. Saishin Igaku 44: 373–374 (in Japanese)
7. Suzuki T (1969) Studies on immunological diagnosis of anisakiasis: Especially on analysis and purified antigens. Saishin Igaku 44: 375–377 (in Japanese)
8. Suzuki T (1968) Studies on immunological diagnosis of anisakiasis. 1 analysis of antigens by the electrophoretic method. Jpn J Parasitol 17: 213–220 (in Japanese)
9. Suzuki T, Shiraki T, Otsuru M, Ishikura H (1979) Studies on the immunological diagnosis of anisakiasis. II Intradermal test with purified antigens. Jpn J Parasitol 19: 1–9 (in Japanese)
10. Shiraki T, Suzuki T, Otsuru M, Sato Y, Kenmotsu M, Asaishi K (1973) Experiments for the application of fluorescent antibody method to histological diagnosis of anisakiasis 2. Antigenic analysis larva, especially on the cuticular antigen. Jpn J Parasitol 22: 141–145 (in Japanese)
11. Suzuki T, Ishida K, Asaishi K, Nishinoz C (1976) Studies on the immunodiagnosis of anisakiasis 5. Analysis of criteria on intradermal and indirect hemagglutination test by means of radioimmunoassay. Jpn J Parasitol 25: 17–23 (in Japanese)
12. Hayasaka H, Ishikura H, Miyagi H, Ueno T, Utsumi A, Sato K (1969) Immunological studies on anisakiasis 1. Its intradermal test. J Clin Surg Soc 29: 81–87 (in Japanese)
13. Ishikura H (1969) Occurrence of anisakiasis and its clinical presentation Saishin Igaku 24: 357–365 (in Japanese)
14. Hayasaka H, Mizugaki H, Asaishi K, Takagi R, Iwano H, Ishikura H, Aizawa M (1970) Seroimmunological responses on intestinal anisakiasis especially its Sarles' Phenomenon. Minophageu Med Review 15: 100–106 (in Japanese)
15. Hayasaka H, Ishikura H, Mizugaki H, Ueno T, Utsumi A, Sato K, Saeki H, Asaishi K, Iwano H (1971) Experimental immunological analysis of host responces on anisakiasis. Saishin Igaku 26: 1786–1800 (in Japanese)
16. Aizawa M (1969) Host immunological responces on anisakiasis. Saishin Igaku 24: 367–372 (in Japanese)
17. Kikuchi K, Toyokawa O, Sato H, Natori T, Ishikura H, Aizawa M (1970) Immunopathological studies on experimental anisakiasis Minophagen Medical Review 15. 54–58 (in Japanese)

18. Toyokawa O, Nakamura K, Ishiyama H, Yokota H, Kikuchi K (1969) Immuno-pathologic studies on experimental anisakiasis. Hokkaido J Med Sci 44: 97–104 (in Japanese)
19. Tyokawa (1972) Host immunopathological responces in experimental anisakiasis. Hokkaido J Med Sci 47: 285–265 (in Japanese)
20. Tozuka M (1974) Human anisakiasis 3. Epidemiology. Fishes and anisakiasis. Koseisha Koseikaku, Tokyo, Japan, pp. 44–57 (in Japanese)
21. Asaishi K, Nishino C, Ebata T, Tozuaka M, Hayasaka H, Suzuki T (1980) Studies on the etiologic mechanism of anisakiasis. Gastroenterol Jpn (1) 15: 120–127, (2) 15: 128–134
22. Nishino C, Asaishi K, Tozuka M, Hayasaka H, Suzuki T (1974) Epidemiological studies on anisakiasis. J Jpn Clin Surg Soc 35: 171–174 (in Japanese)
23. Suzuki T, Shiraki T, Otsuru M (1969) Studies on the immunological diagnosis of anisakiasis. II Isolation and purification of *Anisakis* antigens. Jpn J Parasitol 18: 232–240 (in Japanese)
24. Asaishi K, Nishino C, Tozuka M, Hayasaka H, Otsuru M, Sato Y, Suzuki T, Yoshida A, Kishimoto T (1975) Epidemiology on anisakiasis; especially comparative aspect in Hokkaido and in Okinawa Prefecture Nippon Igishinpo 2676: 30–34 (in Japanese)
25. Kikuchi Y, Ueda T, Yoshiki T, Aizawa M, Ishikura H (1967) Experimental immuno-logical studies of anisakiasis. Igsku no Ayumi 62: 731–736 (in Japanese)

Passive Hemagglutination Test (Boyden)

K. Asaishi, C. Nishino, and H. Hayasaka

Introduction

The etiological mechanism of anisakiasis involves an anaphylactic as well as an Arthus reaction in the digestive tract [1,2]. Cell-mediated immune reaction must also be considered in the establishment of an allergic condition in experimental anisakiasis [1]. To carry out immunological studies on intestinal anisakiasis, indirect hemagglutination (IHA) tests were conducted on anisakiasis patients and controls.

Material and Methods

Preparation of Antigen

The antigen used in the present work was a purified antigen, eluted by the method described by Suzuki, namely hemoglobin(Hb) of the *Anisakis* larva [3]. This antigen was prepared from *Anisakis simplex* larva (Fig. 1), collected from the viscera of mackerel or cod. The worms were washed several times in a normal saline solution and then finally in distilled water. The worms were chopped into small pieces and homogenized in 0.005 M phosphate buffered saline (PBS), pH 7.4 by stirring for 24 hours at 4°C. The homogenate was centrifuged for 30 minutes at 26,000 g, and the supernatant, a perienteric fluid of *Anisakis* larva was dialysed with distilled water at 4°C and then fractionated by salting out with ammonium sulfate. The fraction was precipitated by 60–80% ammonium sulfate, gel-filtrated on a Sephadex G-200 gel-column and chromatographed on a DEAE-cellulose column. Fraction II, the fraction of *Anisakis* larva hemoglobin was lyophilized and stored at −60°C. In order to recognize this isolated protein, polyacrylamide gel disc electrophoresis of *Anisakis* larva hemoglobin and the immunoelectrophoretic pattern developed with anti-Fraction II rabbit serum were carried out [4].

Indirect Hemagglutination (IHA) Test

The preparation of sensitized sheep red blood cells was undertaken according to the method of Boyden [5–6] and is shown in Fig. 2.

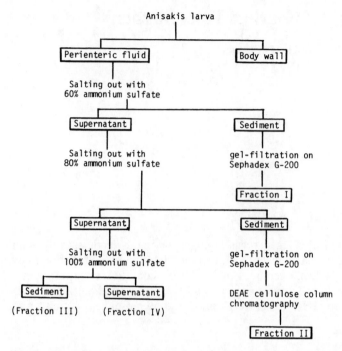

Fig. 1. Procedure of fractionation of *Anisakis* antigen. Fraction II which was precipitated with 60–80% ammonium sulfate, eluted by Sephadex G-200 gelfiltration and 0.15 M Nace in DEAD-cellulose column chromatography was shown to be a specific antigen of *Anisakis* larva

Fresh sheep red blood cells were washed with phosphate buffered saline (PBS) pH 7.2, 3 times. A 2.5 ml sample of a 3% suspension in PBS was added into the same volume of diluted tannic acid solution with 10^5 fold PBS. This suspension was then rotated end-over-end for 15 minutes in cold water and centrifuged at 2500 rpm for 5 minutes and washed with PBS.

A 2.5 ml sample of the 3% tannate sheep red blood cells in saline was mixed with the same volume of *Anisakis* larva hemoglobin dissolved in PB at pH 6.2 (antigen concentration 100 μg/ml). This suspension was rotated end-over-end for 15 minutes at 37°C and centrifuged at 2500 rpm for 5 minutes, the serum and diluted by PBS pH 7.2.

Sensitized sheep red blood cells (0.75%) were used for the indirect hemagglutination test. Dilution of antiserum was carried out by the microtiter method. Namely, 0.025 ml of inactivated antisera were diluted with normal rabbit serum, form 4 to 128 fold, using a dilutor and then dropped into microplate holes.

The same volume of sensitized sheep red blood cells was dropped into these microplate holes, using a dropper. Judgement of reaction was made 3 to 4 hours later. Based on Suzuki's criteria standards [7], when a reaction to 16 fold diluted serum was seen, the case was judged as positive.

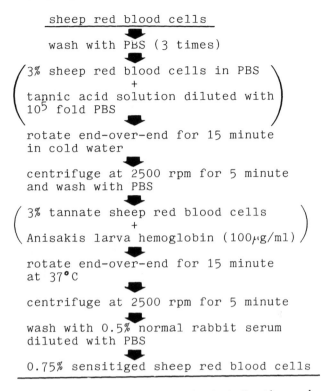

Fig. 2. Preparation method of sensitized sheep red blood cells for the indirect hemagglutination test

Epidemiologic Study [2]

The following subjects were studied during a two year period, from 1974 to 1975: 42 cases of acute anisakiasis patients, a group of 2077 inhabitants residing in Hokkaido ranging in age from 20–82 years of age and 246 high school students from 16–18 years of age.

Results

Fraction II, purified antigen of *Anisakis* larva was a brownish red colored protein. In order to recognize this isolated protein, disc electrophoresis was carried out (Fig. 3), which showed, this purified antigen to be identical with *Anisakis* hemoglobin previously described by Suzuki [1]. Immuno-electrophoretic patterns developed with antibody hemoglobin of *Anisakis* larva serum were revealed (Fig. 4). In reactions with this purified antigen serum, only one precipitation band was seen in the Anisakis antigen of whole worm extracts.

The photograph of the IHA test, using a microplate is shown in Fig. 5. As a result of IHA tests, it was noted that 38 (90.5%) out of 42 anisakiasis patients showed a positive reaction on 16-fold or more diluted serum. Twelve cases

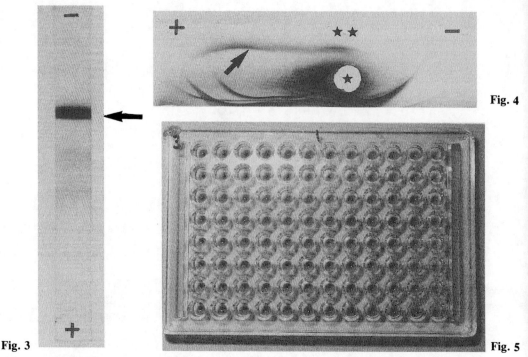

Fig. 3. Polyacrylamide gel disc electrophoresis of purified antigen, hemoglobin of *Anisakis* larva

Fig. 4. Immuno-electrophoretic pattern developed with antibody hemoglobin of *Anisakis* larva serum Arrow: hemoglobin of *Anisakis* larva, *: whole worm extract of the *Anisakis* larva, **: anti-Fraction II serum

Fig. 5. Photograph of the indirect hemagglutination test using a microplate

(28.6%) showed a reaction to 256-fold or more to the diluted serum. A positive reaction was seen in 36.6% of the inhabitants and 19.5% high school students. No significant difference was seen between males and females for the positive reaction of IHA tests. Likewise, no significant difference was seen among the age levels of the general inhabitants.

Discussion

We conducted an investigation into the presence of antibodies in the Hokkaido area, based on the opinion that the cause of anisakiasis is an allergic reaction brought about by penetration of the digestive tract wall with the *Anisakis* larvae [8–9]. In an attempt to determine the etiologic mechanism of anisakiasis, we sensitized the rabbits with whole worm extract and the hemoglobin of the *Anisakis* larva [4].

Passive Hemagglutination Test (Boyden)

A remarkable antibody production was recognized in rabbits administered the hemoglobin by intraperitoneal or subcutaneous injections than in those with the whole worm extract of the *Anisakis* larva. When the degree of antibody production was estimated by the IHA titer, the highest degree was shown intraperitoneally, the intermediate degree was in the subcutaneously injected rabbits and the lowest was in the rabbits injected into the submucosal part of the stomach [9]. This indicated that a sensitized state might be produced when the larva penetrate the wall of the digestive tract and enter the intraperitoneal vavity. This state is more detectable and a highly sensitized state might occur. Numerous immunological studies on anisakiasis have been performed, however, these all used antigens that were crude extracts of the worm, leading to abundant cross reactions. A specific antigen from *Anisakis* larvae is therefore necessary, and Suzuki discovered that hemoglobin of the *Anisakis* larva is such a specific antigen [3] and thereafter this Hb was employed as the antigen in the indirect hemagglutination test of anisakiasis.

Ninety percent of patients showed a positive IHA test reaction, and about 36% of the inhabitants showed the same reaction. Inhabitants in fishing industrial areas showed a high positive rate to IHA tests, while inhabitants of farming areas showed a low positive rate, which may be related to the number of times raw fish is eaten. The fact that inhabitants of Hokkaido showed a higher positive rate compared with those of other districts to IHA test [6], suggests a rise in incidence of anisakiasis.

Numerous reports have indicated the involvement of humoral antibody and cellular immunity reaction in the etiology of anisakiasis. In the future, clarification and elucidation of anisakiasis, including the role of cellular immunity needs to be investigated.

References

1. Asaishi K, Nishino C, Totsuka M, Hayasaka H, Suzuki T (1980) Studies on the etiologic mechanism of anisakiasis. Immunological reactions of digestive tract induced by *Anisakis* larva. Gastroenterologia japonica 15: 120–127
2. Asaishi K, Nishino C, Totsuka M, Hayasaka H, Suzuki T (1980) Studies on the etiologic mechanism of anisakiasis. Epidemiologic study of inhabitants and questionaire survey in Japan. Gastroenterologia japonica 15: 128–134
3. Suzuki T. (1971) Immunodiagnosis of anisakiasis, with special reference to purification of specific antigen. Chinese J Microbiol 4: 217–231
4. Asaishi K (1974) Antigenic analysis of *Anisakis* larva and application of fluorescent antibody technique to histological diagnosis of anisakiasis (in Japanese). Sapporo Med J 43: 104–120
5. Boyden SV (1951) The adsorption of proteins on erythrocytes treated with tannic acid and subsequent hemagglutination by anti-sera. J Exp Med 93: 107–120
6. Nishino C (1977) Epidemiological studies on anisakiasis Sapporo Med J 46: 73–88 (in Japanese)
7. Suzuki T, Ishida K, Ishigooka K, Doi K, Otsuru M, Sato Y, Asaishi K, Nishino C (1975) Studies on the immunological diagnosis of anisakiasis. 5. Intradermal and indirect hemagglutination tests and histopathological examination of biopsied mucous membranes on gastric anisakiasis. Jpn J Parasitol 24: 184–191 (in Japanese)
8. Sato Y, Yamashita T, Otsuru M, Suzuki T, Asaishi K, Nishino C (1975) Studies on the etiologic mechanism of anisakiasis. 1. The anaphylactic reaction of digestive tract to the worm extracts. Jpn J Parasitol 24: 192–202 (in Japanese)

9. Asaishi K et al. (1978) Studies on the etiologic mechanism of anisakiasis. 2. Antibody production and histological changes of digestive tract induced by injection of the insolbilized worm extracts. Jpn J Parasitol 27: 65 (in Japanese)

Immune Adherence (IA), Sarles Phenomenon (SP) and Diffusion Chamber Method (DC)

H. Ishikura, Y. Kikuchi, O. Toyokawa, H. Hayasaka, and K. Kikuchi

Introduction

Immune adherence (IA) is an immune response between the antigen, the raw *Anisakis* larva kept under 37.0°C and the patient sera as the antibody, in addition to the frozen powder compliment of guinea pig and human O-type erythrocyte.

Immune-leuco-adhesion (ILA) is another method immune adherence done between raw *Anisakis* larva kept under 37.0°C and immunized abdominal cells sensitized by *Anisakis* larva in the peritoneal cavity of animals (the antibody), in addition to compliments or not. As the result of this method the immune abdominal cells stick to the surface cuticula of raw worm under microscopic observation. This original method was invented by a group in the Department of Pathology, School of Medicine, Hokkaido University, and is called "Hokkaido Univerity-style ILA."

Sarles phenomenon (SP) was first noted by Sarles in 1939. The antigen used in this method is raw thread or hookworm larvae kept under 37.0°C for up to 24 hours, with immunized animals sera as the antibody. This results in a precipitation adherence phenomenon around the os, the anus and an opening of the excretory organ. Studies of SP using *Anisakis* larva was first tried by Morishita and Nishimura (1968, 1969) [3,4] in Japan, followed by other researchers

Table 1. Sarles phenomenon for several allergic diseases (Observation 12 hours later)

Kind of disease	No. of cases	Concentration of patients' sera				
		4x	8x	16x	32x	64x
Intestinal anisakiasis	2	1	2	2	1	1
Provable int. anisakiasis	7	4	2	3	2	0
Ascariasis	2	0	1	0	0	0
Bronchial asthma	11	3	2	0	0	0
Urticaria	1	0	1	0	0	0
Habitual raw fish eater	1	1	0	1	1	0
Healthy man	4	0	0	0	0	0

using experimental animals [5,6] or sera from human intestinal anisakiasis patients [8].

IA and SP are both precipitation tests, but SP is easier than IA and possible to be put into practice by the clinician as well, only requiring the worm to be kept for four days in the incubator.

Diffusion chamber method (DC) has been done only in animal experiments [2,5,6,8] and is used to show cell mediated immunity. In this method the chamber must be put into the abdominal cavity by laparotomy, or tied with a string inset into the stomach of subject, undergoing oral administration for several hours, making it difficult to use this method for human beings.

Immune Adherens (IA) and Immune Leucoadhesion (ILA)

Toyokawa experimented with this method as follows [2]: Five raw larvae were given orally to a guinea pig five times a week, then 2 ml of somatic antigen was injected into the abdominal cavity. In the experiment on rats, at first somatic antigen added adjuvant was injected subcutanously, then five raw larvae were injected into the abdominal cavity three times a week, and finally 2 ml of somatic antigen was injected into the abdominal cavity. The *Anisakis* larvae were collected from Alaska pollack caught in the sea near Iwanai district in winter, with approximately 100 pieces of raw larvae homogenized by 20 ml physiological saline water.

Production method of abdominal cells

(a) normal abdominal cells of guinea pig: 3 ml of 1% glycogen was injected into the abdominal cavity of the normal guinea pig and five days later the abdominal cavity was washed out using 80 ml of Hanks Solution. This solution was centrifuged and the precipitate mass was concentrated until the grade of concentration was 5×10^6 per 1 ml.

(b) immunized abdominal cells of guinea pig: In this case, the production method is almost the same as the above (a) method, but the first injection into the abdominal cavity used somatic *Anisakis* antigen instead of 1% glycogen.

(c) the case experiments of rats: The production method of abdominal cells is almost the same as the case of guinea pigs, but the quantity of injected solution is different, that is, both 1% glucogen and somatic antigen is 1 ml and Hanks solution 40ml.

Experimental technique (the case of ILA test). 1 ml floating solution of abdominal cells, an additional 0.5 ml five times diluted compliment and two pieces of the raw larvae were taken into a flat angle tube for use with phase contrast microscopic observation incubated under 37.0°C and observed regularly from four hours later by microscopy.

Results of the Experiment (Table 2). In IA the human O-type erythrocyte stuck to the surface of the larvae equally and the contact couldn't be broken even by the movement of the larvae.

In ILA, adhesion was increasingly reinforced by the existence of compliment. With the positive ILA contrast test (no compliment) rate 41 %, while the test with compliment was 89%. This adhesion phenomenon looked like one layer at first, but as time passed, grew gradually to multiple layers or a large irregular agglome rate mass (Figs. 1, 2).

Table 2. Immune-leuco-adhesion in guinea pigs (Results 4 hours later)

Kind of levy cells	Normal P.C.	Immune P.C.
Without component	(+++) 0 (+ +) 0 (+) 0 (±) 2 (−) 8	(+++) 0 (+ +) 4 (+) 9 (±) 2 (−) 17
Positive rate	0%	41%
With component	(+++) 0 (+ +) 4 (+) 7 (±) 7 (−) 10	(+++) 7 (+ +) 30 (+) 20 (±) 5 (−) 2
Positive rate	39%	89%

P.C.: Peritoneal cells, Reactions grade: (+++): severe, (+ +): middle, (+): slight, (±): suspected, (−): negative

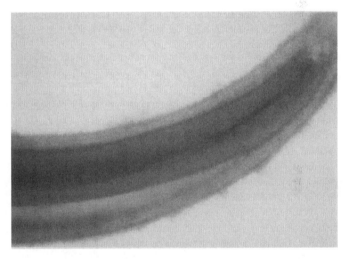

Fig. 1. ILA test (+), A layer of abdominal cells sticks to the surface of the cuticle, and the tissue cells of the larva degenerate

Judgment criteria:
  (−) ------ the precipitate mass didn't stick to the surface of the worm. All normal abdominal cells of guinea pig didn't stick.
  (±) ------ partial layer adhesion in the surface of cuticle
  (+) ------ a diffuse layer of adhesion
  (−)∼(−)- thick-layered ∼ or ∼ accumulate and massive precipitation

The response in rat experiments was slow in comparison with guinea pigs, and judgment was difficult because the non-specific cell agglutinate or adhesive re-

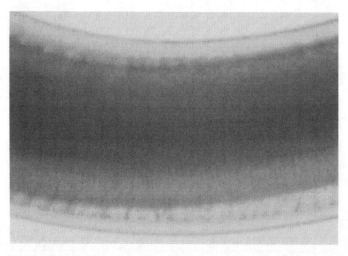

Fig. 2. ILA test (−), No such change as in Fig. 1 of the larva inserted into the hole in the stomach of non-treated animals

sponse in rats which broke out stronger than in guinea pigs, however the tendency of the above described responses were the same in guinea pigs and rats.

Sarles' Phenomenon

Experiments have been carried out on rabbits [3,7,8], and rabbit guinea pigs but only Hayasaka Ishikura et al. have tested using the patient's sera [7,8].

The larva (as the antigen) has been administered orally and subcutanously as well as being injected into the abdominal cavity or somatic antigen given intravenously. Sera taken from several animals with added compliment was intermixed with raw larvae grown under 37°C for three or four days in the hole-slide-glass, and observed by microscope (Fig. 3). Immune sera was diluted multiply researcher and used according to their protocols. Hayasaka et al. decided it appropriate to judge by a 16 times dilution, 12 hours later [7], and done by the size of a deposit around the os, the anus and the opening of excretory organ (Fig. 4).

Some subphenomena were observed at this test, with the recognition of the holdback ecdysis phenomenon of the raw larvae compared with the contrast test [3] and also, the sera which was immunized intensely didn't always respond powerfully under the condition of higher concentration.

It was also reported that the experiment using complement showed a more intense response, and that a feathery mass gathered around the opening of the excretory organ of larva within 2 hours before the Sarles phenomenon appeared (this phenomenon is called "Larval precipitate test") then becoming an irregular scaled form [5]. In this stage the movement of the larvae became slow (this phenomenon is called "Larval immobilization test"). The larvae under this condition was taken into saline where their mobility recovered normally. Larval precipitation (LP) and Larval immobilization (LIB) also appeared in LA and

Fig. 3. SP test, 32-times diluted patients' serum and *Anisakis* larva cultivated under 37°C for 3 days are put into a hole-glass, contained with cover glass, and observed at intervals

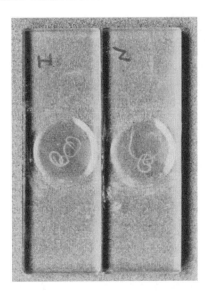

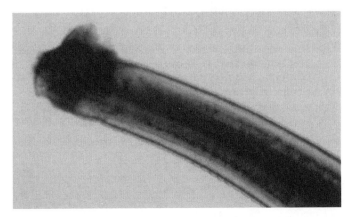

Fig. 4. SP test, 32-times diluted serum, 24 hours later, a strong precipitate product sticks around the mouth of the larva

ILA. The formation of antigen-antibody complex (precipitable mass) and the catching phenomenon of raw larva (immobilization phenomenon) are caused by the reaction of soluble antigens and is one of the host-control responses, which if continued for a long time would cause to the larva die out. These responses are also removed with the collaboration of cell-mediated immunity.

Research done using humans involved the following subjects [7]: 2 cases intestinal anisakiasis confirmed by intestinal reaction; 7 cases of regional ileitis which was possibly anisakiasis; 2 cases of *Ascaris lumbricoides* possessor; 11 cases of asthma bronchiale; one case of urticariasis; one customary raw fish ingester and 4 cases of healthy-looking men who didn't eat raw fish (as controls). Sera was then diluted 16 times of the testee's serum 12 hours following contact between the raw larva and the testee's serum. The positive rate was as follows: Intestinal anisakiasis was 100 %; clinicallly possibe intestinal anisakiasis (regional ileitis) was 42.8%; the customary raw fish ingester was 100 %; the other cases such as the roundworm possessor and healthy men who didn't eat raw fish were all 0% (Table 1).

The studies of the above cases were examined in vitro only, though other research has found the living larva which accompanied the Sarles phenomenon around the opening of the anus and excretory organs of the patient's intestinal wall [10,11].

Diffusion Chamber Method (DC)

This method was tried in order to investigate cell mediated immunity by Aizawa, Kikuchi, Toyokawa (using guinea pigs), Hayasaka, and Ishikura (using rabbits), and supplemented by Suzuki who observed that several cells adhered to the surface of the chamber membrane.

The chamber was put into the abdominal cavity by Aizawa, Toyokawa and Kikuchi, but into the stomach by Hayasaka and Ishikura, all used the HA-type (pore size 0.45μ) chamber. The membrane of these chambers allows soluble antigen such as immunoglobulin to pass through, but not cells, therefore the nature of humoral antibody and that cell mediate immunity could be analyzed clearly.

Material
1. Fresh raw *Anisakis* larvae
2. Abdominal cavity of normal guinea pig
   Abdominal cavity of immunized guinea pig
3. normal abdominal cells (lymphoid cells) of guinea pig
   sensitized abdominal cells (immunized lymphoid cells) of guinea pig
4. Frozen powder guinea pig's complement made by the Hokkaido Institute of Publich Health

Combinate Condition of materials

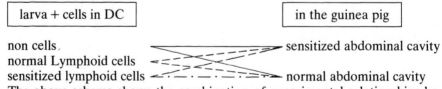

The above schema shows the combination of experimental relationships between the animals whose abdominal cavity were used and the materials which were put into the chamber.

Normally raw larvae put into the abdominal cavity of immunized guinea pigs were killed within 24 hours, but larvae put into the abdominal cavity of normal guinea pigs with the chamber only slowed down their movement after 3–5 days (Table 3). This was caused by the infiltrated fibrin mass, which is not always dependent on immune response, though the infiltration response for the immunized animals was severe (Fig. 5).

Fibrin is included in the host's immune products, larval excretory products and also the antigen-antibody complex, with its reaction being one of the most

Table 3. Larval lesion due to diffsion chamber method (Results 5 days later in guinea pigs)

Kind of levy cells	In the sensitized A.C.		In the normal A.C.	
	Dead larvae	Immobilization	Dead larvae	Immobilization
Non cells	1/6	5/6	1/6	1/6
Non immune P.C.	3/8	4/8	1/8	3/8
Immune P.C.	7/14	7/14	6/14	8/14

A.C.: abdominal cavity, P.C.: peritoneal cells, No. of mumerator is the number of dead or immobilized larvae, No. of denominator is the number of larvae in the diffusion, chamber.

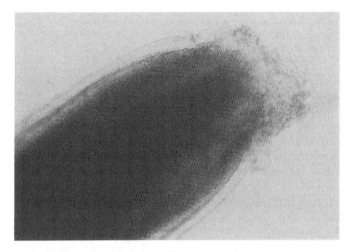

Fig. 5. DC method, oral precipitate reaction in the diffusion chamber

important host defense mechanisms. In the immunized animals, the immune abdominal cells and the raw larva, the oral precipitate mass is hard to leave, (this phenomenon is the same as the SP) (Fig. 6). Furthermore the larval ingestive organs were also damaged (this response is called the intestinal precipitate), and is apt to happen in the case of reinfected intestinal anisakiasis.

In the abdominal cavity of normal guinea pigs, the raw larva and immune lymphoid cells were put with DC, the mobility of the larva slowed down 34% died within 3 days, and 80% within 5 days, caused by cell mediated immunity. This response was more severe than that of the solitary serum antibody, and gave the same result as the combined serous and cell mediated immunity, showing the importance of cell mediated immunity.

Experiments with DC subcutaneously or intraperitoneally have been conducted [7,8], in which adhesion of a large quantity of macrophages was observed, with lymphocyte and neutrophil cells gradually growing to form a granuloma. The chamber has also been placed the intragastric lumen, where it was

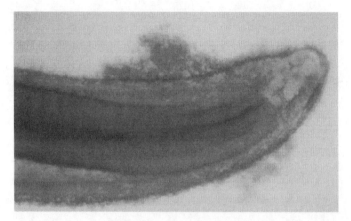

Fig. 6. DC method, a lump of cells sticks near the anus of the larva, and a layer of cells sticks to the surface of the cuticle

observed that neutrophil cells adhered more than intraperitoneally, and in the early stage, adhesion lymphoid cells were recognized [7,8].

In another experiment [9], three pieces of raw larvae were enclosed in the chamber and put into the abdominal cavity of a guinea pig. In the normal guinea pig control a foreign-body reaction occurred, but the immunized guinea pig with the chambered larvae enclosed in the intra-abdominal cavity, showed eosinophil and a few macrophages adhesion onto the chamber membrane surface in an associated foreign-body reaction. However, when the *Anisakis* larva antigen was injected intracutaneously, eosinophil and neutrophil cell adhesion increased, and in these cases the eosinophil cell adhesion was high, but there were few lymphoid cells.

Eosinophilic macrophages increased when immune serum and immune abdominal cells were introduced and immunized passively, with the cell adhesion increasing especially when the immune-soaked cells and the immune serum were put in at the same time. These experiments have all been used to prove that cell-mediated immunity occurred.

Conclusion

Immune Adherence and Sarles' Phenomenon are research methods into the precipitation reaction against raw larva in vitro, while the Diffusion Chamber method is a suitable test to prove cell mediated immunity, which is concerned with the analysis of pathogensis in anisakiasis. IA and SP have been shown to occur in human anisakiasis, and can both be carried out easily by the clinician because of the very simple testing technique. Laboratory raw larvae were bred at room temperature in physiological saline solution for three or four days, but as antigen used for these immune responses were not *Anisakis* specific it was impossible to classify the relative anisakis antibody. Therefore in further research we must pay attention to the cross reaction between *Anisakis simplex* antibody and other anisakidae antibodies.

References

1. Aizawa M (1972) Host response in Anisakiasis. Jpn J Parasitol 17: 255–257 (in Japanese)
2. Toyokawa O (1972) Host immunoligical responses in experimental anisakiasis. Hokkaido J Med Sci 47: 259–265 (in Japanese with English abstract)
3. Morishita Y, Nishimura T (1968) Sarles, phenomenon on *Anisakis* larvae. Jpn J Parasitol 17: 266 (in Japanese)
4. Morishita Y, Nishimura T (1969) Sarles, phenomenon and desheathing inhibition on *Anisakis* larvae, especially in cases of hyper-and reinfections. Jpn J Parasit 18: 355–356 (in Japanese)
5. Aizawa H (1969) Host immunological responses on Anisakiasis. Saishin Igaku 24: 367–372 (in Japanese)
6. Kikuchi K, Toyokawa O, Nakamura K, Ishiyama H, Yokota H, Satoh H, Natori T, Ishikura H, Aizawa H (1970) Immunopathological studies on experimental anisakiasis. Minophagen Medical Review: 54–58 (in Japanese)
7. Hayasaka H, Mizugaki H, Asaishi K, Takagi R, Iwano H, Ishikura H, Aizawa M (1970) Seroimmunological responses on intestinal anisakiasis—especially Sarles phenomenon. Minophagen Medical Review 15: 100–106 (in Japanese)
8. Hayasaka H, Ishikura, Mizugaki H, Ueno T, Utsumi A, Satoh K, Saeki H, Asaishi K, Iwano H. (1971) Experimental immunological and lysis of host responses on Anisakiasis. Saishin Igaku 26: 1786–1800 (in Japanese)
9. Suzuki T, Shiraki T, Kenmotsu M, Otsuru M (1970) Studies on the cell reaction appearing in inflammatory focus on anisakiasis. Minophagen Med Review 15: 93–99 (in Japanese)
10. Inoue Z, Shimizu N, Yoshida Y, Fujii T, Fujita T (1974) Clinical studies on 6 cases of intestinal anisakiasis—particularly 2 cases of intestinal anisakiasis with skip lesions. Clin Surg 29: 808–814 (in Japanese)
11. Fukushima H, Yuge S, Yamakawa Y, Adachi T et al. (1975): A case report of intestinal anisakiasis removed the living worm. J Jpn Soc Clin Surg 36: 721–725 (in Japanese)

Ouchterlony Test and Immunoelectrophoresis

M. Tsuji

In recent years, several laboratories have used immuno-diffusion tests for the diagnosis of anisakiasis. This involved the application of immunoelectrophoresis after preliminary examination by means of the Ouchterlony method, with precipitin bands classified electrophoretically.

Ouchterlony technique. A 0.1% saline worm extract was used as an antigen, and 0.9% agarose in pH 8.2 of veronal buffered saline was employed for the plates. The buffer solution was prepared from 160 grams of sodium veronal dissolved in distilled water to make 10 liters, adding 220 ml of 1N hydrochloric acid to bring the pH up to 8.2. Glass plates (7.5 × 2.5 cm) covered with 3 ml of 0.9% agarose were heated at 85–90°C, and the agar layer allowed to solidify, making two wells with different diameters of 5 mm for the antibody and 2 mm for the antigen. The distance between these two wells was set at 3 mm, and anti-serum was poured into the large well and antigen into the small well. Incubation was done in a moist chamber at room temperature for 12 hours, then at 4°C for a 48 hours period. When the antigen and antibody have diffused to meet each other, several bands at which the relative concentrations permit a precipitate to be found are formed, each corresponding to one antigen-antibody system. After the precipitation bands have developed sufficiently, the plates are washed for 3 days in a physiological solution mixed with a veronal buffered saline, which is changed daily. The plates are then dried and stained by Amido-black 10B.

In immunoelectrophoresis, glass plates (8 × 8 cm) covered with 10 ml of 0.9% agarose were placed in the electrophoretic apparatus so that the filter paper of Whatman No. 1 contacts were immersed in the liquid with a veronal buffered saline solution (pH 8.2, ionic strength 0.05) of the electrode compartments. A saline extract of 0.1% antigen is poured into the well, and the current adjusted to 20 ± 2 volts/8 cm length within a gel, and applied for 3 hours. After electrophoresis is terminated, the serum is concentrated to 1/3 of its original volume, filled to the trough and incubated in a moist chamber for 3 days in the same procedure as Ouchterlony [4].

Immunoelectrophoretic cross reactions between *Anisakis* and other helminths with immunized rabbit sera have been previously described [5]. Some common bands of nematodes do exist, with the strongest reactions observed between the antigen and its homologous anti-sera. After the immunoelectrophoretic absorption technique, band No. 6 which is slightly curved and found in the middle of the antigen well and antibody trough on the negative side of the electrode was

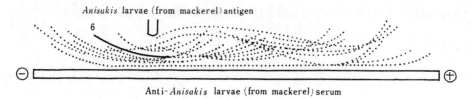

Band No. 6 : Specific for the genus *Anisakis*
Dotted lines : Common bands with other genus antigens

Fig. 1. Antigenic structure and specific band of genus *Anisakis*

recognized as the specific band of genus *Anisakis* (Fig. 1), and was detected in both gastric and intestinal anisakiasis cases. Cross reactions in the immuno-diffusion tests were performed on 12 sero-positive *Anisakis* antigen, cases resulting in antigens of 6 other kinds of helminths being found (Table 1). Nine cases out of 12 showed 1 to 2 bands with *Ascaris suum* female antigen, the 9 cases also displayed 1 to 3 bands with *Toxocara canis* female antigen, 6 cases with *Ascaris suum* male antigen and 3 cases with the antigen of *Dirofilaria immitis* showed 1 to 2 bands, but the antigens of *Fasciola hepatica* and *Taenia saginata* did not show any reaction with those sera in Ouchterlony. In immunoelectrophoresis, 10 cases out of 12 showed 1 to 3 bands with *Ascaris suum* female antigen and 9 cases with the antigen of *Toxocara canis* female showed 1 to 3 band, but the antigen of *Fasciola hepatica* were negative. No cross reaction with trematode and cestode antigens in the sera of sero-positive cases with *Anisakis* antigen were observed in either Ouchterlony or immunoelectrophoresis.

Table 1. Cross reactions in immuno-diffusion tests for sero-positive cases with *Anisakis* antigen

0.1 % NaCl extract antigens	1	2	3	4	5	6	7	8	9	10	11	12	
Ouchterlony													
Anisakis larvae	2[a]	6	2	2	4	3	5	4	3	4	6	2	12/12
Ascaris suum (F)	0	2	1	1	1	0	2	1	1	2	1	0	9/12
Ascaris suum (M)	0	1	1	0	1	0	2	0	0	1	1	0	6/12
Toxocara canis (F)	0	3	1	1	1	1	1	1	0	2	1	0	9/12
Dirofilaria immitis	0	2	0	0	1	0	0	0	0	0	1	0	3/12
Fasciola hepatica	0	0	0	0	0	0	0	0	0	0	0	0	0/12
Taenia saginata	0	0	0	0	0	0	0	0	0	0	0	0	0/12
Immunoelectrophoresis													
Anisakis larvae	3	6	3	2	5	3	6	4	3	4	7	2	12/12
Ascaris suum (F)	1	3	2	1	2	0	2	1	1	2	2	0	10/12
Toxocara canis (F)	0	3	1	1	2	1	2	1	0	2	2	0	9/12
Fasciola hepatica	0	0	0	0	0	0	0	0	0	0	0	0	0/12

[a] Numbers of bands.

Ouchterlony Test and Immunoelectrophoresis 185

As a routine examination 247 samples from patients who had eosinophilia and/or gastro-intestinal complaints after raw fish intake were tested by Ouchterlony and immunoelectrophoresis. A total of 140 samples out of 247 (56.7%) were positive for *Anisakis* antigen, and of the 140, there were 18 with rebound tenderness in the lower part of the abdomen or lower abdominal pain 1 to 3 days after eating raw mackerel, indicating a diagnosis of intestinal anisakiasis. Six out of the 18 cases were examined periodically, with all of the serological tests becoming negative on days 32 to 125. Determination of a complete cure for anisakiasis is very difficult, and reinfection with cannot be excluded among the patients. However, the numbers of precipitin bands in the patients Ouchterlony and immunoelectrophoretic tests show a tendency to decrease as time passes, and become negative within 18 months.

Cross reaction studies of helminthic antigens with several immune diseases have shown that antibodies which precipitated with nematode antigens were detected by Ouchterlony and immunoelectrophoresis in the sera of some patients with inflammatory bowel diseases (Table 2) [6–7]. The serum concentration of *Ascaris suum* protein from patients with helminthiasis and gastro-intestinal diseases was measured by a reliable and sensitive radio-immunoassay [1,3] with high concentrations observed in sera from patients with ulcerative colitis and Crohn's disease, but almost all patients with other gastro-intestinal diseases were within the range observed for controls. The etiology and pathogenesis of inflammatory bowel disease are still unknown. Recently, *Ascaris suum* protein antigenic substance has been found in intact rat and human colonic mucosa, leading to speculation that the findings of *Ascaris suum* protein antigenic substance in sera of patients with inflammatory bowel diseases reflects a

Table 2. Results of Ouchterlony in the sera of ulcerative colitis patients by several helminthic antigens

Antigen	No. exam.	No. posit.
A. suum (F)	123	29
A. suum (M)	120	33
T. canis	122	28
D. immitis	123	41
Anisakis larvae	123	28
Nematodes	123	47 (38%)
F. hepatica	123	17
F. elongatus	123	6
Trematodes	123	18 (15%)
D. latum	70	9
D. caninum	123	20
T. saginata	76	10
Cestodes	123	23 (19%)
Total	123	47 (38%)

186 M. Tsuji

cellular product released from colonic mucosa during active inflammation cross-reactive with nematodes protein [2]. However, other interpretations of this interesting finding cannot yet be ruled out, with the pathogenetic significance of the inflammatory bowel disease remaining to be clarified.

In conclusion, Ouchterlony and immunoelectrophoresis tests are very useful for the diagnosis of anisakiasis and the criteria of cure, by periodical observation of antibody titers. Immuno-diffusion tests should be conducted simultaneously with several helminthic antigens.

References

1. Tanaka K, Miyachi Y, Tsuji M, Miyoshi A (1978) Radioimmunoassay for *Ascaris* specific protein and its clinical approach to gastro-intestinal diseases. Jpn. J. Gastroenterol 75: 1832–1839 (in Japanese)
2. Tanaka K, Kawamura H, Tohgi N, Tsuji M, Hirabayashi N, Yamada H, Miyachi Y, Miyoshi, A (1981) The analysis of immunologically similar substance with *Ascaris suum* specific protein in rat colon mucosa. Jpn. J. Gastroenterol 78: 1606–1612 (in Japanese)
3. Tanaka K, Kawamura H, Tohgi N, Tsuji M, Miyachi Y, Miyoshi A (1983) The measurement of *Ascaris suum* protein by radioimmunoassay in sera from patients with helminthiasis and with gastrointestinal diseases. Parasitology 86: 291–300
4. Tsuji M (1974) On the immunoelectrophoresis for helminthological researches. Jap J Parasitol 23: 335–345 (in Japanese)
5. Tsuji M (1987) General remarks, Serological and Immunological studies on gastric anisakiasis, Gastric anisakiasis in Japan, Springer, Tokyo. p. 89–95
6. Tsuji M, Kimura K (1979) Immuno-serological reaction with nematodes antigens in patients sera of ulcerative colitis. Rinsho Kensa 23: 927–932 (in Japanese)
7. Tsuji M, Yokogawa M (1974) Immunological diagnosis of helminthic infections. In Proceedings of the SEAMEO/Tropical Medicine and Technical Meeting, Harinasuta C (ed) pp. 180–196

Immunodiagnosis for Anisakiasis with Detection of IgE Antibody to Human Anisakiasis by Enzyme-Linked Immunosorbent Assay

Y. Takemoto, M. Tsuji, and Y. Iwanaga

Studies on the production of reaginic antibodies in infections of *Anisakis* larvae in man, have shown that allergic reactions caused by infection of *Anisakis* larvae were due to Type-I allergic reactions in experimental animals [1], while larval re-infection was expected to induce an allergic especially Type-I reaction. Therefore the diagnosis of anisakiasis by enzyme-linked immnosorbent assay (ELISA) has used the values of IgE in patient sera.

0.1% NaCl extract of *Anisakis* larvae was used as the antigen, with sera obtained from 66 patients complaining of abdominal pain after eating raw fish, including 28 cases in which the *Anisakis* larvae were detected morphologically. Twenty-nine sera which were negative for any antigens of helminths by Ouchterlony were used as controls and also did not indicate any leukocytosis and eosinophilia.

ELISA was performed in polystylene tubes (13×72 mm), with the optimal serum dilution found to be $1:30$ in phosphate buffered saline (PBS). For coating procedures, 0.5 ml of antigen with a protein concentration of 20 μg/ml in carbonate buffer (pH 9.6) was added to each tube, then incubated at 4°C overnight and washed five times with PBS.

Sera diluted with 0.02M PBS (pH 7.3) containing 0.5% BSA and 0.05% Tween 20 (PBS/BSA/T) were then added to the tubes, followed by incubation at 37°C for 2 hours and then washed five times with PBS. After washing, 0.5 ml peroxidase-labelled rabbit anti-human IgE ($1:1,000$ dilution) conjugated in PBS/BSA/T was added and incubated at 37°C for 2 hours. The excess conjugate was removed by washing five times with PBS, and then added into each tube to react with 0.5 ml of substrate solution prepared by dissolving 0.4% o-phenylenediamine containing 0.012% H_2O_2 in McIlvain buffer. After incubation at 37°C for 30 minutes in a dark room, the colour reaction was stopped by the addition with 0.5 ml of 3.67N-H_2SO_4. The absorbance in each tube was read as 492 nm.

Specific IgE values of anisakiasis were measured as follows;

$$A = (\bar{X} - B) \times \frac{0.229}{Sn - B} \times 1000$$

A: Specific IgE values
$\bar{X}$: The mean of absorbance values of samples in OD_{492}
B: Blank value
Sn: Absorbance value of the standard sample for the nth measurement
0.229: Absorbance value of $S_1 - B$

Table 1. Values of *Anisakis* specific IgE in sera from patients.

		Number of cases	M ± SE[b]
Control		29	64 ± 6
Patients with abdominal pain after eating raw fish			
	Ouchterlony (+)[a]	41	93 ± 9
	Ouchterlony (−)	25	82 ± 10
	Total	66	89 ± 7
Patients with detected larvae			
	Ouchterlony (+)	15	110 ± 15
	Ouchterlony (−)	13	81 ± 11
	Total	28	97 ± 9

[a] Result with *Anisakis* larva antigen by Ouchterlony
[b] Mean ± Standard error

Ouchterlony was done according to the techniques of Tsuji (1974) on 0.9% agarose L in veronal buffered saline (pH 8.2) [2]. With anisakiasis specific IgE values in patients sera show in Table 1. In 66 patients 41 suffered from abdominal pain after eating raw fish and were positive for Ouchterlony, and IgE values of these positive patients were significantly higher than that of the control sera. On the other hand, 15 out of 28 patients in which larvae were detected by surgical operation were positive for Ouchterlony, and they also showed higher IgE values than that of the control sera. Although IgE values were negative for Ouchterlony positive cases, these values were significantly higher when compared with the control sera.

Examination of specific IgE values in the sera of anisakiasis, 6 out of 28 patients which had larvae detected were tested. Two cases were already positive for Ouchterlony at the time when the presenting symptoms occurred, though IgE values were still lower (Fig. 1). However, the IgE values of these two cases increased after 12 and 50 days from the presenting symptoms. Another four cases were not significantly changed in IgE values though Ouchterlony became positive.

In another series, the values of *Anisakis* specific IgE in patients sera with a high total of IgE (100–23,000 IU/ml) were examined in 25 sera, which also showed negative results with all helminthic antigens by Ouchterlony. The average of the *Anisakis* specific IgE was 69 ± 9 (mean ± standard error), not a significant result compared with that of the control sera (Table 2). It was therefore demonstrated that *Anisakis* antigen used in this study reacted with *Anisakis* specific IgE, indicating that the Type-I allergic ansakiasis reaction was related to *Anisakis* specific IgE in the patients sera by reinfections.

In immunodiagnostic studies of anisakiasis using ELISA, in 7 out of 8 cases in which larvae were detected values of IgA were increased, but 2 out of 6 cases of IgE increased patient sera were decreased afterward [3], but the specific IgE values were changeable in relation to the symptoms of patients. In particular, IgE values were different with primary and secondary infections, suggesting that

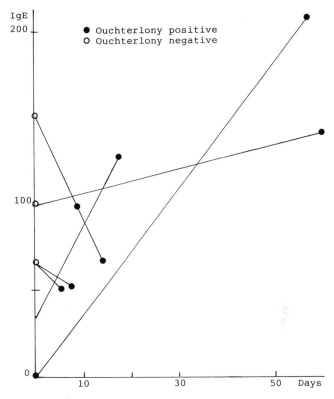

Fig. 1. Changes of *Anisakis* specific IgE values in the sera of anisakiasis

Table 2. Values of *Anisakis* specific IgE in sera with high total IgE

No. of sera[a]	Total IgE (IU/ml)	Specific IgE	No. or sera	Total IgE (IU/ml)	Specific IgE
1	23,184	30	15	2,685	38
2	17,952	61	16	2,600	95
3	12,000	93	17	2,263	170
4	6,500	137	18	2,251	44
5	5,535	82	19	2,000	50
6	5,150	0	20	1,770	30
7	4,500	117	21	1,664	83
8	4,300	30	22	1,400	39
9	4,000	185	23	1,300	64
10	3,467	6	24	1,000–2,000	15
11	2,950	65	25	1,700–1,900	65
12	2,950	38			
13	3,000	111	Average	n = 25	69 ± 9
14	2,800	71	Control	n = 29	64 ± 6

[a] All cases showed negative results with helminthic antigens by Ouchterlony

190   Y. Takemoto et al.

IgE antibodies had different antigenicities according to the primary or secondary infections.

Semi-determination of *Anisakis* larvae crude antigen specific IgE in human serum was performed by enzyme linked immunosorbent assay (ELISA) in order to study the relationship between anisakiasis and anaphylaxis. Using the Ouchterlony method, significantly higher values of specific IgE were obtained from the sera with precipitin bands of *Anisakis* larvae crude antigen than from the control sera, with especially high values obtained from the sera of anisakiasis patients.

To study the role of crude antigen for ELISA coating in immunodiagnosis, a crude antigen was fractionated into six parts on a Sephadex G-200 column. Antigen determinant fractions of sera from five patients were investigated by ELISA, and were shown to be different according to the individual sera.

Finally, it seems possible to diagnose anisakiasis by measurement of specific IgE values detected in serum of primary and secondary infections using more purified antigens.

Summary

The detection of specific *Anisakis* IgE antibodies in human sera was employed for the immunodiagnosis of anisakiasis by enzyme–linked immunosorbent assay ELISA with values of *Anisakis* specific IgE in patients sera which were positive for the Ouchterlony method significantly higher than that of the control sera.

Determination was made for changes of specific IgE values in the sera of six patients whose *Anisakis* larvae were detected by surgical operation. The values of two cases were lower though Ouchterlony was found to be positive at the time when the presenting symptoms occurred. These 2 cases, however, had their IgE values increase after 12 and 50 days. The other four cases had negative Ouchterlony results at the time of the first examination, but became Ouchterlony positive 5–65 days later. The values of IgE in the sera detected as both negative and positive for Ouchterlony were not significantly changed.

References

1. Sato Y, Yamashita T, Otsuru M, Suzuki T, Asaishi T, Nishino C (1975) Studies on the etiologic mechanism of anisakiasis. 1. The anaphylactic reaction of digestive tract to the worm extracts. Jpn J Parasitol 24: 192–202 (in Japanese)
2. Tsuji M (1974) On the immunoelectrophoresis for helminthological researches. Jpn J Parasitol 23: 335–345 (in Japanese)
3. Yoshimura H, Kondo K, Onishi Y, Akao N (1983) Studies on immunodiagnosis of the diseases by heterotopic parasitism of helminthes. Report for Scientific Research (No. 56750159) for the Ministry of Education, pp. 13–27 (personal publication, in Japanese)

Detection of Cellular Immunity by Migration Inhibition Test on Rabbits and Guinea Pigs Immunized with *Anisakis* Larval Antigens

Y. KIKUCHI, H. SAEKI, and H. ISHIKURA

It is well documented that cell-mediated immunity (CMI) plays an important role in the protection of the host against parasite infections. Some earlier workers detected the development of CMI from several Protozoa [1–3], Schistosoma [4–6] or Trichina worm [7], Echinococcus infections [8–10] and others [11,12] by the appearance of delayed type hypersensitivity skin reactions and/or CMI in vitro reactions.

Although several immunological investigations of anisakiasis [13–15] have been reported, only a few papers have discussed mechanisms of cell-mediated immunity to anisakiasis [16], and no reports have investigated CMI to *Anisakis* larval antigens quantitatively by macrophage migration inhibition test. In previous in vivo studies [14] on skin or digestive tract reactions against antigens of *Anisakis* larvae, an immediate and a delayed type of reaction were observed. These reactions were elicited by different types of antigens: soluble or insoluble parts of *Anisakis* larvae, respectively, which were extracted by saline from larval homogenate. The histological findings of digestive tracts affected by *Anisakis* larva seem to show allergic reactions of the Arthus type (acute phase) and delayed type (chronic or granuloma phase) [13], possibly indicating that cellular immunity plays a role in the chronic granulomatous phase of anisakiasis.

In this paper, cell-mediated immunity, especially in vitro macrophage migration inhibition reaction (MI-reaction) [17], is described according to Saeki's data [16] using experimental anisakiasis of guinea pigs and rabbits.

Guinea pigs (Hartley) and rabbits (closed colony) of both sexes were immunized with whole antigens prepared from frozen and dried *Anisakis simplex* larvae (type I) after washing with saline. The extraction method of the half-purified antigens was as follows: 1) extracted antigens: suspension was prepared by Veronal buffered saline (VBS antigen), Unger solution (SOM antigen) or 0.85% saline (PSS antigen) after extraction by ether 2) metabolic antigen (ES antigen): after live larvae were kept in saline for 4-days the saline supernatant was centrifuged and dialyzed with distilled water, followed by freezing and drying. These antigens were filtrated with Milipore filter (pore size 0.25 μ) before use. Antigenic concentration was determined by Lowry's method [18]. The animals were subcutaneously sensitized with whole antigens with complete adjuvant twice in a week and then used one week after the last injection of antigens. Other animals were subcutaneously sensitized with whole antigens without adjuvant 3 times a week and finally with a booster injection of antigens one week before sacrificing.

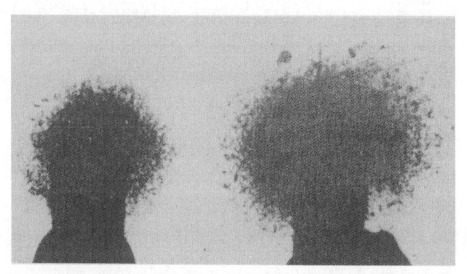

Fig. 1. MI test by peritoneal guinea pig macrophages sensitized by whole *Anisakis* larval-antigens. Right: control MI test without antigens in culture chamber, left: experimental MI test added 25 mg/ml of VBS antigen in culture chamber

The method of skin reaction was as follows; 0.02 ml of various antigens in PBS (200 mg/ml) was injected intradermally in the back of the guinea pigs and rabbits and then the dermal reaction was measured chronologically. The peritoneal cells of the guinea pigs, which contain macrophages and lymphocytes, were washed out by heparinized PBS 4 days after injection with 20–30 ml of 20% Nutrose (Nakarai Kagaku Co. Jpn.) in PBS. The collected macrophages were washed 3 times with PBS. The alveolar macrophages of the rabbits were collected by washing the lungs through the trachea with heparinized PBS and the cell suspension was prepared by centrifugation after 3 washes.

Macrophage migration inhibition (MI) assay included the following two methods: 1) **direct method** (to detect sensitized lymphocytes which mediate migration inhibition factor, MIF); after the final washing and resuspending of the cells in a final concentration of 10^7/ml, the cells were packed into hematocrit capillaries which were sealed by flame at one end. After centrifugation at 800 rpm for 1 minute, these capillaries were cut at the liquid-cell interface. The MI test was performed in a small culture chamber which were filled with MEM culture medium containing 10% FCS. For the experimental group, test antigens were added at required concentrations. After 48 hours culture at 37°C in 5% of CO_2 saturated condition, the migrated area of cultured cells was measured microscopically in two dimensions and compared with control chambers with no test antigens (Figs. 1 and 2). 2) **indirect method** (to detect MIF induced by sensitized lymphocytes); lymphocytes from sensitized animals were cultured with *Anisakis* antigens in vitro for 48 hr, the culture supernatant collected and centrifuged at 3,000 rpm for 30 min. The MI test used macrophages of unimmunized normal animals and culture supernatant of sensitized experimental and/or normal control lymphocytes, with the migrated area measured by the same method as the direct one.

Detection of Cellular Immunity by Migration Inhibition Test

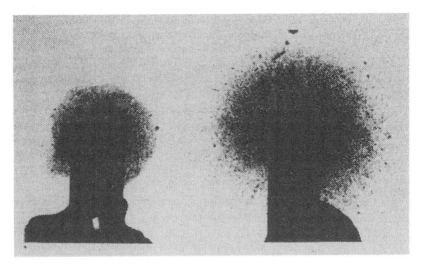

Fig. 2. MI test by alveolar rabbit macrophages sensitized by whole *Anisakis* larva antigens. Right: control MI test without antigen in culture chamber, left: experimental MI test with 25 mg/ml of VBS antigen in culture chamber

Calculation of migration index; the average migration area of triple chambers should be calculated as follows:

$$\frac{\text{Migration area in antigen-added chamber}}{\text{Migration area in antigen-less chamber}} \times 100$$

Results: The direct method of the MI test on alveolar macrophages from sensitized rabbits indicated positive inhibition by various values (Table 1). When guinea pigs were immunized with various antigens with or without adjuvant, peritoneal macrophages showed marked inhibition in the MI test (Table 2). The MI phenomenon of macrophages from sensitized guinea pigs revealed a dose–response relationship such that when 5–50 mg/ml of VBS, SOM and PSS antigens were used, significant differences were observed in MI values, (Fig. 3), however, the macrophages of normal unsensitized animals did not show inhibition. When rabbits were sensitized with three kinds of antigens with adjuvant, no differences were observed in the MI assay (Fig. 4). There were no significant

Table 1. Migration index of alveolar macrophages from sensitized rabbits

In vitro antigen	Dose mg/ml	Migration index (%)					Aver. ± SD
		Exp. 1	Exp. 2	Exp. 3	Exp. 4	Exp. 5	
VBS	25	36.8	9.3	12.7	44.8	45.6	29.8 ± 17.6
	10	62.3	20.8	15.1	67.1	60.4	45.2 ± 25.0
SOM	25	38.2	5.0	14.2	46.2	49.2	30.6 ± 19.8
	10	49.3	21.9	14.2	65.6	60.4	42.3 ± 23.0
ES	25	38.5	6.1	11.4	41.9	48.0	29.2 ± 19.1
	10	49.9	5.1	15.0	65.6	60.1	39.1 ± 27.4

Table 2. Migration index of peritoneal macrophages from sensitized guinea pigs

In vitro Antigen	Dose mg/ml	Migration index (%) Exp. 1	Exp. 2	Exp. 3	Exp. 4	Exp. 5	Exp. 6	Aver. + SD
VBS	50	41.0			29.9	49.3		40.1 + 19.4
	25	49.7			39.0	65.5		51.4 + 10.9
SOM	50		44.4		29.0		60.2	44.5 + 22.1
	25		47.9		38.1		61.6	49.2 + 16.7
PSS	50			41.8		58.0	62.2	54.6 + 15.3
	25			48.0		52.1	69.0	56.4 + 15.7

Fig. 3

Fig. 4

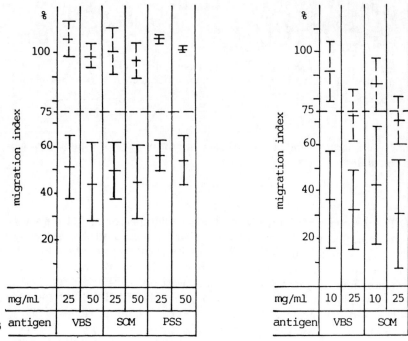

Fig. 3. Migration index of peritoneal macrophages from normal (——) and sensitized (——) guinea pigs

Fig. 4. Migration index of alveolar macrophages from normal (——) and sensitized (——) rabbits

parallel relationships between MI values and sedimentation reaction serum antibody levels, however the maximum erythema reaction, 24–48 h after antigen presentation, were in parallel with the MI test, especially when VBS antigen were used in the guinea pigs after antigen presentation (Fig. 5). There was no such relationship between the values of skin reaction and macrophage migration inhibition in the rabbit.

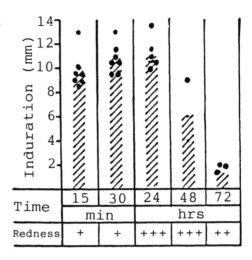

Fig. 5. Skin reaction of sensitized guinea pigs by VBS antigen

Table 3. Indirect migration inhibition test by peritoneal macrophages from normal guinea pigs

In vitro Antigen	Dose mg/ml	Migration index (%)			Aver. + SD
		Exp. 1	Exp. 2	Exp. 3	
VBS	50	58.6	64.4	56.4	59.8 + 5.8
SOM	50	57.6	65.2	57.5	60.1 + 6.2

On the indirect method of MI test by the spleen cell supernatant from sensitized guinea pigs, the MI assay using normal macrophages was markedly inhibited (Table 3), except in rabbits, compared with the supernatant from normal spleen cells, indicating that the lymphocytes of guinea pigs sensitized with *Anisakis* antigens in vitro produced macrophage migration inhibition factor (MIF). In the indirect MI assay, the effects of human MIF against macrophages of guinea pigs indicated no species-specificities in general, thus the clinical status of Anisakiasis could be assessed by the indirect method.

Discussion

The clinical course and histopathological findings of gastric and/or intestinal anisakiasis show two phases; a fulminant and mild form. The fulminant form is observed as a type I and/or type III allergic reaction with extensive edema, fibrinoid swelling in the submucosa and angitis-like lesions. On the other hand, it is suggested that especially from the second through the fourth stage, these histopathological findings show host reaction against parasitic antigens by eosinophilia with destructive worms in the center of these lesions [13]. Analyses have been made in host immune reactions against larval antigens clinically [19] and experimentally [20] using humoral antibodies such as immunoelectrophoresis, sedimentation reaction, hemagglutination reaction and immunofluorescein method. Although there are a few reports of cell-mediated immune reaction to anisakiasis, there are very few on skin reactions [21], diffusion chamber method or, immune adherence [20]. Also, though the role of cell-mediated immunity has been studied in diseases, Anisakiasis has not been explained quantitatively in this respect. For example, in leishmaniasis [2,3], shistosomiasis [6], trichinosis [22] and anisakiasis, delayed hypersensitivity has already been observed by skin reaction, and the defense mechanism against larval reinfection has been investigated experimentally by cell-mediated immunity, such as passive transfer or blast formation, using lymphoid cells in guinea pigs [8], rats [5], mice [2,3] and others [9,11,12].

A few reports of macrophage migration inhibition assay discussing cell-mediated immunity in amoebiasis [1], trichinosis [7] and shistosomiasis [4] have been published. Macrophage migration inhibition factor(MIF) is one of the lymphokines proposed by Dumonde in 1969 [23], and is produced by sensitized T cell lineages detectable in culture supernatant only when sensitized T cells are cultured with the same antigens. The molecular weight of MIF has been reported [24] to be 25,000. The migration inhibition mechanism has been explained as followed; when MIF receptors on macrophages, made of α-L-fucose become bound, membrane adhesiveness is elevated and the motility of the macrophages is depressed by aggregation and clumping between macrophages. The migration inhibition assay index, using antigens such as VBS, SOM and PSS antigen, indicates significant dose-dependent inhibition taking part in the immune phenomenon, especially cell-mediated immunity for the development of anisakiasis. On the other hand, no relationship between serum antibody level and MI index was noted, while there was a strong relationship between the delayed-type skin reaction and the MI test using peripheral blood of shistosomiasis patients [12]. A significant relationship between delayed-type skin reaction and the in vitro MI test in guinea pigs has been found, but not in rabbits.

In Anisakiasis, the major role of cell-mediated immunity in vivo could be explained as the defense mechanism against the antigen of infected worms. Since the chemical nature of parasitic antigens is very complicated, parasitic infection can be considered as xenogeneic transplantation with the in vivo reaction corresponding to a rejection reaction by cell-mediated immunity. MIF and other kinds of lymphokines could interact with macrophages in the affected lesion and the immune reaction to parasitic infection depending on both the life cycle and structures of parasites. In *Anisakis* larva migrans in man, cell-mediated immunity takes several days to kill larvae, so *Anisakis* larvae could have considerable action as pathogens. In our previous report, reinfected *Anisakis* larvae in rabbits died earlier than in the primary infection and were also highly destructed in mice infected with *Trichinella spiralis* [22].

The significance of cell-mediated immunity in Anisakiasis seems to be essentially as a rejection mechanism against parasites acting as foreign bodies and it is suggested that allergic tissue damage by cell-mediated immunity could control the pathological status of parasitic disease.

References

1. Haq A, Sharma A, Ahamad S (1984) Increased macrophage migration inhibition factor production in hamsters sensitized by amoebic antigen and glycan. Parasitic Immunology 6: 391–396
2. De Rossell RA, Bray RS, Alexander J (1987) The correlation between delayed hypersensitivity, lymphocyte activation and protective immunity in experimental murine leishmaniasis. Parasite Immunology 9: 105–115
3. Fahey JR, Herman R (1981) Relationship between delayed hypersensitivity response and acquired cell-mediated immunity in C57BL/6J mice infected with *Leishmania donovani*. Infection and Immunity 49: 447–451
4. Stephen W, Boros DL, David CS (1983) Regulation of granulomatous inflammation in murine schistosomiasis. 11. T suppresser cell-derived, I-C subregion-encoded soluble suppressor factor mediates regulation of lymphokine production. J Exp Med 157: 219–230
5. Auriault C, Balloul J, Pierce RJ, Damonneville M, Sondermeijer P, Capron A (1987) Helper T cells induced by a purified 28-kilodalton antigen of *Schistosoma mansoni* protect rats against infection. Infection and Immunity 55: 1163–1169
6. Lewis FA, Winestock J, James SL (1987) Macrophage activation as an immune correlate to protective immunity against Schistosomiasis in mice immunized with an irradiated, cryopreserved live vaccine. Infection and Immunity, 55: 1339–1345
7. Palmas C, Conchedda M, Bortoletti G, Gabriele H (1985) In vitro cellular immune response in mice and rabbits immunized with *Trichinella spiralis* antigen. Parassitologia 64: 216–222
8. Phillips SM, Fox EG (1984) Immunopathology of parasitic disease: a conceptual approach. Contemp Top Immunobiol 12: 421–461
9. Vuitton DA, Lassegue A, Miguet JP, Herve P, Barale T, Seilles E, Capron A (1984) Humoral and cellular immunity in patients with hepatic alveolar echinococcosis. A 2 year follow-up with and without flubendazole treatment. Parasite Immunology 6: 329–340
10. Al-Kahalidi NW, Barriga OO (1986) Cell-mediated immunity in the prepatent primary infection of dogs with *Echinococcus granulosus*. Veternary Immunology and Immunopathology 11: 73–82
11. Blundell-Hasell SK (1974) Cellular immunity to *Nippostrongylus brasiliensis* in the rat. 11. Influence of infection dose on the production of migration inhibitory factor in vitro. Int Arch Allergy 47: 95–101
12. Green BM, Gbakima AA, Albiez, Taylor HR (1985) Humoral and cellular immune responses to *Onchocerca volvulus* infection in humans. Reviews of Infectious Disease 7: 789–795
13. Kikuchi Y, Ishikura H, Kikuchi K, Hayasaka H (1989) Pathology of gastric anisakiasis. Gastric Anisakiasis in Japan. Epidemiology, Diagnosis, Treatment. Ishikura H, Namiki M (eds) Springer, Tokyo, pp. 117–127
14. Kikuchi Y, Ueda T, Yoshiki T, Aizawa M, Ishikura H (1967) Experimental immuno-pathological studies of intestinal anisakiasis. Igaku No Ayumi 62: 731–736 (in Japanese)
15. Kojima K, Koyanagi T, Shiraki K (1966) Pathological studies of anisakiasis (parasitic abscess formation in gastrointestinal tracts). Jpn J Clin Med 24: 134–143 (in Japanese)
16. Saeki H (1975) Studies on cell-mediated immunity in experimental anisakiasis. J Sapporo Medical College 44: 309–322 (in Japanese)
17. George M, Voughan J (1962) In vitro cell migration as a model for delayed hypersensitivity. Proc Soc Exp Med 111: 514–521
18. Lowry OH, Roserough NJ, Farr AL, Rondall RJ (1956) Protein measurement with Folin phenol reagent. J Biol Chem 193: 265–275

19. Akao N, Yoshimura H (1989) Latex agglutination test for immunodiagnosis of gastric anisakiasis. Gastric Anisakiasis in Japan. Epidemiology, Diagnosis, Treatment. Ishikura H, Namiki M (eds) Springer, Tokyo, pp 97–102
20. Kikuchi K, Toyokawa O, Nakamura K, Ishiyama H, Yokota H, Sato H, Natori T, Ishikura H, Aizawa M (1970) Immunopathology of experimental anisakiasis. Minophagen Medical Review 15: 54–58 (in Japanese)
21. Saeki H, Mizugaki H, Ishikura H, Hayasaka H (1972) Immunological studies on Anisakiasis 11. Participation of immune response in host-tissue reaction and destruction of parasite bodies. Hokkaido J Med Sci 47: 541–550 (in Japanese)
22. Larsh JE Jr, Weatherly NF (1974) Studies on delayed (cellular) hypersensitivity in mice infected with *Trichinella spiralis* 1X Delayed dermal sensitivity in artificially sensitized donors. J Parasitology 60: 93–98
23. Dumonde DC, Wolstencroft RA, Panayi GS, Matthew M, Morley J, Howson WT (1969) "Lymphokines": Non-antibody mediators of cellular immunity generated by lymphocyte activation. Nature 224: 38–42
24. David JR, Schlossman SF (1968) Immunochemical studies on the specificity of cellular hypersensitivity. J Exptl Med 128: 145–1458

Measurement by ELISA of *Anisakis*-Specific Antibodies of Different Immunoglobulin Classes in Paired Sera of Gastric Anisakiasis

N. AKAO

Introduction

Anisakiasis is a common disease among Japanese people who eat raw marine fish such as mackerel, squid, and cod. Accordingly, an accurate infection rate is unclear. From January 1985 to February 1988, 384 sera were received for immunological test, of which thirty-three were parasitologically proven cases. Parasites from the remainder could not be detected with gastro-endoscopy, although their symptoms were strongly suspicious of invasion by *Anisakis* larva in the gastrointestinal wall. Therefore, serological testing is an important tool for the diagnosis of this disease.

Previous workers reported that raw marine fish were widely consumed in Japan; therefore, sensitization to *Anisakis* antigen commonly existed in the Japanese [1], and a high percentage of normal individuals were found to have "background" antibody levels, confusing the interpretation of serological results. In this paper, an enzyme-linked immunosorbent assay (ELISA) with a horseradish peroxidase (HRP) conjugated protein A was employed to determine the specific antibodies of different immunoglobulin classes against *Anisakis* antigen.

Materials and Methods

Antigen. Larval somatic antigen of *Anisakis simplex* was prepared by the methods described previously [2], in which the second stage larvae were collected from mackerel (*Pneumatophorus japonicus*), were washed thoroughly with phosphate buffered saline (PBS, pH 7.2), and were then frozen and dried. These worms were pulverized with mortar and pestle, resuspended in PBS, then centrifuged at 10,000 xg for 60 min, with the resulting supernatant recovered and lyophilized.

Sera of patients and control. Specific antibodies to *Anisakis* antigen were determined on the following four groups: A) 30 parasitologically proven gastric anisakiasis, B) 30 clinically suspected cases, C) 30 people aged 40 to 60, who often eat raw marine fish, D) 30 healthy females at the age of 19 and 20. In a follow-up study, the sera from 8 proven cases of the group A and 6 females of the group D were taken one month after the first examination. ELISA titer was calculated for each test sample as follows;

$$P/N \text{ ratio} = \frac{OD_{510} \text{ of test serum} - OD_{510} \text{ of background}}{OD_{510} \text{ of control serum} - OD_{510} \text{ of background}}$$

Control serum consisted of the pooled sera of 28 adult males who had no antibody to *Anisakis* antigen by Latex agglutination test [2].

Procedure of protein A-ELISA. Specific antibodies of different immunoglobulins were determined with ELISA using HRP conjugated protein A derived from *Staphyloccocus aureus* (Cappel, CA, USA), the plate (Cook #1-220-24) then sensitized with the antigen (20 μg/ml in carbonate buffer, pH 9.6) at 37C overnight. Test serum was diluted 1:800 with PBS supplemented with 1% bovine serum albumin (PBS-BSA), and anti-human IgG (heavy chain specific), IgM and IgA were purchased from Cappel Products (CA, USA). These second antibodies were diluted 1:500 in PBS-BSA. One hundred μl of third antibody, HRP conjugated protein A, were added to each well, and incubated for 1hr at 37C. After washing with PBS-Tween (0.5% Tween 20 in PBS), substrate solution containing 0.5 mg/ml of O-phenylenediamine supplemented with 0.003% H_2O_2 in 0.05 M citrate phosphate buffer, pH 5.0 was added each well, and the reaction stopped with 50 μl of 8N H_2SO_4 in each well.

Results and Discussion

Antibody responses and mean levels of antibodies in proven cases, suspected cases, high risk group, and healthy control group are shown (Fig. 1), (Table 1). It was of interest to note that IgA antibody was raised in 8 (26.7%) cases in group A and 12 (40.0%) in group B, a significant increase. On the other hand, no significant elevation of IgA antibody was observed in group D, while some individuals in group C had relatively high P/N ratio's of IgA antibody.

As to IgM antibody, one proven case showed high P/N ratio (P/N $\geqq$ 2.1). The distributions of the antibodies and the mean antibody levels of IgG and IgM in group C were almost the same as in group D, and elevation of IgG antibody was seen in one case of group A, with similar results noted in group B. The level of IgG antibody of group B was as low as the level of the high or poor risk group.

To evaluate IgA antibody in *Anisakis* infection, 8 sera of the proven case were taken one month after the first examination, and their specific antibodies measured by Protein A-ELISA. The IgA antibody increased markedly compared to IgG or IgM, with the exception of one case, which had shown a high IgA antibody at the first examination (Fig. 2).

The IgM antibody levels of some proven cases was raised in the second examination to the same degree as the IgG antibody level found one month after

Table 1. The results of ELISA of *Anisakis*-specific antibodies of three immunoglobulin classes in the sera of the four groups

Group	IgG	IgM	IgA
A	1.15 ± 0.27	1.10 ± 0.28	1.77 ± 0.77
B	1.30 ± 0.52	2.08 ± 1.17	3.43 ± 3.28
C	0.97 ± 0.31	1.19 ± 0.42	1.18 ± 0.42
D	0.75 ± 0.25	1.36 ± 0.43	0.86 ± 0.19

Measurement by ELISA of *Anisakis*-Specific Antibodies

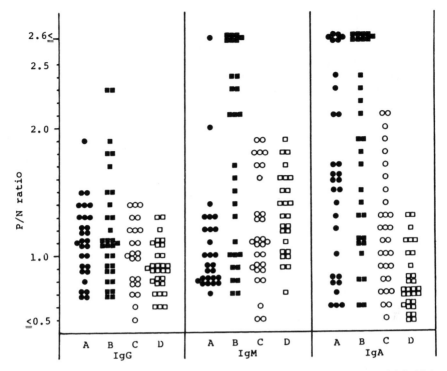

Fig. 1. Distribution of specific antibody titers in serum of proven (●), suspected (■), high risk group without symptoms (○), and control (□)

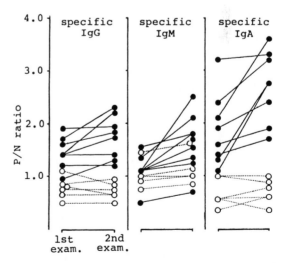

Fig. 2. Changes of specific antibody titers in paired sera of proven cases (●), and control (○)

the first examination. It has been documented that detection of specific antibody, especially that of IgM, is essential to understand the time course of infection in some parasitic diseases [3]. Generally, IgM antibody to antigen can be detected in serum before the appearance of IgG antibody, however, the present results showed that IgM antibody rose together with IgG antibody in the patients sera at the 2nd examination. This data suggested that determination of IgM antibody was not a reliable index of current infection with *Anisakis* larva. In contrast, the proven and suspected cases showed a good IgA antibody response against *Anisakis* antigen, suggesting the parasite may primarily stimulate an immune reaction in the gastro-intestinal wall of the host.

It is argued that dimeric IgA in mucus secretion plays an important role in the prevention of intestinal pathogens such as *Trichinella spiralis*, from invading host tissue [4], however, serum IgA exists as a monomeric. The function of serum IgA antibody has not been clearly understood; however, this antibody may act as an effective barrier against parasitic infection at the gastro-intestinal phase, and IgA-mediated antibody dependent cell mediated cytotoxcity (ADDC) might be involved in the destruction of third-stage larvae of *Nippostrongylus braziliensis* [5].

Few studies have been made on the value of diagnosis of serum IgA antibody level in parasitic infection. In some strains of mice multiply infected with *Nematospiroides dubius*, a fourfold increase of IgA antibody has been observed in comparison with uninfected mice [6], while Trophozoites of *Giardia muris*, parasitized on the intestinal mucus membrane of infected mice, also stimulated their local immune system, and IgA antibody was detected in their sera by solid-phase RIA [7]. Furthermore, a prolonged IgA response was observed in the patients with *T. spiralis* [8]. The relationship between *Anisakis* and immunoglobulins, particularly IgA in sera of anisakiasis patients has remained unsolved, however, our study by means of protein A-ELISA on paired patients sera suggests that *Anisakis* infection may provide a potent stimulus for the systemic synthesis of IgA antibody. Based on our results, it is considered likely that the measurement of IgA antibody has a role in the diagnosis of human anisakiasis.

Type I anaphylaxis reaction appears to be involved in *Anisakis* infection, with IgE antibody in the sera of patients with gastric anisakiasis rapidly raised after onset [9–11]. Further investigation into immune responses involving the different classes of immunoglobulins in sera are required to further clarify the entity of human anisakiasis.

References

1. Suzuki T, Ishida K, Ishigooka K, Doi K, Otsuru M, Sato R, Asaishi K, Nishino C (1975) Studies on the immunological diagnosis of anisakiasis. 5. Intradermal and indirect hemagglutination tests, and histopathological examination of biopsied mucous membranes on gastric anisakiasis. Jpn J Parasitol 24: 184–191 (in Japanese)
2. Akao N, Yoshimura H (1988) Latex aggulutination test for immunodiagnosis of gastric anisakiasis. In: Ishikura H, Hayasaka H (eds) Advances of gastric anisakiasis in Japan (in press)
3. Krahenbuhl JL, Remington JS (1982) The immunology of toxoplasma and toxoplasmosis. In: Cohen S, Warren KS (eds) Immunology of parasitic infections 2nd ed., Blackwell Scientific Publications, Oxford, London, pp. 356–421

Measurement by ELISA of *Anisakis*-Specific Antibodies

4. Crandall RB, Crandall CA (1972) *Trichinella spiralis*: Immunologic response to infection in mice. Exp Parasitol 31: 378–398
5. Befus D, Bienenstock J (1984) Induction and expression of mucosal immune responses and inflammation to parasitic infections. Contemporary topics in immunobiology Vol. 1 In: Marchalonis, JJ (ed) Immunobiology of parasites and parasitic infections. Plenum Press, New York, pp. 71–108
6. Williams DJ, Behnke JM (1983) Host protective antibodies and serum immunoglobulin isotypes in mice chronically infected or repeatedly immunized with the nematode parasite *Nematospiroides dubius*. Immunology 48: 37–47
7. Anders RF, Roberts-Thomson IC, Mitchell GF (1982) Giardiasis in mice: analysis of humoral and cellular immune responses to *Giardia muris*. Parasite Immunol 4: 47–57
8. Knapen FVan Franchimont JF, Verdonk AR, Stumpf J, Undeutsh K (1982) Detection of specific immunoglobulins (IgG, IgM, IgA, IgE) and total IgE levels in human trichinelosis by means of the enzyme-linked immunosorbent assay (ELISA). Am J Trop Med Hyg 31: 973–976
9. Desowitz RS, Rayborne RB, Ishikura H, Kliks MM (1985) The radioallergosorbent test (RAST) for the serological diagnosis of human anisakiasis. Trans R Soc Trop Med Hyg 79: 256–259
10. Tachibana M, Yamamoto Y (1966) Serum anti-Anisakis IgE antibody in patients with acute gastric anisakiasis. Jpn J Diges Dis 83: 2132–2138 (in Japanese)
11. Nakata H, Tachibana M, Sakamoto Y, Morita M, Okazaki K, Yamamoto Y, Yamamoto Y, Ito K (1986) Analysis of antigens defined by anti-Anisakis larvae IgG and antibodies in sera of patients with gastric anisakiasis. Jpn J Diges Dis 83: 2456 (in Japanese)

Detection of Anti-*Anisakis* Antibody of IgE Type in Sera of Patients with Intestinal Anisakiasis

Y. YAMAMOTO, H. NAKATA, and Y. YAMAMOTO

Introduction

Intestinal anisakiasis had been little understood when Ishikura [1,2] described its clinical, pathological and immunological aspects. Following this, about 150 cases of intestinal anisakiasis were reported by 1974 [2,3] in which patients mostly suffered from intestinal obstruction which required surgery. Swollen and hemorrhagic small intestine lesions were demonstrated with an *Anisakis* larva's head penetrating into the mucous membrane. Colonic anisakiasis, however, has been infrequently reported, with only 20 cases reported by 1985 [2–6].

In many case of intestinal anisakiasis, it was very difficult to pre-operatively establish the diagnosis. Only in Hasegawa's report [6] were *Anisakis* larvae recognized endoscopically in the large intestine, but it was not ascertained clinically whether the larvae caused intestinal anisakiasis or were only present incidentally. Because of infrequent endoscopic examination, serological diagnostic procedures are very important for the clinical diagnosis of intestinal anisakiasis. We have attempted to measure serum anisakis-specific antibody of IgE isotype by radioallergosorbent test (RAST) using tissue extracts of *Anisakis* larvae (type 1) as antigen, to evaluate whether RAST is useful diagnostic test for intestinal anisakiasis [17].

Materials and Methods

1. Blood samples. Sera were obtained successively from two patients with intestinal anisakiasis and stored at $-20°C$.
2. *Anisakis* antigens. *Anisakis simplex* larvae collected from various fishes were homogenized in PBS by Polytron (Kinematica Co.). A soluble antigenic extract was prepared after centrifuging at 20,000 G for 1 hour.
3. Assay of anti-anisakis IgE antibody. Anti-anisakis IgE antibody was measured by radioallergosorbent test (RAST), according to Miyamoto's method [7]. In this paper disks (Toyo Filter Paper Co.) of 4 mm in diameter were activated and coupled with *anisakis* antigens (1 mg/ml), then incubated with 0.1 ml of 1/100 or 1/1,000 diluted serum overnight at room temperature and washed with PBS containing 0.1% Tween 20. Disks were next incubated with 0.05 ml (over 50,000 CPM) of ^{125}I-rabbit anti-human IgE (Daiichi Isotope) overnight at room

206   Y. Yamamoto et al.

temperature and washed with the same buffer. They were counted by gamma-counter and each sample assayed in triplicate.

High-titered sera (from patients of acute gastric anisakiasis) were used for generating a calibration curve and a highest-titer was assigned arbitrarily as 10,000 units of specific antibody, against which all sera tested and calculated for their content of *Anisakis* antibodies of IgE type.

4. SDS-PAGE and immunoblotting. Sodium dodecyl sulphate-polyacrylamide gel electrophoresis (SDS-PAGE) of *Anisakis* extracts were performed according to Laemmli [8] in a 7.5% separation gel and a 3% stacking gel. The antigenic extracts were prepared at a concentration of 2 mg/ml, diluted 1/1 with SDS-dye cocktail (125 mM Tris-HCl, pH6.8 containing 4% SDS and 10% beta-mercaptoethanol) and warmed at 60°C for 10 min. The samples were then run at a concentration of 20 micrograms/3 mm-sample well width, electrophoresis being completed in 1.5 hours, after which, one part of gel was stained with Coomassie brilliant blue R-250.

The electrophoretic blotting was carried out as described by Towbin et al. [9], with antigens transferred to a nitrocellulose membrane using an Electrotransfer Blotting Apparatus (Marysol Ltd.) for 4 hours at 4–10°C. The nitrocellulose membrane was soaked in Tris buffered saline (TBS, pH8.0) containing 8% BSA and 0.3% Tween 20 for 1 hour, and then in TBS containing 10% rabbit-serum and 0.1% BSA for 1 hour for quenching of non-specific adsorption. The membrane was then cut into strips, numbered and incubated individually with 5.0 ml of a 1/10 or 1/20 diluted serum, rocking overnight at 4°C. The strips were washed with TBS 5 times each for 5 min, and incubation with ^{125}I-rabbit anti-human IgE was carried out overnight at 4°C, with subsequent washings done as described above. IgE binding bands were visualized autoradiographically by using a New RX film (Fuji Film), the optimal exposure time ranging between 16 to 32 hours.

To assign a molecular weight to each radioactive band, a calibration curve was plotted by using standard molecular weight markers which were run simultaneously.

Case reports

Case 1. T.M. (Fig. 1) A 44 year old woman suddenly had abdominal pain 6 hours after ingestion of raw fish. On hospital admission, examination revealed a temperature of 37.5°C, tenderness in the epigastrium, a white blood cell count of 8,700, positive serum C-reactive protein, and plain film of the abdomen revealing many intestinal fluid levels. She underwent an operative laparotomy the next day, with the preoperative diagnoses of small intestinal obstruction.

A small amount of yellowish-brown ascites were noted in the abdominal cavity. A 20 cm length of jejunum, from 360 cm to 380 cm of Treitz's ligament, was indurated and hemorrhagic on the serosa, with oral-sided intestinal dilatation up to 100 cm of Treitz's ligament. Resection of a 40 cm-long piece of jejunum was performed including the indurated 20 cm-long lesion, where the intestinal wall was thickened and the lumen was narrowed and obstructed by stagnant inflammatory excretion and debris (Fig. 2).

On gross appearance, the mucous membrane of the narrow portion had thickened Kerckring folds, was edematous and partly eroded, but no *Anisakis* larva

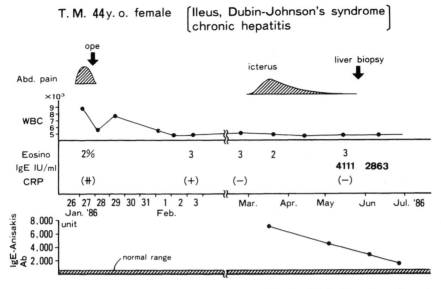

Fig. 1. Clinical course of Case 1

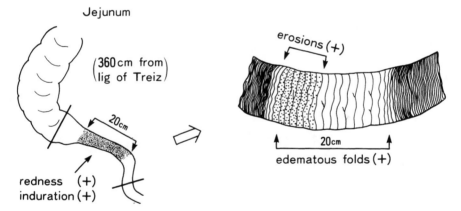

Fig. 2. Schema of resected jejunum (Case 1)

were discovered (Fig. 2). Microscopic findings revealed epithelial erosions, slightly edematous change with eosinophilic infiltration in the mucosal layer (Fig. 3a), and severe edema with massive infiltration of eosinophils in the submucosa (Fig. 3b). Pathological diagnosis was acute nonspecific inflammation with severe eosinophilic infiltration, and the clinical course after admission is shown (Fig. 1).

Case 2. T.Y. (Fig. 4) A 45 year old man had epigastralgia and heart burn a day after eating raw fish. On admission, examination revealed an elastic, hard mass in the right lower quadrant of the abdomen, with laboratory findings showing a

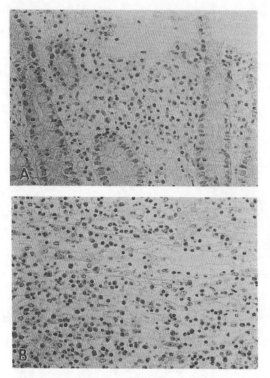

Fig. 3. Microscopic findings of the jejunum (Case 1) **A** Note epithelial erosions, and edema with eosinophilic infiltrations in the mucosal layer. **B** Note massive eosinophilic infiltrations and edema in the submucosa

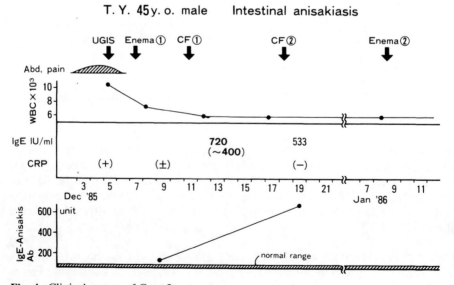

Fig. 4. Clinical course of Case 2

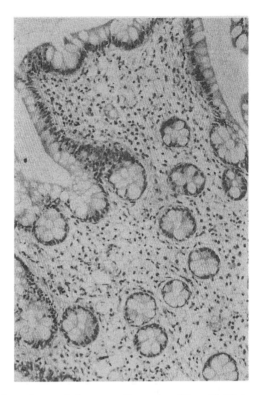

Fig. 5. Microscopic findings of biopsied specimen of the ascending colon (Case 2). Note edematous mucosa with moderately increased eosinophilic infiltrations

leukocytosis of 10,700, positive CRP and positive occult fecal blood. Barium-meal and barium-enema studies revealed a normal stomach and small intestine, but luminal narrowing with irregular mucosal surface in the middle 1/3 of the ascending colon. Colonofiberscopic findings showed inflamed and edematous mucosa with multiple erosions, and the biopsied specimen had acute non-specific inflammation with moderate infiltration of eosinophils in the mucosa. The clinical course after admission is shown (Fig. 5).

Results

1. RAST assay. CPM vs stepwise dilutions of a high-titered serum from a patient with acute gastric anisakiasis (10,000 units) was plotted for generating a calibration curve (Fig. 6).

In case 1, the titers of serum anti-*Anisakis* IgE antibodies were measured as 7,000, 4,500, 3,500, 2,800, 1,500 units on the 60th, 106th, 120th, 140th and 154th day from onset, respectively (Fig. 1). In case 2, the titers were measured as 75 units on the 6th day and 610 units on the 16th day from onset (Fig. 4).

2. SDS-PAGE and immunoblotting. Two sera (one serum from case 1, measured as 7,000 units of IgE-*Anisakis* antibody and the other from case 2, mea-

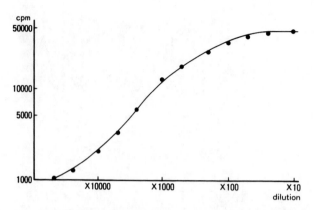

Fig. 6. Dilution curve of serum anti-*Anisakis* IgE antibody

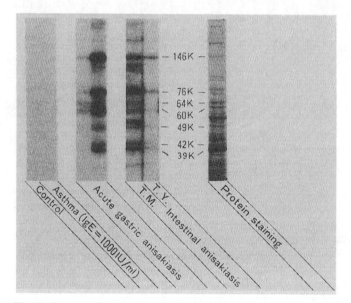

Fig. 7. Immunoblotting of *Anisakis* larva extracts by sera of patients with intestinal anisakiasis (Case 1 and 2)

sured as 610 units) were analysed by Western blotting. Sera of acute gastric anisakiasis with titers of 1,800 and 7,400 units were also analysed as controls. Multiple bands of 146k, 76k, 64k, 60k, 49k, 42k and 39k (kilodaltons) were visualized autoradiographically with sera of case 1 and 2, which were similarly observed with two sera of acute gastric anisakiasis (Fig. 7).

Discussion

It is widely accepted that serum total IgE levels are high in human helminthic infections [10]. In the experimental *Nippostrongylus brasiliensis* infection of the mouse, potentiation of anti-hapten IgE response, and potentiation of non-specific IgE production were observed, with carrier-specific helper T cells mediating the latter process [11,12]. However in human intestinal anisakiasis, total serum IgE was not confirmed to be elevated clinically, and parasite-specific antibody of IgE type has never been assayed, though in acute gastric anisakiasis patients, IgE anisakis antibody has been measured by radioallergosorbent test (RAST) [13], and ELISA [14–16]. *Anisakis* simplex-specific IgE antibody has been reported in all sera of 5 patients with parasitologically confirmed and clinically suspected anisakiasis [13], and specific IgE antibody was increased in 6 (75%) of 8 patients sera in comparison with the sera before the illness [14]. Specific IgE antibodies (n = 28) showed significantly higher values than those from control serra (n = 29) [15], while anti-*Anisakis* IgE antibodies were detected in 4 (80%) of 5 sera of patients 3 to 4 weeks after onset but none (0%) of 2 sera on the first day of illness [16].

We also reported by using RAST [17,18] that single or serial measurements of anti-*Anisakis* IgE antibodies were useful in the diagnosis of acute gastric anisakiasis.

In single assays (Fig. 8), 17 of 20 patients (85%) with acute gastric anisakiasis showed high titers ranging 30 to 3,000 units and 3 of 9 patients (33%) with *Metagonimiasis yokogawai* infection and 1 of 7 patients (14%) with allergic diseases (3 with bronchial asthma, 4 with allergic rhinitis) showed slightly higher titers (30–54 units). In Nankoku city where acute gastric anisakiasis is prevalent, 18 of 70 healthy general inhabitants (26%) and 9 of 29 patients (31%) with

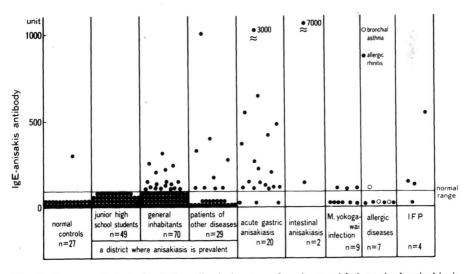

Fig. 8. Serum anti-*Anisakis* IgE antibody in sera of patients with intestinal anisakiasis (Case 1 and 2) and other diseases

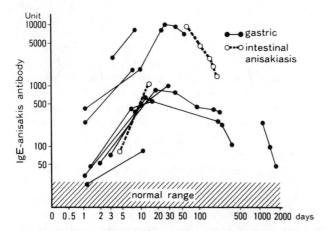

Fig. 9. Serial measurements of anti-*Anisakis* IgE antibody (Case 1 and 2)

miscellaneous diseases (peptic ulcer, chronic gastritis, gall stone etc.) showed high levels, ranging from 30 to 1,000 units. They had not had any episodes of severe abdominal pain suggesting of intestinal anisakiasis before, but none of 49 junior high school students in the city showed abnormal levels. In 27 staff members (normal controls), only one (4%) showed a high titer, who had experienced no episodes of anisakiasis.

The cross-antigenicity of *Anisakis* homogenate to other Nematode extracts has been reported [19], which may explain the slightly high titers observed in sera of patients with Metagonimiasis, and the high titers demonstrated in sera of healthy inhabitants might result from other unknown Nematode infections, or these people may have experienced one or more latent *Anisakis* infections.

In the serial measurements in acute gastric anisakiasis (Fig. 9), specific IgE antibody in sera of patients showed mostly high titers (27–500 units) or partly normal (0–26) on the 1st–3rd day of illness, which increased rapidly to their maximal levels on the 30–60 day (500–10,000 units), and stayed at the maximal levels up to the 6–8 months, decreasing very gradually.

Though the rapid increase of specific IgE antibody may be a secondary phenomenon to *Anisakis* infection, it is noteworthy that the specific IgE antibody was detected in most cases in the earliest stage of the illness (on the 1st to 3rd day), suggesting that the very early specific IgE reaction may be a secondary response and acute gastric anisakiasis means a re-infection, clinically associated with allergic reactions in the stomach. Investigation of specific IgG, IgM and other antibodies will shed more light on the pathogenesis of acute gastric anisakiasis.

On the contrary, unlike the patients with acute gastric anisakiasis, the high titers shown in healthy general inhabitants and patient-centrols, did not change or slightly decreased during the next 1 to 24 weeks (Fig. 10), which may suggest that the sero-positive subjects or patients without acute gastric anisakiasis may have experienced one or more latent *Anisakis* or other Nematode infections.

Serial measurements of IgE *anisakis* antibody revealed that in case 1 (small intestinal anisakiasis) the 7,000 u. titer on the 60th day of illness decreased gra-

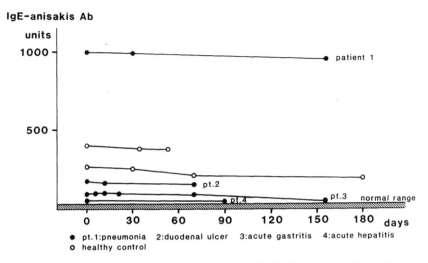

Fig. 10. Serial measurements of anti-*Anisakis* IgE antibody in sero-positive subjects without overt anisakiasis

dually to 1,400 u. by the 154th day, and in case 2 (colonic anisakiasis) the titer increased rapidly from 75 u. on the 6th day to 610 u. on the 16th day. These changes seems to be similar to those observed in acute gastric anisakiasis (Fig. 9).

The serial response of the *Anisakis* specific IgE in the clinical course of intestinal anisakiasis is similar to that observed in the course of acute gastric anisakiasis, and to catch a rapid increase in IgE *Anisakis* antibody in the early stage of the illness is thought to be very useful for the diagnosis of intestinal anisakiasis.

Moreover, IgE response to *Anisakis* larvae was qualitatively analysed by using the immunoblotting method. In the two patients with intestinal anisakiasis, IgE response to large numbers of antigens (146k, 76k, 64k, 60k, 49k, 42k, 39k-proteins) were demonstrated, and the antigens detected in sera from intestinal anisakiasis were mostly identical to those detected in sera from acute gastric anisakiasis (Fig. 9). To identify each of these antigens and to determine whether *Anisakis*-hemoglobin [19] is implicated as one of the target-antigens will be part of the on-going research [20,21].

In intestinal anisakiasis, specific IgE response in the early phase may also be a secondary phenomenon to *Anisakis* infection, with further elucidation on the role of specific IgE antibody in the pathogenesis of intestinal anisakiasis required.

Conclusion

Anti-*Anisakis* antibody of IgE isotype has been detected in sera of two patients with intestinal anisakiasis using the RAST assay and specific antibodies analysed by Western immunoblotting. We concluded that:

214 Y. Yamamoto et al.

a) In two cases of intestinal anisakiasis, anti-*Anisakis* IgE antibody rapidly increased in the early 1–2 weeks, and gradually decreased through the late 8–22 weeks of the illness. The time-response of anti-*Anisakis* IgE antibodies was very similar to that seen in acute gastric anisakiasis.

b) Through the qualitative analysis of *Anisakis* antigens detected in sera from intestinal anisakiasis patients, the IgE response against a large numbers of antigens was confirmed. Each of these antigens was mostly identical to those detected in sera from acute gastric anisakiasis.

c) Serial measurements of serum anti-*Anisakis* IgE antibody were very useful in the diagnosis of intestinal anisakiasis as well as acute gastric anisakiasis.

References

1. Ishikura H, Hayasaka H, Kikuchi Y (1967) Acute regional ileitis at Iwanai in Hokkaido, with special reference to intestinal anisakiasis. Sapporo Med J 32: 183–196
2. Ishikura H (1968) Clinical and immunopathological studies on anisakiasis. Hokkaido Med J 43: 83–99 (English abstract)
3. Iwano H, Ishikura H, Hayasaka A (1974) Epidemiological study on anisakiasis in Japan during recent five years. Geka Shinryo 16: 136–1342 (in Japanese)
4. Oshio T, Nishii H, Harada T, Usuya N, Ogawa K (1973) A case of anisakiasis in the sigmoid colon. Geka Shinryo 15: 207–210 (in Japanese)
5. Nishikawa M, Horie Y, Takeda H, Kaga K, Hiyoshi Y, Iwanaga Y, Gomyoda M (1981) A case of colonal obstruction due to Anisakis infection. Jpn J Gastroenterol 78: 154 (in Japanese)
6. Hasegawa H, Miyagi S, Otsuru M (1985) Anisakiasis confirmed by endoscopic examination of the large intestine. Jpn J Parasitol 34: 37–40
7. Miyamoto T, Mano K, Ito K, Tomiya Y, Horiuchi Y (1973) Radioallergosorbent test (RAST) using paper disc. Arerugy 22: 584–593 (English abstract)
8. Laemmli UK (1970): Cleavage of structural proteins during the assembly of the head of bacteriophage T4. Nature 227: 680–650
9. Towbin H, Staehelin T, Gordon J (1979) Electrophoretic transfer of proteins from polyacrylamide gels to nitrocellulose sheets: Procedure and some application. Proc Natl Acad Sci USA 76: 4350–4354
10. Araki T, Nakazato H, Ikoma K (1976) Studies on the immunity in parasitic diseases. 1. Serum IgE levels in helminthiasis and those changes after treatment. Jpn J Parasitol 25: 153–160 (English abstract)
11. Kojima S, Ovary Z (1975) Effect of *Nippostrongylus brasiliensis* infection on antihapten IgE antibody response in the mouse. 1. Induction of carrier specific helper cells. Cell Immunol 15: 274–286
12. Kojima S, Ovary Z (1975) Effect of *Nippostrongylus brasiliensis* infection on antihapten IgE antibody response in the mouse. 2. Mechanism of potentiation of the IgE antibody response to a heterologous hapten-carrier conjugate. Cell Immunol 17: 383–391
13. Desowitz RS, Raybourne RB, Ishikura H, Kliks MM (1985) The radioallergosorbent test (RAST) for the serological diagnosis of human anisakiasis. Transactions Roy Soc Trop Med Hyg 79: 256–259
14. Yoshimura H (1983) Studies on the immunological diagnosis of diseases caused by heterotopic (migrating) helminthic infections. Reports of Research Works supported by Grants-in-aids for Scientific Research from the Ministry of Education, Science and Culture of Japan in 1982 (56570159) (in Japanese)
15. Takemoto Y, Tsuji M (1985) Detection of *Anisakis* larvae crude antigen specific IgE by means of enzyme–linked immunosorbent assay. Arerugi 34: 403–410 (English abstract)

Detection of Anti-*Anisakis* Antibody of IgE Type 215

16. Takahashi S, Sato N, Sato T, Takami T, Ishikura H, Mukaiya M, Yajihashi A, Tsurushiin M, Hayasaka H, Kikuchi K (1986) Detection of anti-*Anisakis* larvae antibodies using micro–ELISA method. Igaku no ayumi 136: 691–692 (in Japanese)
17. Yamamoto Y, Tachibana M, Okazaki K, Sakaeda H, Yamamoto Y (1984) IgE-*Anisakis* antibody in the sera of patients with acute gastric anisakiasis. Jpn J Gastroenterol 81: 1489 (in Japanese)
18. Tachibana M, Yamamoto Y (1986) Serum anti-*Anisakis* IgE antibody in patients with acute gastric anisakiasis. Jpn J Gastroenterol 83: 2132–2138 (English abstract)
19. Tsuji M (1974) On the immunoelectrophoresis for helminthological researches. Jpn J Parasitol 23: 335–345 (English abstract)
20. Suzuki T, Shiraki T, Otsuru M (1969) Studies on immunological diagnosis of anisakiasis. 2. Isolation and purification of *Anisakis* antigen. Jpn J Parasitol 18: 232–240 (English abstract)
21. Nakata H, Yamamoto Y, Yamamoto Y (1990) Analysis of antigens defined by anti-*Anisakis* larvae antibodies of IgE and IgG type in the sera of patients with acute gastrointestinal anisakiasis. Jpn J Gastroenterol 87: 762–770 (English abstract)

Development of Monoclonal Antibodies Reacting with *Anisakis simplex* Larvae

S. TAKAHASHI, A. YAGIHASHI, N. SATO, and K. KIKUCHI

Anisakiasis is a common disease in Japan, since people eat raw fish as sushi and sashimi. Sushi is also becoming very popular in the United States and in some European countries with anisakiasis found in these places also, although the frequency is much lower when compared to Japan. The diagnosis of ansakiasis can be made from the history of eating raw fish, in addtion to physical findings, though such a final clinical diagnosis is not easy even with the development of gastrofiberscopical examination of patients. Furthermore, it is known that this disease becomes more complicated when it continues as a chronic from [1], with lesions frequently consisting of various sized granuloma formations with different degrees of fibrosis and inflammatory cells [2]. It is also more difficult to correctly diagnose anisakiasis of the small intestines, since it is usually difficult to see the whole length of intestines in the fiberscopical examinations.

The establishment of serodiagnosis using intestinal and gastric anisakiasis patients sera is obviously important, not only from the clinical point of view but also for investigating the immunobiological profile of the pathological development of anisakiasis. These approaches have been attempted and reported by several laboratories, however, it has been difficult to obtain a successful result with respect to specificity. That is, the assay system cross-reacts with sera from patients infected with other parasites, though it is reasonable to anticipate that monoclonal antibodies (mabs) reacting specifically against *Anisakis simplex* larvae could break through this problem.

We developed such mabs by hybridizing HAT sensitive mouse myeloma cell NS-1 with spleen cells of mice immunized with *Anisakis simplex* larvae, namely An1 through An7 [3]. These mabs could react specifically with *Anisakis simplex* larvae except An6, which also reacted weakly with *Ascaris suum*, (Table 1), and they did not react with *Pseudoterranova decipirens* larvae, *Toxocara cati*, *Trichinella spiralis*, *Echinococcus multilocularis*, and *Dirofilaria immitis*. Table 2 summarizes the localization of antigens detected by mabs in frozen sections of *Anisakis simplex* larvae, and indicate that these mabs could recognized different antigenic epitopes present on *Anisakis simplex* larvae. Therefore, it seems that mabs could be a powerful tool to dissect and analyze the immunobiological development of anisakiasis and the roles of each specific antigen detected by each mab.

Among antigens detected by mabs, excretory-secretory (ES) antigen seems important from an immunobiological point of view because it may add to the pathological development of anisakiasis, with An1, An2 and An6 reacting with

Table 1. The reactivity of monoclonal antibodies against various parasites and human tissues

Par. \ MoAb	An1	An2	An3	An4	An5	An6	An7	5A5	13C6	14B2
Anis.	+	+	+	+	+	+	+	+	+	+
Asc.	−	−	−	−	−	±	−	+	+	+
Pt.	−	−	−	−	−	−	−	+	+	−
T.C.	−	−	−	−	−	−	−	nd*	nd	nd
T.S.	−	−	−	−	−	−	−	nd	nd	nd
E.M.	−	−	−	−	−	−	−	nd	nd	nd
D.I.	−	−	−	−	−	−	−	nd	nd	nd
Hum.	−	−	−	−	−	−	−	nd	nd	nd
Ig	IgGI	IgGI	IgM	IgGI	IgM	IgGI	IgM	IgA	IgGI	IgGI

Par.: Parasites and human tissues, Anis.: *Anisakis simplex* larvae, Asc.: *Ascaris suum*, Pt.: *Pseudoterranova decipiens*, T.C.: *Toxocara cati*, T.S.: *Trichinella spiralis*, E.M.: *Echinococcus multilocularis*, D.I.: *Dirofilaria immitis*, Hum.: Human tissues. *: not determined. Ig: isotype of monoclonal antibodies

Table 2. Summary of the localization of antigens detected by monoclonal antibodies in frozen sections of *Anisakis simplex* larvae

MoAb	muscle	pseudocoel	R-cell	intestine	E-S antigen
An1	+	−	+	−	+
An2	+	±	+	+(m)	+
An3	+	±	±	−	−
An4	+	±	+	±	−
An5	+	+	−	−	−
An6	+	−	±	+(c)	+
An7	−	−	+	+(m)	−

+ : positive, − : negative, m: membrane, c: cytosole, R-cell: Renette cell

ES antigen on the frozen section of *Anisakis simplex* larvae, although only An2 could react with this antigen when produced and secreted into the supernatant within 48 hr of larvae culture (Fig. 1). ES antigen seems to very rapidly be denatured, losing the determinant detected by An2. The antigenic epitopes recognized by An1 and An6 already appear to be destroyed, and these two mabs could not react with ES antigen in the culture supernatant of *Anisakis simplex* larvae. This data suggests that An2 is a powerful mab for establishing a specific serodiagnosis system for anisakiasis, and using micro-ELISA method, we are now further developing this specific system.

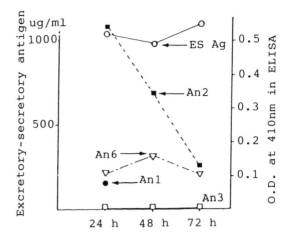

Fig. 1. The reactivities of monoclonal antibodies against ES antigen in micro-ELISA. An1 (●), An2 (■), An3 (□) and An6 (▽). Protein content in ES antigen was determined by the method of Lowry et al. (○)

References

1. Ashby BT, Appleton PJ, Dawson I (1964) Eosinophilic granuloma of gastro-intestinal tract caused by herring parasite *Eustoma rotundatum*. BMJ 1: 1141–1145
2. Tanaka J, Torisu M (1978) *Anisakis* and eosinophil. I. Detection of a soluble factor selectively chemotactic for eosinophils in the extract from *Anisakis* larvae. J Immunol 120: 745–749
3. Takahashi S, Sato N, Ishikura H (1986) Establishment of monoclonal antibodies that discriminate the antigen distribution specifically found in *Anisakis* larvae type I. J Parasit 72: 960–962

Serodiagnosis of Intestinal Anisakiasis Using Micro-ELISA—Diagnostic Significance of Patients' IgE

S. Takahashi, A. Yagihashi, N. Sato, and K. Kikuchi

Introduction

It is known that anisakiasis may develop in patients who have eaten raw fish such as sushi and sashimi, with the *Anisakis* larvae being the etiological parasite in this disease [1]. It first enters the gastric lumen, then penetrates gastric mucosa, localizing most often in the stomach, though, it can enter the small intestine as well, where the diagnosis is often more difficult [2]. This parasite also produces chronic granulomatous lesions which need to be differentiated from benign or malignant gastro-intestinal tract tumors.

The pathological development of anisakiasis is also not known in detail, though it is generally considered that acute anisakiasis could occur in patients who have already been sensitized by *Anisakis* larvae. Furthermore, a large part of the immunobiological aspects of developing granulomatous lesions of this disease remain to be elucidated.

To investigate the disease process and aspects of host immune responses against *Anisakis simplex* larvae, patients' antibody production using micro-enzyme linked immunosorbent assay (ELISA) was studied, and IgG, A and M (IgGAM), and IgE against *Anisakis simplex* larvae antigen comparatively assessed.

Materials and Methods

Anisakis simplex larvae antigen. This parasite was homogenized in PBS, and the supernatant obtained after centrifugation at 3,000 rpm for 10 min.

Patients' sera. Patient A suffered from acute anisakiasis one month before serum sampling. He was diagnosed as chronic gastrointestinal anisakiasis, with granulomatous lesions in the gastrointestinal areas confirmed histologically. Patient B suffered from acute anisakiasis on month before serum sampling as well, but was not found to have any granulomatous lesions.

Micro-ELISA. Approximately 50 ng protein content of *Anisakis* larvae antigen was applied to each microtiter plate well (Immulon 2, Dynatech). The plates were incubated at 37 C for 1 h, washed with PBS, then treated with 10% BSA for 1 h to inhibit background activity. The patients' sera at various dilutions with

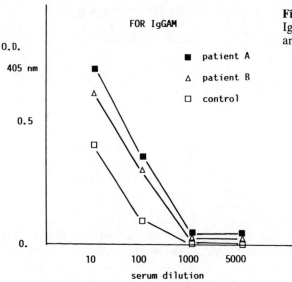

Fig. 1. The reactivity of patients' IgGAM against *Anisakis* larvae antigen in micro-ELISA

PBS were then applied, incubated at 37 C for 1 h, then were extensively washed by PBS, and 1,000 × diluted peroxidase-conjugated goat anti-human IgGAM or anti-human IgE applied to the wells. They were also washed by PBS and 150 microgram/ml of 2,2'-azinobis (3-ethylbenz-thiazolinesulfonic acid) diammonium salt (Sigma) was added. A buffer for this reaction was 0.05M sodium citrate, pH 4.0, with 0.01% H_2O_2. O.D. was counted at 405 nm by ELISA counter (MR6,000, Dynatech).

Results and Discussion

The sera from patients A and B was diluted at 10, 100, 1000 and 5000 × with PBS, applied to the micro-ELISA plates. The IgGAM of patient A obviously reacted with *Anisakis simplex* larvae antigen (Fig. 1), as did patient B. However, serum from a control who had not eaten raw fish also showed relatively high reactivity.

The reactivity of IgE from these patients is shown (Fig. 2), clearly demonstrating that the control IgE did not react with *Anisakis simplex* larvae antigen, while IgE from patients A and B reacted highly with the antigen. This data indicates that detecting IgE against *Anisakis simplex* larvae antigen by micro-ELISA could provide a highly useful diagnostic tool.

As the diagnosis of intestinal anisakiasis is difficult for physicians [2], the titration of patient IgE reacting with *Anisakis simplex* larvae antigen could be beneficial for the exact diagnosis of this particular disease. The titration of patient IgGAM may also contribute to the clinical diagnosis, but the background activity to the antigen was relatively high, though this should be reduced more by technical improvements.

The serodiagnostic examination of anisakiasis patients is very important in understanding the developmental process of this disease [3], and these

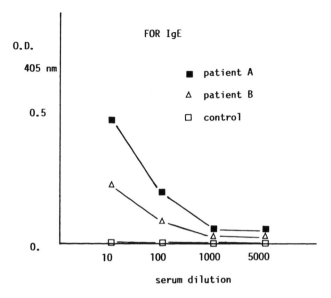

Fig. 2. The reactivity of patients' IgE against *Anisakis* larvae antigen in micro-ELISA

approaches may clarify the immunobiological aspects of intestinal anisakiasis. Currently, we are developing more specific serodiagnostic assay systems using monoclonal antibodies that will hopefully react specifically against *Anisakis simplex* larvae antigen [4].

References

1. Matthews EB (1984) The source, release and specificity of *Anisakis* simplex larvae. J Helminth 58: 175–185
2. Pincus GS, Coolidge C (1975) Intestinal anisakiasis: first case report from north America. Am J Med 59: 114–120
3. Maizels RM, Phillip M, Ogilvie BM (1982) Molecules on the surface of parasitic nematodes as probes on the immune response in infection. Immunol Rev 61: 109–136
4. Takahashi S, Sato N, Ishikura H (1986) Establishment of monoclonal antibodies that discriminate the antigen distribution specifically found in *Anisakis* larvae (type 1). J Parasit 72: 960–962

Mechanism of Eosinophilia in Parasitic Infection with Special Emphasis on the Eosinophil Chemotactic Lymphokines Directed Against Different Maturation Stages of Eosinophils

Y. NAWA, M. OWHASHI, and H. MARUYAMA

Abstract

In this review, we have demonstrated three major facets of the eosinophilic mechanism in parasitic infections. Firstly, eosinophilia is primarily a matter of cell differentiation and/or maturation from hemopoietic stem cells. During infections with tissue-invading parasites, large numbers of pluripotent hemopoietic stem cells are generated, and mobilized to extramedullary hemopoietic sites such as the liver, where they become mature eosinophils in response to the increased demand.

Secondly, mechanisms of eosinophil mobilization from the site of production to circulation or to the inflamed site were reviewed, with chemotactic reactivity of eosinophils from various compartments examined, and a variation seen with their stages of maturation. Eosinophils obtained from bone marrow (BM-Eo) showed high chemotactic reactivity against the mast cell-derived eosinophil chemotactic factor of anaphylaxis (ECF-A), whereas those obtained from the peritoneal cavity (PEC-Eo) did not, although both BM-Eo and PEC-Eo responded equally well with parasite-derived, complement-derived, or lymphocyte-derived ECFs. Therefore, the use of different maturation stages of eosinophils is critically important for understanding the mechanisms of eosinophil mobilization.

Thirdly, by using BM-Eo and PEC-Eo as indicators for in vitro chemotaxis, ECF lymphokines directed against BM-Eo and against PEC-Eo were isolated separately. Thus, these two distinctive types of ECF lymphokines can be used as one of the differentiation/maturation markers of eosinophils. In addition, when BM-Eo were cultured with ECF lymphokine selective to PEC-Eo, they became reactive to ECF lymphokine selective to PEC-Eo, suggesting that ECF lymphokine selective to PEC-Eo is not only a chemoattractant but also has an eosinophil differentiation activity.

From these results, eosinophil production and differentiation/maturation should be critically considered for studying the mechanisms of eosinophilia in parasitic infections.

Introduction

In discussing the mechanisms of eosinophilia in parasitic infections, three different points should be considered; 1) accelerated eosinophil production in bone

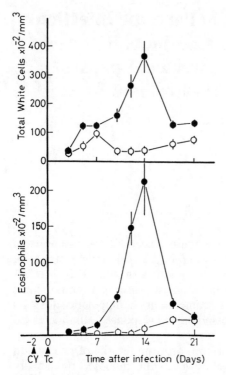

Fig. 1. Kinetic changes of total white cell counts (top) and eosinophil counts (bottom) in W/W^v (○) and +/+ (●) mice after cyclophosphamide treatment and *T. canis* infection. Mice were given an intraperitoneal injection with 200 mg/kg CY and, 2 days later, they were infected with 1,000 *T. canis* eggs. Vertical bar: SE of the mean from 5 mice (from ref. 27 with permission)

marrow and other extramedullary hemopoietic organs such as the liver and spleen, 2) release or mobilization of eosinophils from the site of eosinophilopoiesis into the circulation, 3) emigration of eosinophils from the circulation to the extravascular inflamed site. The mediation of tissue eosinophilia on the basis of lymphokine-mediated mechanisms has been revented by Dr. Hirashima et al. [52], so this article, focuses on the production and release of eosinophils from the site of eosinophilopoiesis.

Accelerated Eosinophil Production

Eosinophils are minor white blood cell components in normal animals, which increase rapidly in number during infections with tissue-invading helminths. They are, like other blood cells, derived from pluripotent hemopoietic stem cells. Thus, WBB6F$_1$ W/W^v mice, which are known to be deficient in hemopoietic stem cells, show a poor eosinophil response upon stimulation with the combination of cyclophosphamide-treatment and *Toxocara canis* infection (Fig. 1) [26]. Similarly, the granulopoietic response to endotoxin in irradiated or nonirradiated W/W^v mice is sluggish and subnormal compared to that in +/+ mice [6], and the poor neutrophil response of W^v/W^x mice to a grafted neutrophilia-inducing, colony-stimulating factor-producing tumor has been re-

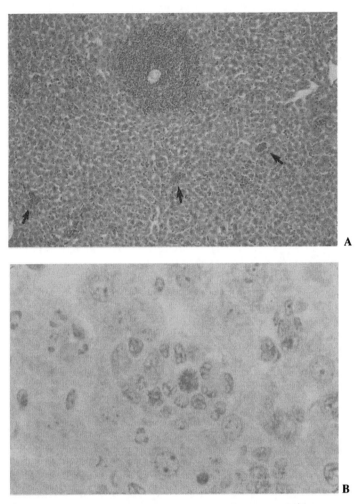

Fig. 2. Hemopoietic foci observed in the liver of *S. japonicum*-infected mice. **A** shows closely associated five typical foci of eosinophil lineage. **B** is a high power view demonstrating mitotic figures in the single focus (Fig 2A from ref. 22 with permission)

ported [43]. These results indicate that, regardless of the type of white blood cells, their differentiation is primarily determined by the level of pluripotent hemopoietic stem cells.

Extramedullary Eosinophilopoiesis

Although bone marrow is the major site of hemopoiesis in normal adult animals, extramedullary hemopoiesis is often associated with increased demand from disorders such as severe anemia or tissue inflammatory reactions. Extramedullary myelopoiesis of eosinophils has been described histologically in the liver of experimental murine schistosomiasis mansoni [7,10,15]. Recently we have confirmed these observations during the course of *Schistosoma japonicum* infection in mice (Fig. 2) and demonstrated further that the number of pluripotent hemopoietic stem cells measured by spleen colony assay is substantially increased in

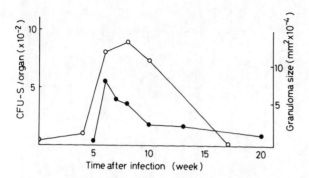

Fig. 3. Kinetic changes of the number of pluripotent hemopoietic stem cells (○), which were measured by spleen colony assay (Fu-S), in the liver of *S. japonicum*-infected mice. Also shown are the kinetic changes of granulomatous lesions in the lover (●) (modified from ref. 22 with permission)

the liver around the time of the acute stage of eosinophil-rich granulomatous response against deposited eggs (Fig. 3) [22]. Similar but more prominent liver eosinophilopoiesis and the accumulation of hemopoietic stem cells were observed in *T. canis*-infected mice (Maruyama et al., submitted for publication). These results indicate the possible importance of extramedullary myelopoiesis as the source of eosinophils in response to the increased demand, and that infections with tissue-invading parasites are extremely powerful stimuli for eosinophilopoiesis, even promoting extramedullary production.

Humoral Factors Involved in Eosinophilopoiesis

The directional differentiation from pluripotent stem cells towards eosinophil lineage is, like other blood cell types, under the influence of humoral factors. Such factors involved in myelopoiesis are generally called myelopoietin, growth/differentiation factor, or colony-stimulating factor (CSF). Specifically concerning eosinophilopoiesis, a wide range of humoral mediators such as eosinophilopoietin [21], eosinophil colony-stimulating factor (Eo-CSF) [24,28], or eosinophil differentiating factor [42] have been reported. Eosinophilopoietin is a low molecular weight peptide probably containing 5–10 amino acids, first detected in vivo in the serum from eosinophil-depleted animals, and then in the serum from *Trichinella spiralis*-infected rats. Related to eosinophilopoietin, studies using the in vitro liquid culture system of mouse bone marrow cells have shown the presence of an eosinophil growth stimulating factor (Eo-GSF) in the media conditioned by *T. spiralis*-infected mouse spleen cells upon stimulation with *T. spiralis* antigen [1,41]. Physicochemical and functional similarities of eosinophilopoietin and Eo-GSF was further confirmed by these workers [1]. Apart from eosinophilopoietin or Eo-GSF, Eo-CSF was detected by the semisolid softagar culture system, which was first established independently by Pluznik and Sachs [40] and by Bradley and Metcalf [8] for the clonal growth/differentiation of granulocyte-macrophages. Metcalf [24] reported the factor-dependent clonal growth/differentiation of murine eosinophils terming this factor Eo-CSF, the major source of which was media conditioned by spleen cells stimulated with

Mechanism of Eosinophilia in Parasitic Infection

pokeweed mitogen [20,23]. In the generation of eosinophil colonies from human bone marrow or peripheral blood cells, human placenta conditioned medium was most commonly used as the Eo-CSF source [28], and both murine and human Eo-CSF have an apparent molecular weight of 30,000–50,000 and are physicochemically separable from GM-CSF [9,28].

Apart from the factor-dependent eosinophil growth/differentiation described, the human promyelocytic leukemia cell line, HL-60 cells, can also differentiate into eosinophils under a slightly alkaline culture condition without the addition of any particular growth/differentiation factors [12]. If such a phenomenon is applicable to normal cells, at least a certain stage of eosinophil maturation is factor-independent, and this point needs further research and clarification.

Role of T Lymphocytes

Since the possible importance of lymphocytes on the mediation of eosinophilia was first reported [2], T lymphocytes have been considered as necessary partici-pants in the series of events leading to accelerated eosinophil production, with some of the eosinophilopoietic factors listed above apparently produced by T cells. Eosinophilia occurs in BALB/c nu/+ mice, but not in nu/nu littermates, after pretreatment with cyclophosphamide followed by immunization with key-hole limpet hemocyanin (KLH) incorporated in complete Freund's adjuvant [48]. T cell dependence of eosinophilia is also supported by the fact that T cell depleted mice fail to mount an eosinophil response to *T. spiralis* larvae and that this failure can be restored by thymus grafting [49], as well as reports that *S. mansoni*-infected nu/+ mice show significantly greater eosinophilia than nu/nu mice [39]. Two models for parasite-induced eosinophilia have been proposed [48]; (1) parasites may stimulate the elaboration of a T cell product that is not normally seen when T cells are stimulated by other antigens. (2) parasites may cause the elaboration of 2 signals; one, a T cell-dependent promoter of eosi-nophilopoiesis, and another that acts on the progenitor cell compartment, ex-panding it or making it receptive to the T cell signals.

Against previously reported T cell-dependent eosinophilia, it has recently been found that, after *T. canis*-infection, the magnitude of the major peak of peripheral blood eosinophilia observed at around day 10 of infection was compa-rable between nu/+ and nu/nu mice, although the small second peak, which was observed in nu/+ mice on day 28, was not observed in nu/nu mice [45]. Thus, both T cell-dependent and independent eosinophilia were elicited in *T. canis*-infected mice. Thymus-independent eosinophilia induced by a non-parasite anti-gen (KLH) was also reported recently by using congenitally athymic rnu/rnu rats [4].

Eosinophil Mobilization

Eosinophils are, like other blood cells, generated from stem cells in the bone marrow under the action of specific molecular regulators [9], released into the circulation, and then reach a tissue compartment or inflamed site. Thus, the distribution of eosinophils in the body can be divided into three major compart-ments; bone marrow, vascular and tissue compartments [3]. When the mecha-nisms for the mobilization of eosinophils are considered, two different steps

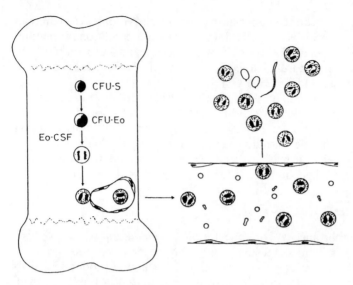

Fig. 4. Schematic diagram of the three major compartments of eosinophils, bone marrow, vascular and tissue compartment

should be distinguished (Fig. 4); 1) from bone marrow and other extramedullary eosinophilopoietic compartments to the vascular compartment, and 2) from the vascular compartment to tissue compartments or inflamed sites. In spite of the extensive work on humoral mediators of eosinophilotaxis, the role of these factors on the two different steps of eosinophil mobilization has never been fully discriminated.

Eosinophil mobilization from the site of production to the vascular compartment. The factors controlling this step are poorly understood [3]. Although an eosinophil releasing factor has been reported in a series of passive transfer experiments involving plasma from rats 12–24 h after a single injection of *T. spiralis* larvae [44], whether this eosinophil release was from bone marrow or from the marginating pool of the vascular compartment was not critically studied [5]. Furthermore, the physicochemical nature of the eosinophil releasing factor has not been clarified. Apart from the eosinophil releasing factor [44] both the parasite-derived high molecular weight ECF [29] and the host mast cell-derived low molecular weight ECF [30], probably ECF-A, were detected in the serum of acute stage of murine schistosomiasis. Since both of these ECFs were chemotactic to eosinphils obtained from bone marrow (data not shown), they could be possible candidates for the factors which mobilize eosinophils from the site of production to the vascular compartment, also indicating that the use of different maturation stages of eosinophils is important to evaluate the biological role of ECFs. This point will be discussed in subsequent sections.

Eosinophil mobilization from the vascular compartment to the tissue compartment. In terms of the accumulation of eosinophils at the site of inflammatory reactions caused by parasite infections, various parasite species such as *Anisakis* [47], *Ascaris* [46], *Schistosoma* [18,19,31], *Spirometra* [17], or *Fasciola* [16] possess ECF activity, some of which have been isolated and characterized physi-

Mechanism of Eosinophilia in Parasitic Infection   231

cochemically. Additionally various host-derived ECFs such as mast cell-derived ECF-A, complement-derived ECF, and lymphocyte-derived ECF are, in one way or another, involved in the mediation of tissue eosinophilia [51]. In parasitic infections, the generation, production and/or release of these host-derived ECFs is obviously dependent on the antigenic stimuli of the parasites. Splenic T lymphocytes [36] and granuloma T cells [32], reported to produce and release ECF lymphokine upon stimulation with the specific antigen. All these parasite- and host-derived ECFs are known to act as chemoattractants causing directional migration of eosinophils from the vascular to the tissue compartment, and at least some of them can be detected in the circulation possibly acting as a releasing factor for eosinophils at the site of production. This possibility should be examined by using naive eosinophils as the indicator for chemotaxis assays in vitro.

Chemotactic Reactivity of Eosinophils from Various Compartments

The use of different maturation stages of eosinophils seems to be important to analyze the mechanism of eosinophil mobilization from the site of production to the inflammatory sites via the circulation. Recently we have found that eosinophils obtained from bone marrow (BM-Eo) could be considered as naive to an array of chemoattractants, whereas those obtained from the peritoneal cavity (PEC-Eo) seemed to be already functionally modified during circulation or migration [26]. Thus, although both BM- and PEC-Eo respond equally well to various chemoattractants such as ECF lymphokine, complement-derived ECF, or parasite-derived ECF, the reactivity to ECF-A was markedly different between them (Fig. 5). Unresponsiveness of PEC-Eo to ECF-A could be explained by chemotactic deactivation [13,14,50], because a low molecular weight ECF-A-like substance was detected in the ascitic fluid of cyclophosphamide-treated, *T. canis*-infected mice [26]. Functional heterogeneity of eosinophils has also been reported in that only 'hypodense' eosinophils could mediate high levels of IgE-dependent schistosomula killing [11], while data we have (unpublished observation) revealed that BM-Eo were heavier than PEC-Eo in Percoll density gradient centrifugation.

Heterogeneity of ECF Lymphokine

Since chemotactic reactivity of eosinophils varies, depending upon their maturation/differentiation lineage, the use of different maturation stages of eosinophils as an indicator for the detection of ECF lymphokine would allow the physicochemical and/or functional heterogeneity of ECF lymphokines to be depicted. For this purpose, we have used eosinophils obtained from bone marrow and the peritoneal cavity of cyclophosphamide-treated, *T. canis*-infected mice as the indicator cells. In addition, chemotactic reactivity of peripheral blood eosinophils obtained from mice treated by the same methods were also examined.

When ECF activity in the conditioned medium of antigen-specifically stimulated *S. japonicum*-infected mouse spleen cell culture, which was known to attract BM-Eo [36], was tested against BM- and PEC-Eo, this conditioned medium showed dose-dependent ECF activity against PEC-Eo as well. After gel-chromatography on Sephadex G-75, an apparent molecular weight of ECF-

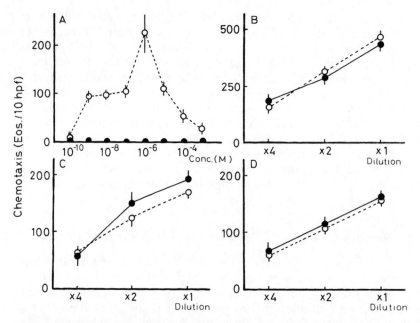

Fig. 5. Chemotactic reactivity of eosinophils obtained from bone marrow (○) or peritoneal cavity (●) of cyclophosphamide-treated, *T. canis*-infected mice to various chemoattractants. A: Synthetic ECF-A, B: soluble egg antigen (250 μg/ml original stock) of *S. japonicum*. C: Con A-stimulated spleen cell conditioned medium. D: Zymosan-activated guinea pig serum. Chemotactic reactivity is expressed as a mean count ± SE of migrated eosinophils in 10 high power field of triplicate assays (from ref. 26 with permission)

lymphokine recognized by BM-Eo was 15,000, whereas that by PEC-Eo was 30,000. By DE52 anion-exchange column chromatography, ECF-lymphokine reactive to BM-Eo was eluted at around 0.14 M NaCl concentration, whereas that recognized by PEC-Eo was eluted at around 0.1 M NaCl concentration. After isoelectric focusing, however, ECF activity against BM- and PEC-Eo were detected at the same position, approximately pH 3.6 [37]. From these results, two types of ECF lymphokines were separately purified by the combination of DE52 anion-exchange chromatography, Procion Red Agarose affinity chromatography, and SW 3000 high-pressure liquid chromatography [38]. After these steps of purification, ECF directed against BM-Eo is shown as a relatively weak, broad single band in the region of about 10,000 dalton, whereas that against PEC-Eo is shown as a sharp single band of 46,000 dalton on SDS-PAGE (Fig. 6).

When specificity of these two isolated ECFs was tested against BM-Eo, PEC-Eo, and circulating Eo, ECF directed against BM-Eo could attract only BM-Eo, whereas that directed against PEC-Eo could attract not only PEC-Eo but also circulating Eo. Synthetic ECF-A, which was used as a standard chemoattractant, was chemotactic against both BM- and circulating-Eo but not against PEC-Eo.

Since lymphokines are, in general, known to have multidirectional effects, we have postulated that our ECF lymphokine preparations might alter the chemo-

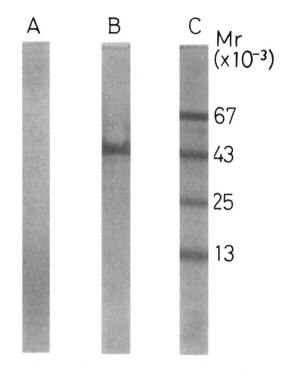

Fig. 6. SDS-PAGE analysis of isolated ECF lymphokine. ECF lymphokine directed against BM-Eo (BM-ECF-L)(**A**) and that directed against PEC-Eo (PEC-ECF-L)(**B**) were isolated from the media conditioned by spleen cells from mice infected with *S. japonicum* by a combination of anion-exchange chromatography on DE52, affinity chromatogaphy on Procion Red agarose, and high-performance liquid chromatography. Two kinds of ECF lymphokines and molecular weight standards were electrophoresed on 7.5% SDS-PAGE (from ref. 38 with permission)

tactic reactivity of BM-Eo. To test this possibility, BM-Eo were cultured in the presence of the each type of isolated ECF lymphokine for 4 days and their chemotactic reactivity examined against two types of ECF lymphokine and synthetic ECF-A (Table 1). When BM-Eo were cultured with ECF lymphokine selective to PEC-Eo, they became reactive to ECF lymphokine selective to PEC-Eo, and although they retained chemotactic reactivity against synthetic ECF-A, they lost reactivity against ECF lymphokine selective to BM-Eo. Incubation of BM-Eo with ECF lymphokine selective to BM-Eo did not alter the reactivity.

Regulation of ECF Lymphokine Production

Granulocyte-macrophage colony-stimulating factor (GM-CSF) has been detected in the sera of murine schistosomiasis japonica [34], and also produced by splenic T lymphocytes of *S. japonicum*-infected mice [32]. Recently GM-CSF has been considered not only as a myelopoietin, but also displays various macrophage regulatory functions [25], and is likely to be involved in the regulation of eosinophilia. When isolated intact granulomas of *S. japonicum*-infected mice

Table 1. Chemotactic reactivity of eosinophils obtained from bone marrow after incubation with eosinophilotactic lymphokine

Cultured with	Chemotactic activity against			
	BM-ECF-L	PEC-ECF-L	ECF-A	PBS
(−)	57.3 ± 10.7	8.0 ± 3.8	56.7 ± 7.0	6.0 ± 1.4
BM-ECF-L	66.6 ± 8.7	17.4 ± 5.1	50.0 ± 1.4	8.6 ± 4.5
PEC-ECF-L	6.7 ± 1.6	62.7 ± 2.2	52.7 ± 4.4	10.0 ± 1.4

Eosinophil-rich bone marrow cells (4×10^6 cells/ml, 50% eosinophils) were cultured in the presence of either eosinophil chemotactic lymphokine selective to bone marrow eosinophils (BM-ECF-L) or to peritoneal exudate eosinophils (PEC-ECF-L). Four days after culture, the cells were washed and their chemotactic reactivity against BM-ECF-L, PEC-ECF-L, or synthetic ECF-A was examined. Phosphate-buffered saline (PBS) served as a negative control of the chemoattractant. Each figure represents mean ± SE of migrated eosinophils in 10 high power fields of the triplicate assays [from ref. 38 with permission].

were cultured under the presence of GM-CSF, which was partially purified from the media conditioned by spleen cells of *S. japonicum*-infected mice, significant augumentation of ECF lymphokine production was observed (Fig. 7) [33]. This enhanced ECF lymphokine production was due to the activation of macrophages by GM-CSF. These results show that ECF lymphokine production is under the regulation of another type of lymphokine, GM-CSF, and suggest that the regulatory mechanisms of eosinophilia are, like an immune system, constructed as a complicated network (Fig. 8).

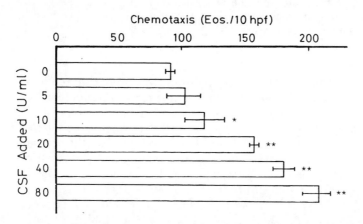

Fig. 7. Effect of granulocyte-macrophage colony stimulating factor (GM-CSF) on ECF production by intact granulomas. Various concentrations of partially purified GM-CSF was added to the cultures of isolated intact granulomas (100 granulomas/ml) of the liver of *S. japonicum*-infected mice. The conditioned media were harvested 24 h after culture and their ECF activity was examined. Background count of eosinophil migration towards various concentrations of GM-CSF preparation or culture medium was less than 10/10 high power field. Horizontal bars represent SE of the mean (*: $p < 0.05$, **: $p < 0.01$ by Student's t-test) (from ref. 33 with permission)

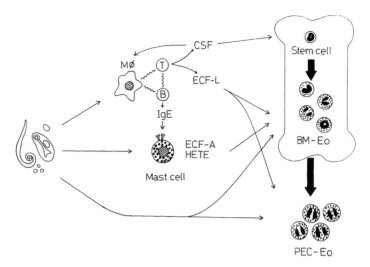

Fig. 8. Schematic diagram of the regulatory mechanisms of the production and mobilization of eosinophils in parasite infections

Conclusion

This article reviews recent advances in the understanding of the mechanisms of eosinophilia occuring during parasitic infection. A rapid development of immunology and hematology has led to the use of various fascinating tools such as different maturational stages of hemopoietic cells or humoral factors involved in the growth/differentiation of hemopoietic cell lineage. Thus, the next direction of research is how and why such mechanisms are triggered by parasitic stimuli, and if eosinophils are powerful effectors of host defence against parasites, then, why should parasites stimulate disadvantageous host responses against themselves?

References

1. Bartelmez SH, Dodge WH, Mahmoud AAF, Bass DA (1989) Stimulation of eosinophil production in vitro by eosinophilopoietin and spleen-cell-derived eosinophil growth-stimulating factor. Blood 56: 706–711
2. Basten A, Beeson PB (1969) Mechanism of eosinophilia. II. Role of the lymphocyte. J Exp Med 131: 1288–1305
3. Beeson PB, Bass DA (1977) Life cycle. In Smith LH Jr. (ed), The eosinophil. Major problems in internal medicine XIV, Saunders, Philadelphia, pp. 3–9
4. Blomjous FJEM, Elgersma A, Kruzinga W, Ruitenburg EJ (1986) Thymus independence of eosinophilia induced by a non-parasite antigen. Int Archs Allergy Appl. Immun 79: 376–379
5. Colley DG, James SL (1979) Participation of eosinophils in immunological systems. In Gupta S, Good RA (eds), Cellular, molecular, and clinical aspects of allergic disorders. Comprehensive Immunology 6, Plenum, New York, pp. 55–86
6. Boggs SS, Wilson SM, Smith WW (1973) Effects of endotoxin on hematopoiesis in irradiated and nonirradiated W/W^v mice. Radiat Res 56: 481–493

7. Borojevic R, Stocker S, Grimaud JA (1981) Hepatic eosinophil granulocytopoiesis in murine experimental schistosomiasis mansoni. Br J Exp Pathol 62: 480–489
8. Bradley TR, Metcalf D (1966) The growth of mouse bone marrow cells in vitro. Aust J Exp Biol Med Sci 44: 287–300
9. Burgess A, Nicola N (1983) Growth factors and stem cells Academic Press, Sydney, pp 43–91
10. Byram JE, Imohiosen EAE, Von Lichtenberg F (1978) Tissue eosinophil proliferation and maturation in schistosome-infected mice and hamsters. Am J Trop Med Hyg 27: 267–270
11. Capron M, Capron A, Dessaint JP, Torpier G, Johansson SGO, Prin L (1981) Fc receptors for IgE on human and rat eosinophils. J Immunol 126: 2087–2092
12. Fischkoff SA, Pollak A, Gleich GJ, Testa JR, Misawa S, Reber TJ (1984) Eosinophilic differentiation of the human promyelocytic leukemia cell line HL-60. J Exp Med 160: 179–196
13. Goetzl EJ, Austen KF (1976) Structural determinants of the eosinophil chemotactic activity of the acidic tetrapeptides of eosinophil chemotactic factor of anaphylaxis. J Exp Med 144: 1424–1437
14. Goetzl EJ, Foster DW, Goldman DW (1983) Receptor-directed modulation of human eosinophil function. In Yoshida T, Torisu M (eds), Immunobiology of the eosinophil, Elsevier, New York, pp. 61–76
15. Grimaud JA, Borojevic R (1972) Mésenchyme et parenchyme hépatique dans la bilharziose expérimentale à *Schistosoma mansoni:* Métaplasie Myéloide. CR Acad Sci Paris 274: 897–899
16. Horii Y, Fujita K, Owhashi M (1986) Partial purification and characterization of eosinophil chemotactic factors from soluble extract of *Fasciola* species. Am J Vet Res 47: 123–126
17. Horii Y, Owhashi M, Ishii A, Bandou K, Usui M (1984a) Leukocyte accumulation in sparganosis: Demonstration of eosinophil and neutrophil chemotactic factors from the plerocercoid of *Spirometra erinacei* in vivo and in vitro. Am J Trop Med Hyg 33: 138–143
18. Horii Y, Owhashi M, Ishii A, Bandou K, Usui M (1984b) Eosinophil and neutrophil chemotactic activities of adult worm extracts of *Schistosoma japonicum* in vivo and in vitro. J Parasitol 70: 955–961
19. Horii Y, Ishii A, Owhashi M (1985) In vitro and in vivo induction of neutrophil and eosinophil chemotactic responses by *Schistosoma japonicum* cercaria. Am J Trop Med Hyg 34: 513–518
20. Johnson GR, Metcalf D (1980) Detection of a new type of mouse eosinophil colony by Luxol-Fast-Blue staining. Exp Hematol 8: 549–561
21. Mahmoud AAF, Stone MK, Kellermeyer RW (1977) Eosinophilopoietin. A circulating low molecular weight peptide-like substance which stimulates the production of eosinophils in mice. J Clin Invest 60: 675–682
22. Maruyama H, Higa A, Asami M, Owhashi M, Nawa Y (1990) Extramedullary eosinophilopoiesis in the liver of *Schistosoma japonicum*-infected mice, with reference to hemopoietic stem cells. Parasitol Res (in press)
23. Metcalf D, Johnson GR (1978) Production by spleen and lymph node cells of conditioned medium with erythroid and other hemopoietic colony-stimulating activity. J Cell Physiol 96: 31–42
24. Metcalf D, Parker J, Chester HM, Kincade PW (1974) Formation of eosinophil-like granulocytic colonies by mouse bone marrow cells in vitro. J Cell Physiol 84: 275–289
25. Moore RN, Hoffeld JT, Farrar JJ, Mergenhagen SE, Oppenheim JJ, Shadduck RK (1981) Role of colony-stimulating factors as primary regulation of macrophage functions. Lymphokines 3: 119–148
26. Nawa Y, Owhashi M, Imai J, Abe T (1986) Chemotactic reactivity of eosinophils obtained from bone marrow and peritoneal cavity of cyclophosphamide-treated *Toxocara canis*-infected mice. Int Archs Allergy Appl Immun 80: 412–416

Mechanism of Eosinophilia in Parasitic Infection 237

27. Nawa Y, Owhashi M, Imai J, Abe T (1987) Eosinophil response in mast cell-deficient W/W^v mice. Int Archs Allergy Appl Immun 83: 6–11
28. Nicola NA, Metcalf D, Johnson GR, Burgess AW (1979) Separation of functionally distinct human granulocyte-macrophage colony stimulating factors. Blood 54: 614–627
29. Owhasi M, Horii Y, Ishii A, Nawa Y (1986a) Detection of high molecular weight eosinophil chemotactic factor in murine schistosomiasis sera. Am J Trop Med Hyg 35: 1192–1197
30. Owhashi M, Horii Y, Ishii A, Nawa Y (1986b) Low molecular weight eosinophil chemotactic factor (ECF) in the serum of murine schistosomiasis japonica. Int Archs Allergy Appl Immunol 79: 178–181
31. Owhashi M, Ishii A (1982) Purification and characterization of a high molecular weight eosinophil chemotactic factor from *Schistosoma japonicum* eggs. J Immunol 129: 2226–2231
32. Owhashi M, Maruyama H, Nawa Y (1986) Eosinophil chemotactic lymphokine produced by egg-associated granulomas in murine schistosomiasis japonicum. Infect Immunol 54: 723–727
33. Owhashi M, Maruyama H, Nawa Y (1987) Granulocyte-macrophage colony-stimulating factor enhances the production of eosinophil chemotactic lymphokine by egg-associated granulomas of *Schistosoma japonicum*-infected mice. Infect Immunol 55: 2042–2046
34. Owhashi M, Nawa Y (1985) Granulocyte-macrophage colony-stimulating factor in the sera of *Schistosoma japonicum*-infected mice. Infect Immunol 49: 533–537
35. Owhashi M, Nawa Y (1986) Granulocyte-macrophage colony-stimulating factor produced by splenic T lymphocytes of mice infected with *Schistosoma japonicum*. Infect Immunol 51: 213–217
36. Owhashi M, Nawa Y (1987a) Eosinophil chemotactic lymphokine produced by spleen cells of *Schistosoma japonicum*-infected mice. Int Archs Allergy Appl Immunol 82: 20–25
37. Owhashi M, Nawa Y (1987b) Eosinophil chemotactic lymphokine produced by spleen cells of *Schistosoma japonicum*-infected mice. II. Physicochemical heterogeneity of eosinophil chemotactic lymphokines selective to bone marrow- or peritoneal exudate-eosinophils. Int Archs Allergy Appl Immunol 83: 290–295
38. Owhashi M, Nawa Y (1987c) Eosinophil chemotactic lymphokine produced by spleen cells of *Schistosoma japonicum*-infected mice. III. Isolation and characterization of two distinctive eosinophil chemotactic lymphokines directed against different maturation stages of eosinophils. Int Archs Allergy Appl Immunol 84: 185–189
39. Phillips SM, Diconza JJ, Gold JA, Reid WA (1977) Schistosomiasis in congenitally athymic (nude) mouse. I. Thymic dependency of eosinophilia, granuloma formation and host morbidity. J Immunol 118: 594–599
40. Pluznik DH, Sachs L (1965) The cloning of normal 'mast cells' in tissue culture. J Cell Comp Physiol 66: 319–324
41. Ruscetti FW, Cypess RH, Chervenick PA (1976) Specific release of neutrophilic- and eosinophilic-stimulating factors from sensitized lymphocytes. Blood 47: 757–765
42. Sanderson CJ, Warren DJ, Strath M (1985) Identification of a lymphokine that stimulates eosinophil differentiation in vitro. Its relationship to interleukin 3, and functional properties of eosinophils produced in cultures. J Exp Med 162: 60–74
43. Sonoda T, Hayashi C, Kitamura Y, Nakano T, Bessho M, Hirashima K, Miyazaki E, Hara H (1984) Poor response of W^v/W^x mice to a grafted neutrophilia-inducing, colony-stimulating factor-producing tumor. Exp Hematol 12: 850–855
44. Spry CJF (1971) Mechanism of eosinophilia. VI. Eosinophil mobilization. Cell Tissue Kinet 4: 365–374
45. Sugane K, Oshima T (1982) Eosinophilia, granuloma formation and migratory behavior of larvae in the congenitally athymic mouse infected with *Toxocara canis*. Parasite Immunol 4: 307–318

46. Tanaka J, Baba T, Torisu M (1979) *Ascaris* and eosinophil. II. Isolation and characterization of eosinophil chemotactic factor and neutrophil chemotactic factor of parasite in *Ascaris* antigen. J Immunol 122: 302–308
47. Tanaka J, Torisu M (1978) *Anisakis* and eosinophil. I. Detection of a soluble factor selectively chemotactic for eosinophils in the extract from *Anisakis* larvae. J Immunol 120: 745–749
48. Vadas MA (1981) Cyclophosphamide pretreatment induces eosinophilia to nonparasite antigens. J Immunol 127: 2083–2086
49. Walls RS, Carter RL, Leuchers E, Davies AJS (1973): The immunopathology of trichiniasis in T-cell deficient mice. Clin Exp Immunol 13: 231–242
50. Wasserman SI, Whitmer D, Goetzl EJ, Austen KF (1975) Chemotactic deactivation of human eosinophils by the eosinophil chemotactic factor of anaphylaxis (38527). Proc Soc Exp Biol Med 148: 301–306
51. Weller PF, Goetzel EJ (1980) The regulatory and effector roles of eosinophils. Adv Immunol 27: 339–371
52. Hirashima M, Hirotsu Y, Hayashi H (1983) Natural mediators of eosinophil chemotaxis in inflammation. In Yoshida T, Torisu M (eds), Immunobiology of the eosinophil, Elsevier, New York, pp 213–227

Antigenicity of the Cuticle with Emphasis on the Immunocytochemical Approach

Y. Takahashi and T. Araki

Abstract

Since the introduction of immunostaining technology, our knowledge of reading and interpretating histological specimens has expanded enormously. This powerful tool allows us to study the in situ localization of the antigen providing new insights into both experimental and clinical immuno-parasitology. However, inherent problems such as false negative and false positive results are always present in spite of technological advancements in resin, antibody and stain enhancement. In this article, we briefly explain current immunostaining techniques, with emphasis on why immunostaining of the cuticle inner-layers is so difficult.

The cuticular surface is the easiest structure for immunostaining due to its open access to antibody and because it can be immunostained without prefixation. Furthermore, number of studies have revealed its antigenicity. However unlike the surface, the inner-layers of the cuticle are problematic during innerlayers immunostaining, with the cuticle acting as a barrier which inhibits the free diffusion of even low molecular weight substances. The most reliable method of enabling the antibody to have access to the inner-layer antigen is by thin sectioning of the cuticle and subsequent immunostaining, but even with this method the available antigen seems to occur preferentially on the cut surface of the cuticle. Such a small amount of antigen is often difficult to detect by means of light microscopy employing flourescence or peroxidase as visual markers. Thus special considerations need to be made in the design and interpretation of cuticular immunostaining, compared to staining of other cell components. Immunogold staining on ultrathin sections is the most reliable and sensitive technique to localize antigen buried in the cuticle inner layers with high resolution. Taking advantage of this method it was shown that the antigenic moieties are distributed in the inner-layers of the cuticle without any regional preference, and the body and hindgut cuticle are similar in antigenicity while the esophagus is different. This technique will open up new ways to investigate the immunological involvement of the cuticle, which can no longer be seen simply as an inert, unobstrusive covering provoking little immune responsiveness.

Introduction

The antigenic property of the cuticle is a major area that needs to be researched and clarified, since it is an extracellular material covering the entire surface of the nematode and the most obvious point of contact between the worm and the host. Four major approaches in the study of the cuticular antigen have been used so far. 1)Immunochemical analysis of the solubilized components of the cuticle [9,12,14,17,18–21] 2) cell adherence test in the presence of a specific antibody [7,9,12,13,18,23,25,26] 3) Complement activation study [11,23] 4) Immunohistochemical staining [2,4,6,9,14,16,24].

Immunohistochemical staining is a powerful technique that allows the study of the topographical antigenic distribution, based on the interaction between the specific antigen and antibody. This technique has been greatly expanded and developed enabling positive identification of tissue constituents. However, like other methods commonly employed by biologists, immunohistochemistry has inherent problems and limitations that must be kept in mind for the design of immunostaining protocols and the interpretation of results. In addition to general immunostaining difficulties, the cuticle presents a unique problem of impermeability. This study is technically concerned with immunostaining of the nematode cuticle from a practical point of view, with most of the report derived from personal experience gained from studies on the antigenicity of *Trichinella spiralis* muscle larvae. We believe there are compositional similarities of the cuticles of *Trichinella* and *Anisakis* and, therefore, the knowledge obtained from the former is applicable to the latter.

The Cuticle Surface Antigen

Because the cuticular surface can be exposed without difficulty to macromolecules, as is the case of the specific first antibody and secondary labeling antibody, it is one of the easiest structures to be studied. Its tough structural composition is an advantage during immunostaining, since it can hardly be destroyed during a regular staining process, and doesn't require prefixation. Although prefixation tends to create free radicals capable of causing nonspecific binding, immunostaining without prefixation yields less false-positive results.

The cuticle surface antigen has been studied using ferritin [2,5,14] and fluorescein [9,14,16[as visual markers. Scanning electron microscopy has also been employed in combination with immunostaining [10], and based on evidence, it is reasonable to conclude that the cuticle surface contains an antigen which is recognized by the host during an infection. The surface appears to be the site of a very interesting and critical group of antigens responsible for immune recognition and parasite vulnerability to lethal immune mechanisms [12, 13] and, yet is able to change antigenicity several times during the parasite's developmental cycle [12]. Investigative attention should be shifted to the topographical distribution of the cuticle antigen, because the nematode cuticle is not only replaced by moults but can also grow in a vectorial fashion from the mid region of the worm during the intermoult period [8,15]. If the new stage-specific antigen is expressed on the mid-region of the cuticle surface, it may have regional preferences as to its antigenicity.

The Cuticle Inner-Layer Antigen

Unlike the surface, the inner-layers of the cuticle are problematic during immunostaining, as the cuticle acts as a barrier inhibiting the free diffusion of even low molecular weight substances [3]. The question that immediately comes to mind is how can first and second antibodies gain access to antigen buried in the cuticle, the inner-layers of which are inaccessible to antibodies unless they are exposed by an unmasking procedure during immunostaining. To our knowledge, the most reliable method allowing the antibody open access to the inner-layer antigen is by thin sectioning of the cuticle followed by immunostaining. This is a popular technique often used to expose antigen located inside membrane-bound structures such as cell cytoplasm, mitochondria, Golgi apparatus and cytoplasmic granules. Once the barrier or membrane is broken by sectioning, antibody has a good chance to bind to the antigen situated within such structures. Even using this method, the available antigen seems to occur preferentially on the cut surface of the cuticle, and such small amounts of antigen are often difficult to detect by light microscopy employing fluorescence or peroxidase as visual markers. However, other structures, such as cytoplasmic granules, stain well because the antibodies available for staining can internally penetrate those structures and bind sufficient amounts of antigen for positive staining at a significant level.

The basic techniques for immunostaining at both light and electron microscopic levels are now described with special emphasis on the cuticle inner-layer antigen with explanation of the occasional difficulty one may encounter in the interpretation of immunostained specimens.

Immunofluorescence

Conventional immunofluorescence (IF) involves tissue freezing, cryosectioning, immunostaining and examination under a fluorescent microscope. This simple method has several advantages in the testing of the antigenicity of the nematode, however, it does not seem to be efficient for the localization of the cuticular inner-layer antigens. IF staining on cryosections clearly shows the cuticular surface stained in a linear pattern and internal organs, such as the stichosome, stained in a granular pattern (Fig. 1), with little doubt as to such results. However, because of the faint immunostaining intensity of the cuticle inner-layers, it is difficult to ascertain whether the immunostaining in the cuticle inner-layers in positive or negative. This frustrating result is simply because IF is not sensitive enough to detect small amounts of antigen on the cut surface of the cuticle.

In the case of a small nematode such as *Trichinella spiralis* one may encounter another problem. The body wall of *Trichinella* consists of the cuticle, hypodermis, and a contractile and a noncontractile part of muscle cells [6], but the resolution given by IF is not clear enough to distinguish such thin layers, and precise localization cannot be determined.

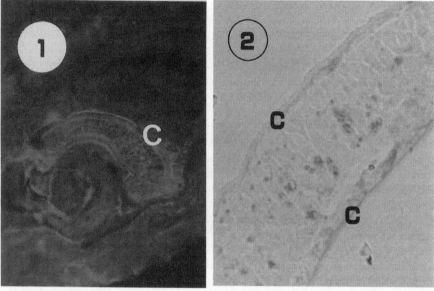

Fig. 1   Fig. 2

Fig. 1. Immunofluorescence. Encysted larvae in the diaphragma are cryosectioned and stained with sera from infected rats. Strong positive staining is shown along the outer surface of the parasite, while further inward there are negative and positive lines. This unique staining pattern likely reflects some morphological characteristics of the cuticle and its neighboring structures. However, lack of resolution does not allow for distinguishing which structure is responsible for positive staining

Fig. 2. Immunoperoxidase at the light microscope level. Acrytron-embedded parasites are sectioned and immunostained with the aid of the avidine-biotine amplifying system. Positive reaction can be identified by the presence of brown deposit of DAB

Immunoperoxidase at the Light Microscope Level

The immunoperoxidase method can be performed on deparafinized sections or on hydropilic-resin sections, such as JB4, Acrytron and LR White. A first antibody labeling is followed by a second antibody labeling. Immunostaining of the positive area can be identified by the end product of the peroxidase reactions, which are indicated by a brown coloration. A method to enhance and improve the reaction's sensitivity is to allow a small quantity of antigen in the tissue to be detected by the same concentration of the antibody. The most successful results in intensifying a positive stain are obtained by exploiting the strong attraction between avidin and biotin (Fig. 2), and for a better morphological orientation, sections can be counterstained with HE or nuclear stained after the immunostaining. Counterstained sections permit a more accurate interpretation than that obtained by IF, e.g., in our *Trichinella* sections the cuticle, stichosome, esophagus, mid- and hindgut, genital primordium, cords, and muscle cells were easily identified by counterstaining. When immunostained, the end product of peroxidase was easily distinguished over the stichocyte, the substances occupying

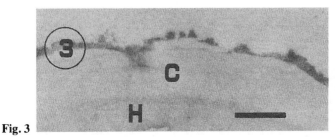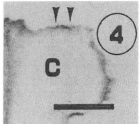

Figs. 3 and 4. Pre-embedding immunoperoxidase method. Immunostained cryosections are processed for embedding in resin and thin sectioned parallel to the glass slide (Fig. 3) or perpendicular to the glass slide (Fig. 4). The outer surface of the cuticle is definitely positive for immunostaining (Figs. 3 and 4), while the inner-layers look negative. However, the cut surface of the cuticle is positive (arrows in Fig. 4). It is on this basis that the cuticular inner-layers are concluded to be antigenic

the esophagus and the midgut as well as glycogen aggregates. Since these structures allow penetration of macromolecules, the antibody for immunostaining passes through the cut surface and reacts with the internally buried antigen, resulting in sufficient intensity for positive immunostaining, however, there were still no convincing results obtained for the cuticular inner-layers simply because of the impermeable nature of the macromolecules.

Immunoperoxidase at the Electron Microscope Level

According to the established method for immunoperoxidase staining at the electron microscope level, the tissue is prefixed, frozen, cryosectioned in 4 μm thick sections, mounted on a glass slide, immunostained using peroxidase as a visual marker, treated with DAB for peroxidase developing and examined under an electron microscope. Two different staining results may be produced depending on direction of the sectioning. When the specimen (immuno-stained 4 μ cryosection) is sectioned perpendicular to the glass slide, the resulting ultrathin sections include the cuticular surface as well as the cut-surface of the cuticle. Both surfaces, when successfully exposed to the antibody, display a positive reaction, while the unexposed inner-layers display a negative reaction (Fig. 4). The immunoperoxidase technique at the electron microscope level seems to be sensitive enough to detect a small amount of antigen on the cut-surface of the cuticle, which cannot be achieved by light microscopy. However, when the specimen is sectioned parallel to the glass slide, the resulting ultrathin sections include cuticular surface and its inner-layers, with the cuticle surface reacting positively while the inner-layers are negative simply because the latter escapes cytochemical detection (Fig. 3). The cut-surface of the cuticle, that is, the exposed inner-layer of the cuticle, is usually out of the section. Both immunoelectron microscope techniques result in essentially the same staining but the staining profiles that appear on electon micrographs are different. Therefore, spatial consideration needs to be made for correct interpretation.

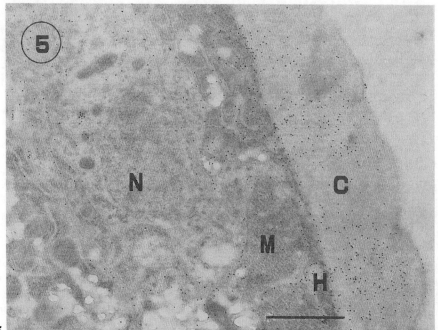

Fig. 5

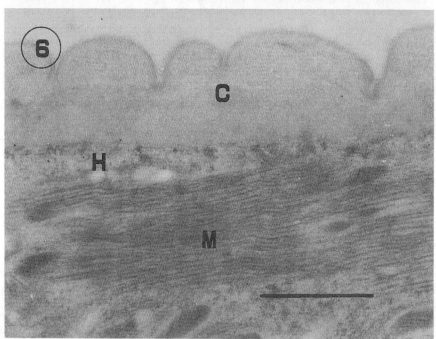

Fig. 6

Antigenicity of the Cuticle

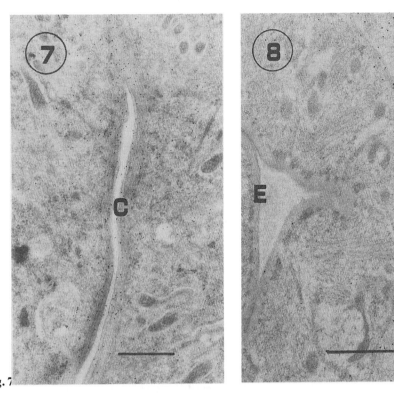

Fig. 7

Fig. 8

Figs. 5–8. Electron micrographs stained by immunogold method. Monomeric colloidal gold particles are distributed over the entire layer of the body cuticle (Fig. 5) and the hindgut cuticle (Fig. 7). Although the number of antigenic moieties involved in immunoreaction on the cut-surface of the cuticle is supposedly small, the immunogold method is sensitive enough to detect such weak reactions. The esophageal cuticle is negative in immunostaining (Fig. 8) suggesting it is endowed with different antigenicity from other cuticles. Thus a high resolution achieved by immuno-gold method enabled the antigenic difference of each cuticle to be revealed.

Immunogold

Immunogold is a more recent technique [1] providing the highest resolution in immunostaining and can be used in both pre-embedding and post-embedding methods. For the study of the cuticular inner-layer antigen, the post-embedding method is preferable. The tissue is fixed, dehydrated, and embedded in hydrophilic resin, ultrathin sections prepared and immunostaining performed on the sections. After the first antibody labelling, a protein A/gold complex is used as the second step in immunostaining. In this staining system, advantage is taken of the ability of the protein A, derived from *Staphylococcus aureus*, to bind to the Fc fraction of IgG and colloidal gold particles. In our experience, the protein A/gold complex gives superior results over the anti-antibody/gold complex, though recent advances in the quality of hydrophilic resin have also brought about excellent antigen availability exposed on ultrathin sections with less or minimal background staining.

	PRE-EMBEDDING	POST-EMBEDDING
VISUAL MARKER	FLUORESCENCE	PEROXIDASE
PROCESS	FREEZING 4-μ CRYO SECTION IMMUNO STAINING	FIXATION EMBEDDING 2-μ SECTION IMMUNO STAINING
3 DIMENTIONAL VIEW		
MICROSCOPICAL OBSERVATION		

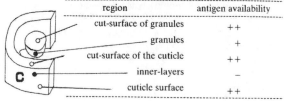

region	antigen availability
cut-surface of granules	++
granules	+
cut-surface of the cuticle	++
inner-layers	−
cuticle surface	++

A schematic illustration showing regional difference in antigen availability. Open circles indicate "open-access" antigen, closed circles indicate internally-buried antigen. C: cuticle, H: hypodermis, M: myofilament, HE: hemolymph, E: esophagus, N: nucleus, G: glycogen

This method allows for the detection of antigenic moieties exposed to the cut-surface of the ultrathin sections, is sensitive enough to pick up very small amounts of antigen, and colloidal gold particles can be visualized against counterstained histology. Therefore, successful staining with the immunogold method results in precise localization of antigen, which cannot be achieved by light microscopy. The disadvantage of this method is that protein A only binds to a certain type of IgG while other types of IgG cannot be detected.

ELECTRON MICROSCOPE	
PRE-EMBEDDING	POST-EMBEDDING
PEROXIDASE	COLLOIDAL GOLD
FREEZING 4-μ CRYO SECTION IMMUNO STAINING ELECTRON MICROSCOPY	FIXATION EMBEDDING ULTRATHIN SECTION IMMUNO STAINING

Summary of Immuno-staining

How the cuticle displays different staining patterns depending on the method employed

Each immuno-staining method and result are briefly summerized in this table. For the purpose of simplification only two components are illustrated, the cuticle (c) which is an impervious layer, and granules (g) as a representative of other common cell organelles which are not impervious.

In "3 Dimensional View", emphasis is made to show antigen availability, the regions where antibody has an access are indicated by half shadow. Note impervious and pervious structures are exposed in a different way.

In "Microscopical Observation", staining pattern of each method is schematically illustrated.

Fluorescence. Immunofluorescence on cryosections, white indicates positive, black indicates negative, and gray indicates week staining.

Peroxidase. Immuno-peroxidase staining followed by DAB reaction, black indicates positive staining, white indicates negative, and gray indicates week staining.

Colloidal gold. Protein A is conjugated with colloidal-gold particles and used as the second layer of staining solution. Dots indicate positive staining area can be exposed to antibody.

We have successfully applied the immunogold method to our study on the cuticle's antigenicity. As shown in Fig. 5, the inner-layers of the cuticle are densely stained without regional preference, and background deposition on the non-tissue area is minimal. The thin extension of the cord cell cytoplasm beneath the cuticle is also positive, however, the nucleus (N), and myofibrils (M) are always negative and act as a good built-in control. High resolution immunoelectron micrography obtained by the gold method provides new insights in the antigenic nature of other cuticles. Dense and uniform staining is shared by the cuticle of the hindgut (Fig. 7), but not the cuticle of the esophagus (Fig. 8). Despite their morphological resemblance, the esophagial cuticle seems to be antigenically different from other cuticles.

Serodiagnostic Potential of the Cuticle Inner-Layer Antigen

The superiority of the immunogold technique, in terms of reproduceability, specificity and sensibility has been confirmed, and this highly reliable technique has been used to evaluate the potential of the cuticular antigen as a serodiagnostic test. Our laboratory has a library of sera taken from patients with a wide variety of nematode infections including ascariasis, enterobiasis, gnathostomiasis and trichinosis, and all of the sera reacted more or less positively with the cuticular inner-layers, suggesting that this antigen is endowed with less specificity. We concluded that for serodiagnosis purposes, the cuticular inner-layer antigen may be used as a "screening" but not as a specific antigen.

References

1. Beesley JF (1985) Colloidal gold probes for parasite antigens. Parasitol Today 1: 145–146
2. Brzosko WJ, Gancarz Z (1969) Immunoelectronoscopic studies on antibody binding to the cuticle of *Trichinella spiralis* larvae. Wiadomosci Parazytologiczne T. XV, Nr 5–6
3. Chen SN, Howells RE (1979) The uptake in vitro of dyes, monosaccharides and aminoacids by the filarial worm *Brugia pahangi*. Parasitology 78: 343–354
4. Crandall CA, Echevarria R, Arean VM (1963) Localization of antibody binding sites in the larvae of *Ascaris lumbricoides var. suum* by means of fluorescent techniques. Exp Parasitol 14: 296–303
5. Despommier DD (1974) The stichocyte of *Trichinella spiralis* during morphogenesis in the small intestine of the rat. In: Kim C (ed) Trichinellosis, Intext Educational Publishers, New York, pp. 239–254
6. Despommier DD, Kajima M, Wostman S (1967) Ferritin-conjugated antibody studies on the larva of *Trichinella spiralis*. J Parasitol 53: 618–624
7. Gadea DL, Moore LA, Oliver-Gonzalez J (1967) Adsorption of globulin to the cuticle of larvae and adults of *Trichinella spiralis*. Am J Trop Med Hyg 16(6): 750–751

Antigenicity of the Cuticle

8. Jungery M, Clark NWT, Parkhouse RM (1983a) A major change in surface antigens during the maturation of newborn larvae of *Trichinella spiralis*. Mol Biochem Parasitol 7: 101–109

9. Jungery M, Mackenzie CD, Ogilvie BM (1983b) Some properties of the surface of nematode larvae. J Helminthol 57: 291–295

10. Kim CW, Ledbetter MC (1981) Detection of specific antigen-antibody precipitates on the surface of *Trichinella spiralis* by scanning electron microscopy. In: Kim CW, Ruitenberg EJ, Teppema JS (eds) Trichinellosis, Reedbooks, Chertsey, England, pp. 65–69

11. Leventhal R, Soulsby EJL (1977) *Ascalis suum*: Cuticular binding of the third component of complement by early larval stages. Exp Parasitology 41: 423–431

12. Maizels RM, Philipp M, Ogilvie BM (1982) Molecules on the surface of parasitic nematodes as probes of the immune response in infection. Immunological Rev 61: 109–136

13. McLaren DJ, Mackenzie CD, Ramaho-Pinto FJ (1977) Ultrastructural observations on the in vitro interaction between rat eosinophils and some parasitic helminths. Clin Exp Immunology 30: 105–118

14. Murrell KD, Graham C (1982) Solubilization studies on the epicuticular antigens of *Strongyloides ratti*. Veterinary Parasitology 10: 191–203

15. Ogilvie BM, Philipp M, Jungery M, Maizeles RM, Worms MJ, Parkhouse RME (1980) The surface of nematodes and the immune response of the host. In: Van den Bossche H (ed) The host Invader Interplay, Elsevier, Amsterdam, pp. 99–104

16. Ogimoto K (1984) Study on immunofluorescence of Japanese strain of *Trichinella spiralis* (Iwasaki strain, Yamagichi 1974) V. Immunoelectron and immunofluorescent microscopic localization of antigen. Hirosaki Med J 36: 283–296

17. Parkhouse RME, Phillip M, Ogilvie BM (1981) Characterization of surface antigens of *Trichinella spiralis* infectivae larvae. Parasit Immunol 3: 339–352

18. Perrudet-Badoux A, Anteunis A, Dunitresucu SM, Binaghi RA (1978) Ultrastructural study of the immune interaction between perioneal cells of larvae of *Trichinella spiralis*. J Reticuloendothel Soc 24 (3): 311–314

19. Philipp M, Parkhouse RME, Ogilvie BM (1980) Changing proteins on the surface of a parasitic nematode. Nature (London) 287: 538–540

20. Philipp M, Parkhouse RME, Ogilvie BM (1981) The molecular basis for stage specificity of the primary antibody response to the suface of *Trichinella spiralis*. In: Kim CW, Ruitenberg FJ, Teppema JS (eds), Trichinellosis, Reedbooks, Chertsey, England, pp. 59–64

21. Philipp M, Worms MJ, McLaren DJ, Ogilvie BM, Parkhouse RM, Taylor PM (1984) Surface proteins of a filarial nematode: a major soluble antigen and a host component on the cuticle of *Litomosoides carinii*. Parasit Immunol 6: 63–82

22. Pritchard DI, Crawford CR, Duce IR, Behnke JM (1985) Antigen stripping from a nematode epicuticle using the cationic detergent cetyltrimethylammonium bromide (CTAB). Parasit Immunol 7: 575–585

23. Stankiewicz M, Jeska EL (1973) Leukocytes and *Trichinella spiralis*. Immunology 25: 827–834

24. Takahashi Y, Uno T, Nishiyama T, Yamada S, Araki T (1988) Immunocytolocalization study of the external covering of *Trinchinella spiralis* muscle larva. J Parasitol 74: 270–274

25. Tam ND, Paradimitriou J, Keast D (1983) The location of antigenic sites on the surface of the nematode parasite *Strongyloides ratii* reactive to antibody-directed cellular cytotoxicity from both macrophages and eosinophils from the natural host. Aust J Exp Boil Med Sci 61: 629–636

26. Vernes A, Poulain D, Prensier G, Deblock S, Biguet J, Wattez A (1974) Trichinose experimentale. III. Action in vitro des cellules peritoneales sensibilsées sur les larves musculaires des premiers stades: Étude preliminaire comparative en microscopie optique et electronique à transmission et balayage. Biomedicine 21: 140–145

Immune Response to *Anisakis* Larvae in Healthy Humans

C. NISHINO, K. ASAISHI, and H. HAYASAKA

Introduction

Van Thiel et al. [1, 2] postulated an allergic reaction as an important etiological factor in the mechanism of anisakiasis, and from subsequent histological studies on patients with this disease and experimental anisakiasis, it is generally considered as an Arthus–type allergic inflammation. However, there have been many cases reported which cannot be explained solely as an Arthus reaction [3]. On the basis of animal studies, the authors have already reported that local anaphylactic reactions in the digestive tract may also be involved in addition to the Arthus–type reaction especially in those showing acute symptoms [4]. Therefore, the course of the disease after infection by *Anisakis* larvae is believed to be closely related to the presence/absence and level of the antibody against *Anisakis* larvae in the infected patient. People living in Hokkaido Japan, an area where the incidence of anisakiasis is high were investigated, for the presence/absence of antibody against *Anisakis* larvae. One of the objectives of this investigation was to forecast the incidence of anisakiasis in both the present and future by analyzing subjects for presence/absence of a history of infection by *Anisakis* larvae, that is, their *Anisakis* sensitization state. Based on the hypothesis that local anaphylactic reactions in the digestive tract, as well as an Arthus reaction, are involved in the etiological mechanism of anisakiasis, we also aimed at detecting antibodies against *Anisakis* larvae.

Thus, both cytotropic antibodies causing local anaphylactic reactions were analyzed by skin testing, and serum antibodies involved in Arthus reactions were analyzed by indirect hemagglutination test (IHA). In addition, the relationship between the skin reaction and serum IgE was investigated by determining the serum IgE level in some of the subjects.

Materials and Method

The following subjects were studied: 37 cases of acute anisakiasis patients, 2,592 healthy adults, 375 high school students and 141 young children.

A specific antigen, namely hemoglobin (Hb) of *Anisakis* larvae, was eluted after the method of Suzuki (Fig. 1) [5].

Skin tests were run on 37 patients, 2,364 healthy adults, 375 high school students, and 141 young children. The concentration of antigen was 125 μg/ml of

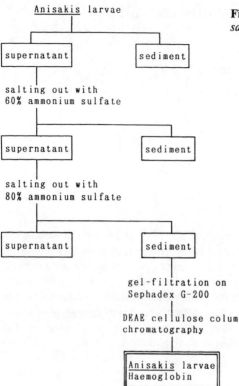

Fig. 1. Preparation of specific antigen, *Anisakis* larvae Hemoglobin (Suzuki 1973 [5])

protein nitrogen. 0.02 ml was injected intracutaneously into the forearm of the subjects, and after 15 minutes, the horizontal and vertical diameters of the wheal and erythema were measured. When the wheal and erythema diameter was 9 mm and 20 mm respectively, the case was judged positive according to Ishizaki's criteria [6].

IHA (Indirect Hemaglutination) tests were conducted on 37 patients, 2,077 healthy adults and 246 high school students. The concentration of antigen was 100 µg/ml and sensitized sheep red cells were made after the method of Boyden [7]. Based on Suzuki's criteria [8], when a reaction to 16 fold diluted serum was seen, the case was judged positive.

Serum IgE was measured in 13 anisakiasis patients and 136 people sampled at randomly. Serum total IgE was carried out by radioimmunosorbent test using Phadebas IgE test kit manufactured by the Pharmatia company, and measurement of specific IgE done by radioallergosorbent test (RAST).

Result

Skin Tests: All 37 patients showed a positive intracutaneous reaction. Healthy adults were positive in 63% (1,491/2,365), high school students 39.3% (110/375), young children 2.1% (3/141).

Immune Response to *Anisakis* Larvae in Healthy Humans

Table 1. Positive Rate of Skin test and IHA test (I)

	Skin test	IHA
Patients of anisakiasis	100.0% (37/37)	89.2% (33/37)
General population (adults)	63.0% (1491/2365)	36.6% (760/2077)
High school students	28.3% (110/375)	19.5% (48/246)
Young children	2.1% (3/141)	

Table 2. Positive rate of skin test and IHA Test (II)

	Skin test	IHA
Fishing villages	75.0% (282/376)	55.7% (49/88)
Farming villages	43.0% (37/86)	16.3% (14/86)

IHA test: 33 out of 37(89.2%) anisakiasis patients showed a positive reaction to 16fold or more diluted serum. Positive reaction was seen in 36.6% (760/2077) of the healthy adults and 19.5% (48/246) of the high school students (Table 1).

No significant difference was seen between male and female positive reactions either in skin testing or IHA. Likewise, no significant difference was seen between age levels of healthy subjects. The population of the fishing villages showed 75.0% (282/376) positive skin tests and 55.7% (49/88) positive IHA tests, while farming villages showed 43.0% (37/86) and 16/3% (14/86) positive (Table 2). Absolutely no correlation was seen between the wheal size of the skin test and IHA titers in either anisakiasis patients or healthy subjects.

In subjects in whom both skin tests and IHA tests were conducted, the following 4 categories were set up an investigated.

Type   I.   skin test positive, IHA test positive
Type II.   skin test positive, IHA test negative
Type III.   skin test negative, IHA test positive
Type IV.   skin test negative, IHA test negative

It is believed that type I, II and III which showed positive in either or both tests are groups which have antibodies to *Anisakis* larvae.

The total IgE value for anisakiasis patients showed a maximum of 5,400 U/ml with a minimal value of 220 U/ml, the mean at 1,009 U/ml. Specific IgE was revealed in 10 out of 13 patients, and a tendency to specific IgE findings was seen in the high value of total IgE. Among the general population, the number of persons showing total IgE value of over 300 U/ml was as follows; Type I 77.8%(28/36), Type II 70.0%(21/30), Type III 50.0%(14/28), Type IV 21.4%(9/42). A clear difference was seen between skin test positive Types I and II and skin test negative Types III and IV (Fig. 2). The positive rate of specific IgE was, Type I 77.8%(28/36), Type II 63.3%(19/36), Type III 7.1%(2/28) and Type IV 2.4%(1/42). A significant difference in specific IgE rate was seen between Types I and II and Types III and IV (Fig. 3). Further, while high measured values were seen in Types I and II, in Types III and IV, even when detected, the values were low. No significant correlation was seen between specific IgE and the diameter of the wheal in the skin test. Serum specific IgE showed a high incidence

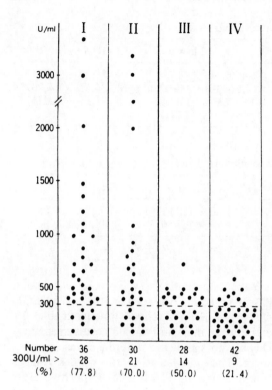

Fig. 2. Distribution of total IgE values in each group. A clear difference was seen between skin test positive types I and II, and skin test negative types III and IV

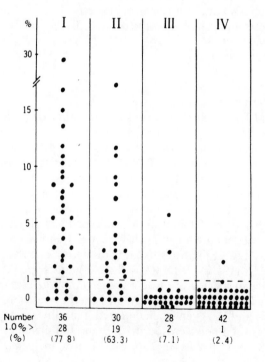

Fig. 3. Distribution of specific IgE values in each group. A significant difference of specific IgE rate was seen between types I and II and types III and IV. In types III and IV even with detected, the values were low

Immune Response to *Anisakis* Larvae in Healthy Humans

(71.7%) within the skin test positive group, while a low incidence (4.1%) was seen in the negative group.

Discussion

All of the patients with anisakiasis showed a positive reaction in the skin test using hemoglobin of *Anisakis* larvae, which is the specific antigen of this parasite. In IHA, as well, 89.2% of the patients were positive. These results indicate that the nature of the disease is an allergic reaction and that *Anisakis* larval hemoglobin is useful as an antigen for the skin test and IHA.

Many healthy subjects were found to be positive in the skin test and IHA. This finding indicates that they were sensitized to *Anisakis* larvae as a result of past larval infections and that the disease is likely to develop if they are re-infected. The positive rate in the tests were higher in the people of fishing areas than those of farming areas and the positive rate increased as age increased. These results, probably reflects the frequency of eating raw fish.

An immediate allergy includes two different types of expression: One is an Arthus–type reaction caused by antibodies in the blood flow (serum antibodies), and the other is a local anaphylaxis in the digestive tract in which antibodies localized in the tissues (cytotropic antibodies) are involved. In the present investigation on healthy subjects, antibodies in the blood flow were detected by IHA, while cytotropic antibodies were detected by the skin reaction, which is the dermal expression of anaphylaxis in the digestive tract. The investigation revealed the presence of four types in the healthy subjects: (1) positive for both cytotropic antibodies and serum antibodies, (2) positive for only cytotropic antibodies, (3) positive for serum antibodies and (4) negative for both antibodies, which corresponds to a division in patients anisakiasis in accordance with etiology, namely whether the reaction was anaphylactic or Arthus type [9].

1) Combination of both reaction type
2) Anaphylactic reaction
3) Arthus reaction type
4) Simple inflammatory reaction to the foreign body type

References

1. Van Thiel PH Kuipess FC, Roskam RT (1960) A nematode parasite to herring, causing acute abdominal syndromes in man. Trop Geogr Med 12: 97–113
2. Van Thiel PH (1962) Anisakiasis. Parasitology 52: 16–17
3. Asaishi K (1974) Antigenic analysis of *Anisakis* larva and application of fluorescent antibody technique to histological diagnosis of anisakiasis. Sapporo Med J 43: 104–120 (in Japanese)
4. Sato Y, Yamashita T, Otsuru M, Suzuki T, Asaishi K, Nishino C (1975) Studies on etiologic mechanism of anisakiasis. 1. The anaphylactic reaction of digestive tract to the worm extracts. Jpn J Parasitol 24: 192–202 (in Japanese)
5. Suzuki T (1973) Immunodiagnosis of anisakiasis, with special reference to purification of specific antigen. Chinese J Medical Microbiol 4: 217–231
6. Ishizaki T (1973) Fundamental studies on the skin test by parasitic antigens and their application. Jpn J Parasitol 22: 13–33 (in Japanese)

7. Boyden SV (1951) The absorption proteins on erythrocytes treated with tannic acid and subsequent hemagglutination by anti-sera. J. Exp Med 93: 107–120
8. Suzuki T, Ishida K, Ishigooka K, Doi K, Otsuru M, Sato R, Asaishi K, Nishino C (1975) Studies on the immunological diagnosis of anisakiasis. 5. Intradermal and indirect hemagglutination tests and histopathological examination of biopsied mucus membranes on gastric anisakiasis. Jpn J Parasitol 24: 184–191 (in Japanese)
9. Nishino C (1977) Epidemiological studies on anisakiasis. Sapporo Med J 46: 73 (in Japanese)

Conclusion

H. ISHIKURA and K. KIKUCHI

This manuscript is a companion volume to the previously published book named Gastric Anisakiasis in Japan.

It has been accomplished by the efforts of many people such as clinicians, parasitologists, oceanographers, fishery research workers, ichthylogists and pathologists etc. They have described the morphology of anisakid larva and surveyed paratenic host fish and squid caught off the seas of Japan. Epidemiology, clinical symptomatology, pathology, diagnostic methods, fundamental research into specific antigens, monoclonal antibodies, eosinophilia and lymphokine of the parasite were made clear by their research. We editors, believe that if you read this book, you will obtain the most recent information regarding studies on intestinal anisakiasis in Japan. However studies on these matters must be pursued in the future. Although extra-gastrointestinal anisakiasis was reported in only 45 cases in Japan, the number of cases in which worms perforate through the intestinal wall is gradually increasing. Such invasion through the abdominal cavity by worms is significant in the analysis of pathogenesis or formation of immunity and the complications of secondary bacterial infection.

Unfortunately it seems that in Japan the study of, and policy for, the prophylaxis of anisakiasis is very slow. Such a policy is very important as in Japan many people eat raw fish, an inveterate national habit when compared with Europe and America. In the Netherlands where this disease was found, the freezing of fish to combat the origin of infection was regulated by law in 1968. However some Japanese medical scholars say this legal regulation will not be realized in Japan. We oppose this opinion, but if legal regulation is impossible, we must make efforts to get rid of worms from fish muscle by using medical instruments such as ultrasonic ray, and laser beam devices and so on. We must think of a way of destroying the worms in the fish muscle if we are unable to remove them.

Every rose—sashimi and sushi—has a thorn—*Anisakis* larva!

The Japanese export of sashimi and sushi should not continue while there is worm contamination, and such contamination must be solved by the Japanese themselves.

Subject Index

Abdominal cavities   5-8, 11, 145
   pain   92, 120, 122, 145, 152, 159, 187, 206
abscess-granuloma   8, 140
   formation type (3rd stadium)   140
accelerated eosinophil production in
   bone marrow   225
acute gastric anisakiasis   5
   ileus   89, 94, 96, 99, 130
   localized enteritis   3
ADDC   202
adhesion   115, 121, 130, 135, 173, 174
adults of *Anisakis*   25, 81
advanced cancer   117
air contrast radiograph   106
Alaska pollack   3, 6, 16, 96, 174
Allotheuthis media   35
amoebiasis   196
An1   217, 218
An2   217, 218
An6   217, 218
An7   217
anaerobic bacteria   124
analysis of allozymes   81
anaphylaxis   190
ancylostomiasis   156
angioatelectasia   159
anisakid larvae   6
Anisakis antigen   8, 188
   hemoglobin   213
   larvae type I DNA   83
     larvae type II   53, 81, 82, 83
   specific IgE   188, 190, 211, 218
   type I larvae   10, 61, 81
     type III   73
anterior extremity   31, 77
   tip of the body   24
anti-*Anisakis* IgE   209, 211, 214
antigen-antibody complex   178

antigenic cross-reactivity   102
anti-hapten IgE   211
anti-human IgG   200
anus   173, 176
appendicitis   92, 94, 107, 116, 119, 122,
   129, 135, 152
A. physeteris   25
arabesque greeling   16
arrow-toothed halibut   16
Arthus phenomenon   121, 191
Arthus type allergy   140, 167, 251
ascariasis   156, 248
Ascaridoidea antigens   160
Ascaris   102, 153, 164, 177, 230
Ascalis suum   184-185, 211
ascites   93, 94, 98, 110, 111, 113, 130, 132,
   135, 206
Asian Pacific waters   34
assymptomatic cases   7, 9, 11, 12, 92
Atlantic herring   34
   salmon   34
Atheresthes evermanni   41-43

B$_{12}$ 98
Bacillus infection   8, 9, 12, 89, 114, 121,
   122, 125, 126, 129, 135, 140
bacterial cultivation   9
Balaenoptera borealis   35
BALB   229
barracoota   54
Bauchin's valve   95, 135
big-eye sardine   16
bleeding   7
bloody stool   93, 148
bluefin tuna (*Thunnus thynnus*)   145
blue whales   36
blunting of the Kerckring fold   102
BM   231, 232

BM-Eo 225, 231-233
B. musculus (blue whales) 36
   brevicauda (pigmy blue whales) 35
boring tooth 23, 31, 45, 48, 73, 75-77
Boyden 252
  method 161
B. physalus 35
Branchiostegus japonicus japonicus
  (sea bream) 54
brownstriped mackerel 16

Calamary squid 54
Calanoida 33
Callorhinus ursinus 35
Capepoda 68
capillaries 139
Caprella septentrionalis 32
catanic hosts 6
C57BL/6-W/W^v mice 226
cell-derived ECF-A 231
cell-mediated immunity (CM1) 174,
  177-180, 191, 196
cellular immunity 162, 167, 191
central high echoic band 117
cetacean 35
Chaetognata 33
C. harengus pallasi 34
chemotherapy 98
chicken halibut 16
Chilean waters 34
circulating-Eo 232
Chirocentrus dorab 71
chromoprotein hemoglobin antigen 161
chub mackerel 16, 25, 34
chum salmon 34
clonorchiasis 156
Cl. pallasi 42
Clupea harengus (North Sea herring) 32-34
cod 152, 199
  eggs 48
codfish 16, 81, 82, 85
coding sequences 85
coelecterata 33
Cololabis saira (saury) 54
colon 110, 209
common mackerel 49, 54
conical boring tooth 24, 77
conservative therapy 119
Contracaecum 78, 81, 82
  genus 68
  larvae 77, 82, 83, 86

  osculatum 42, 43
  sp. 45, 48, 68
  type A 48, 53, 76-78
copepods 36, 71
cords 242
Coryphaena hippurus Linnaeus 54
Crohn's disease 107, 117, 185
cross reactivity 153, 157, 161, 171, 184, 185
crustacea 33, 36
cuticle's antigenicity 247
cuticle inner-layers 239
  antigen 240-241, 245
  surface 239, 241, 243
cuticular structures 73
cysts 121

DAB 243
  reaction 248
DBTS 78, 79
DC 179
DEAR-cellulose chromatography 161
decapoda (crustacea) 33
Decapterus macrosoma Bleeker 63, 68
delayed allergic reaction 8, 161, 162, 191,
  196
Dentex tumifrous 6
denticles 73, 76, 78
dermoid-like features 150
differential diagnosis 107
diffusion chamber (DC) 174, 178, 180, 196
Diofilaria immitis 153, 217
diphyllobothriasis 156
diverticulitis 107
dolphins 35
Dorytenthis bleekeri (calamary squid) 45,
  54
  kensaki (squid) 49
double-contrast study 106
Douglous pouch 113
DOWT 78, 79

ECF lymphokine 225, 231-233, 234
ECF-P 120
ECFs 230
E-CSF 229
echinicoccosis 156
Echinococcus multilocularis 191, 217
echogram 115
edema 8, 107, 130, 133, 135, 137, 139,
  140, 145, 148, 152, 195, 207
eggs 31, 36, 119, 157

Subject Index

E. japonica (Japanese anchovies) 51
ELISA 157, 159, 187, 188, 190, 199, 200, 211
E. nana 23, 24, 33, 34
endoscopy 11, 96
Engraulis japonica 49, 71
enterobiasis 248
enzyme-linked immunosorbent assay (ELISA) 155, 187, 190, 199
Eo 232
Eo-CSF 229
Eo-GSF 228
eosinophils 130, 137, 138, 140, 145, 148, 152, 162, 180, 185, 187, 195, 209, 225, 229, 230, 235
eosinophilic cells 8, 94, 98, 125, 135, 150, 159
E. pacifica 33
erythrocyte sedimentation rate 98
ES antigen 8, 71, 140, 142, 191, 218
E. similis 23, 33
Etrumeus microps (round herrings) 52
teres 61, 68, 71
Euphausia pacifica 16, 23, 24
superba 35
vallentini 16, 33
Euphausiacea (crustacea) 33, 59
euphausiids 23, 36
euphausiid-feeding fish 35
extra-gastro intestinal anisakiasis 7, 129, 145
extramedullary myelopoiesis of eosinophils 227

Fasciola hepatica 184
Fasciolar 230
fascioliasis 156
Fc fration of IgG 245
filariasis 156
fin whales 35
flare 8
flathead 59, 60
flying fish 54
freeze-dried antigen 161
Freund's adjuvant 229
frozen powder guinea pig's complement 178
Fugu rubripes 59
fulminant from 12, 13, 96, 99, 119, 129, 132, 135-136, 137, 140, 142

GA 129
Gadus macrocephalus (pacific cod) 25, 41, 43, 45, 160, 161
morhua (gadoids including) 34
gas 93, 94, 109-111, 122
gastric anisakiasis 3, 10, 61, 68, 107, 119, 140, 164, 212-214
cancer 147
ulcer 148
genomic DNA 81-83, 85
rDNA 85
genus *Euphausia* 24
Globicephala macrorhyncus 82
GM-CSF 229, 233, 234
gnathomiasis 248
Golgi apparatus 241
granulation with black pigments 51
granulocyte-macrophage colony-stimulating factor (GM-CSF) 233

habour seals 35
haddock 34
half-mouthed sardine 16
Halichoerus grypus 35
Hb 171
HE 242
helper T cells 211
hemagglutination test 155, 171
hematocrit capillaries 192
Hemiramphus sajori 54
hemoglobin (Hb) 167
antigen 161, 164
He. otakii 42, 43
herring 16, 33
Hexagrammos otakii 41
Hippoglossoides dubius (plaice) 45
Hippoglossus stenolepis 41-43
Hokkaido University style ILA 173
horse mackerel 34, 49, 54, 111, 160, 221
host-derived ECFs 231
host's immune products 178
HpaII 83
HRP 200
human MIF 195
Hyas araneus 32
Hybond-N 83
hybridization 85, 86
hydropilic-resin sections 242
Hysterothylacium-Contracaecum type B 53

IA 129-131, 174, 180

IA 129-131, 174, 180
IgA 188, 200, 202, 221
IgA-mediated antibody 202
IgE 159, 187, 188, 206, 211-214, 222, 251, 252
  antibodies 190
IgG 200, 202, 221
IgGAM 222
IgM 200, 202, 212, 221
IHA 171, 252, 253, 255
  test 169-171, 253
ILA 177, 174
ileus 9, 107, 109, 111, 125, 130, 131, 135, 148, 152, 161
immobilization phenomenon 177
immune abdominal cells 173
  adherence (IA) 173, 174, 196
immune-leuco-adhesion (ILA) 173, 174
immunoblotting 209
immunodiagnosis 125, 152, 153, 188
immunodiffusion tests 183, 184, 186
immunoelectrophoresis 102, 150, 153, 155, 157, 183, 185-186, 195
immunofluorescein method 195
immunofluorescence (IF) 155, 241
immunogold 245
immunosorbent assay (ELISA) 221
indirect hemaggulation (IHA) test 167, 251
  MI assay 195
internal therapy 90
intestinal caecum 45, 48
  tuberculosis 117
intradermal Boyden reaction 162
ischemic ileitis 107

jack mackerels 33, 57, 59, 60
Japanese anchovies 51, 52
  chub mackerel 16
  euphausiids 23
  pilchard 16
  sardines 27, 51
jumping phenomenon 142

Katsuwonus pelamis 25, 54
Kerckring's folds 109, 206
kobumaki 48
kotsuke 48

L3 73
large-size squid 35

larval immobilization (LIB) 176
  precipitation (LP) 176
latent vitamin B deficiency 98
Lateolabrax japonicus (young bass) 54
latex agglutination 145, 148, 150, 152, 153, 200
Leishmaniasis 196
L-fluctose 196
life cylce of *A. simplex* 24, 31
Li. herzensteini 42
L3 larvae of Terranova type B 75
L4 larva 73, 76
localized Arthus phenomena 121
Loligo forbesi 35
Lowry's method 191
LR White 242
lymph node swelling 115, 116, 135
lymphocyte-derived ECF 225, 231
lymphoma 115

mackerel 45, 48, 57, 59, 71, 81-83, 101, 102, 107, 145, 148, 185, 199
  sashimi 148
macrophages 179, 180, 192, 193, 195, 196, 234
macrophage migration inhibition (MI) 192, 194
    reaction (MI-reaction) 141
marine crustaceans 32
mast cell-derived eosinophil chemotactic factor of anaphylaxis (ECF-A) 225
Meganyctiphanes norvegica 32
Melanogrammus aeglefinus (haddock) 34
Merlangius merlangus (whiting) 34
Merluccius gayi (hake) 34
metagonimiasis 156, 212
  yokogawai 211
MI 192, 193, 196
micro enzyme linked immunosorbent assay (micro-ELISA) 218, 221, 222
mid-region of the cuticle surface 240
MIF 192, 196
mild form 9, 89, 90, 96, 119, 125, 129, 131, 136, 140, 142, 195
mirror-like shape 122
MI test 192-196
  values 194
monoclonal antibodies 13, 160, 164, 217, 223
Mugil cephalus 60
Miller-Abbot tube 90, 99

Subject Index

myeloma cell   217
My. polyacanthocephalus   42

nationwide surveys   3
Nematospiroides dubius   202
Nibea albifiora   59
Nippostrongylus braziliensis   202, 211
niveaus   111
nonspecific IgE   211
normal spleen cells   195
Nyctiphanes australis   33
   couchi   32

Obstructed   206
objective symptoms   93
Ommastrephes sloanei pacificus   45
Oncorhynchus keta (chum salmon)   34
   nerka   34, 43
Osmerus eperlanus morda   96
Ouchterlony' test   145, 148, 150, 152, 153,
   155, 160, 183, 188, 190

pacific cod   25, 45, 48
   halibut   16
   herring   34
Pandalus borealis   24, 33
Pa. olivaceus   43
paragonimiasis   156
Paralichthys olivaceus   41, 54
paratenic host   10, 23, 34, 121, 122
parasite-derived ECF   231
passive cutaneus anaphylaxis (PCA)   162
P. borealis   24
PEC-Eo   225, 231-233
peroxidase-conjugated goat anti-human IgE
   222
            IgGAM   222
Phoca vitulina   35
phytoplanktons   52
pickled mackerel   111
piscivorous fish   35
P. kessleri   24, 33
planktonic animals   33
Platycephalus indicus   60
Pl. azonus   42, 43
Pleurogrammus sp.   160
   azonus   41
Pleuronichtys cornutus   60
   stellatus   42
pluripotent hemopoietic stem cells   227
Pneumatophorus japonicus japonicus

(mackerel)   45, 49, 59
polyacrylamide-gel electrophoresis   83
precipitation tests   174
pre-embedding method   245
prey-predator relationships   33
probable intestinal anisakiasis   3, 13
Prognichthys agoo (flying fish)   54
procedure of protein A-ELISA   200
protein A-ELISA   200, 202
protozoa   191
pseudoterranovasis   162
Pseudoterranova decipiens   13, 42, 43, 164
PSS   196

rabbits   6
[125]I-rabbit anti-human IgE   206
radioallergosorbent test (RAST)   152, 205,
   209, 211, 213
radiography   109, 110, 111, 113
Raphidascaris   59, 63, 76, 78
   type A   76
rDNA   85, 86
reaginic antibodies   187
   reaction   159, 162
RIA   202
rRNA   82, 85
25s rRNA   81-83, 86
[32]P-25s rRNA   83
round herrings   52, 54

Sagittoidea (Chaetognatha)   33
Salmo salar (Atlantic salmon)   34
sardine   16, 45, 49, 61, 66, 68, 71
Sardinops m.   61, 68, 71
Sardinops melanosticus   26, 45, 49, 59, 61
sarles phenomenon (SP)   173, 176, 178, 180
sashimi   53, 147, 152, 153, 217, 221
Sau3AI   83
Saurida wanieso   68
scanning electron microscope   24, 73, 240
schistosoma   191, 230
Schistosoma japonicum   227, 233
schistosomiasis Mansoni   156, 227, 230
Schulz-Dale reaction   121
Scombridae   68
Scomber japonicus   6, 7, 10, 24, 25, 34, 57,
   59, 61, 68, 160
Scomberomorus niphonicus   60, 147
Sculpins   96
Scyphozoa (Coelecterata)   33
Sebastiscus marmoratus   68

Sebastes taczanowskii 41
secondary bacterial infection 92
second-stage larvae of *A. simplex* 33, 36
sedimented antigen 8
Se. iracundus 42
sei whales 35
semisolid softagar culture system 228
Seriola quinqueradiata (young yellow-tail) 54
serodiagnostic examination 217, 222
Se. taczanowskii 43
Se. trivittatus 42
Shimesaba 48
shistosomiasis 196
Sillago japonica (sillago) 54
simple abdominal X-rays 109
S. japonicum 231, 233, 234
skin test 159, 162, 164, 194, 196, 251-253, 255
skipjack tuna 25
skip lesions 8, 10, 130, 135
slim mackerel 16
S. mansoni 229
S. meranosticta (sardines) 49, 51
sockeye salmon 34
soft tumor 130
SOM 71, 161, 162, 196
somatic antigen 160, 161, 174, 176
sonolucent echo zone 110
southern blot assay 83, 85
SP 173, 174, 180
spanish mackerel *(Scomberomorus niphonius)* 147
sparganosis 156
specific *Anisakis* IgE antibodies 190
  antigen 171
  IgE (antibodies) 188, 190, 211-213, 252, 253
  monoclonal antibody 159
Sphyraena schlegeli (barracoota) 54
Spirometra 230
spleen colony assay 227
splenic T lymphocytes 231
squid 16, 45, 49, 53, 54, 60, 152, 199
ST 160-162, 164
  test 159
Staphylococcus aureus 200, 245
starch-electrophoretic method 160
Stenella coeruloalba (dolphins) 35
stereomicroscope 82
subjective complaints 92

surface ultra-structure 24
surumeika squid 54
sushi 153, 217, 221
Synapho-branchus affinis 25
synthetic ECF-A 233

T. adunca 77
Taenia saginata 184
taeniasis 156
T. canis 228, 231
T cell 196, 229
T cell-dependent eosinophilia 229
T. declivis 33
teleosts 33
Teragra chalcogramma (walleye pollock) 7, 10, 24, 27, 34, 43, 45, 68, 96, 160
terminal ileitis 115, 116
  ileum 109, 130, 148
Terranova 43, 59, 81
  dicipines larvae 11
    A 11
  larvae type-C 68
  type A 75
terranovasis 13, 71
thin linear high echoic image 109
Thunnus thynnus orientalis (young tunny) 54
Thyn. genus 68
Thynnascaris sp. 63
  type A 59
  type B 59, 78
  type C 59
Thysanoessa 59
  raschii 32
T. inermis 32
T. japonicus (jack mackerel) 59
T. longicaudata 32
T. longiceps 33
T. lymphocytes 229, 233
Todarodes pacificus (flying squid) 6, 7, 16, 26, 34, 43, 49, 60
  saggittatus 35
Todaropsis eblane 35
total IgE 159, 211, 253
Toxocara 153
  canis 153, 162, 184, 226
  cati 217
toxocariasis 156
T. pacificus 53, 54
Trachurus japonicus (horse mackerel) 6 7, 10, 26, 34, 49, 57

Subject Index

novaezelandiae 33
T. raschii 32, 33
treatment of stomach anisakiasis 49
Trichina worm 191
Trichinella 240, 241
  spiralis 82, 83, 85, 196, 202, 217,
    228-230, 240, 241
Trichinosis 196, 248
Trichiurus lepturus 6
Tris buffered saline (TBS) 206
Trophozoites of *Giardia muris* 202
tunny tuna 16

ulcerative colitis 117, 185
ultrafine abdominoscopy 94
ultrasonic diagnostic 12
ultrasonography 3, 96, 109, 116, 125
Unger solution (SOM antigen) 160, 161,
  191
Upeneus bensasi 68
urticariasis 177

walleye pollock 25, 27, 34, 45
wave-like phenomenon 9
western immunoblotting 210, 213

V.B.S. antigen 160, 161, 194, 196
vegetable plankton 68
ventricular appendix 45, 48
Veronal buffered saline (VBS antigen)
  183, 191

X-ray 3, 12, 14, 90, 92, 94, 96, 99, 111, 113,
  122, 124, 125, 133

yellowfish 152
yellow-tail 54
young tunny 54
young yellow-tail 54

zooplanktons 52